NEW FOODS FOR HEALING

PREVENTION'S®

NEW FOODS
FOR HEALING

Capture the Powerful Cures of More Than 100 Common Foods

By Selene Yeager
and the Editors of

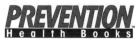

Rodale Press, Inc.
Emmaus, Pennsylvania

Notice

This book is intended as a reference volume only, not as a medical manual. The information given here is designed to help you make informed decisions about your health. It is not intended as a substitute for any treatment that may have been prescribed by your doctor. If you suspect that you have a medical problem, we urge you to seek competent medical help.

Library of Congress Cataloging-in-Publication Data

Yeager, Selene.
    Prevention's new foods for healing : capture the powerful cures of more than 100 common foods, from apricots and bananas to wine and yogurt / by Selene Yeager and the editors of Prevention Health Books.
       p.   cm.
    Includes index.
    ISBN 0–87596–413–3 hardcover
    1. Diet therapy—Popular works.   2. Herbs—Therapeutic use.
    I. Prevention Health Books.   II. Title.
    RM217.Y43   1998
    615.8'54—dc21   97–22468

Distributed in the book trade by St. Martin's Press

2   4   6   8   10   9   7   5   3   1   hardcover

---- OUR PURPOSE ----

*"We inspire and enable people to improve
their lives and the world around them."*

Prevention's New Foods for Healing – Editorial Staff

Editor: Matthew Hoffman

Senior Managing Editor: Edward Claflin

Writers: Selene Yeager with Julia VanTine, Bridget Doherty, Joely Johnson, Kristine Napier, Tom Rinderle

Recipe Editor: Sharon Sanders

Recipe Developer: Virginia Van Vynckt

Book Project Researcher: Christine Dreisbach

Editorial Researchers: Jennifer Barefoot, Tanya H. Bartlett, Elizabeth A. Brown, R.D., Susan E. Burdick, Kelly Elizabeth Coffey, Lori Davis, Carol J. Gilmore, Sarah Wolfgang Heffner, Jennifer L. Kaas, Nicole A. Kelly, Nanci Kulig, Paris Mihely-Muchanic, Deanna Moyer, Kathryn Piff, Linda Rao, Terry Sutton Kravitz, Margo Trott, Teresa A. Yeykal, Shea Zukowski

Senior Copy Editor: Jane Sherman

Copy Editors: Kathryn A. Cressman, David R. Umla

Associate Art Director: Faith Hague

Cover and Book Designer: David Q. Pryor

Illustrator: Kristine Ream

Layout Designers: Karen Lomax, Donna G. Rossi

Manufacturing Coordinators: Patrick T. Smith, Michelle Hill

Office Manager: Roberta Mulliner

Office Staff: Julie Kehs, Bernadette Sauerwine

Rodale Health and Fitness Books

Vice-President and Editorial Director: Debora T. Yost

Executive Editor: Neil Wertheimer

Design and Production Director: Michael Ward

Research Manager: Ann Gossy Yermish

Copy Manager: Lisa D. Andruscavage

Book Manufacturing Director: Helen Clogston

Contents

INTRODUCTION
THE FOOD-FOR-HEALING REVOLUTION

We've been eating a lot of the same foods for hundreds of years. So what's so "new" about *Prevention's New Foods for Healing*?

Quercetin, for one. You've probably never heard of it and neither have most doctors. But you'll know about it now because this exciting "new" substance, found in apples and other fruits, is an amazing heart protector. Or consider lycopene: Found in tomatoes and apricots, it has the ability to dramatically reduce the risk for cancer.

Quercetin, lycopene, flavonoids, sulforaphane, alpha-carotene...these are just a few of the incredibly powerful substances in foods that have the ability to prevent and even stop a host of diseases. And you'll read about them all—from the old-guard vitamins and minerals to the newly discovered natural compounds with tongue-twisting names—in this book. In fact, the editors at *Prevention* Health Books spent more than two years pouring through scientific journals and interviewing hundreds of the country's top food experts to get the best and most recent advice and information on how to take advantage of something we all love to do (eat) to avoid something we all fear (disease). What we discovered amazed us—and it's sure to amaze you, too.

In the following pages, you'll discover that it often takes more than just vitamins, minerals, and fiber to be able to label a food a "healing" food. Many foods also contain an abundance of microscopic healing substances known as phytonutrients. These substances are believed to be so powerful that some scientists are calling them "the vitamins of tomorrow."

The discovery of phytonutrients has changed everything we know about foods. Oats, for example, have long been known to lower cholesterol because of the dietary fiber they contain. But that's not the only reason they protect the heart. Scientists now know that oats contain natural chemicals that are 50 percent more powerful than even vitamin E in reducing the risk of heart disease.

Apples are another food that will surprise you. They've always been thought to be healthy, mostly because they are so chock-full of vitamins and fiber. But it turns out that the quercetin in apples is so strong that one study showed that people who ate one-quarter of an apple a day (along with some onion and tea) had half the risk of heart disease of people who did not.

One of the most exciting discoveries is that some foods can literally stop chemical changes that can lead to cancer. Watercress, for example, has been found to block some of the harmful effects of cigarette smoke.

Scientists have also discovered ways to make the foods that we eat even more powerful. You know, for instance, that beta-carotene (found in carrots, broccoli, and other dark orange and dark green vegetables and fruits) is good for your heart. But scientists have learned that the body can't absorb beta-carotene unless you eat it with a little fat. That's why a drizzle of olive oil or a dab of yogurt on cooked carrots can vastly increase their healing powers.

Garlic also needs a little help. Eat a whole clove and you'll get strong breath, but not a lot of health. Chop it fine, however, and suddenly the protective compounds are released.

And the list of foods and their magical healing powers goes on and on.

As with all *Prevention* Health Books, *Prevention's New Foods for Healing* gives you the information and practical how-to advice that will empower you to take charge of your health—on your own and naturally. We were so determined to deliver you the most up-to-date, authoritative guide to the healing power of food that we made changes in the book right up to press time. So grab an apple and start reading—and eating to your health's content!

The Editors of *Prevention* Health Books

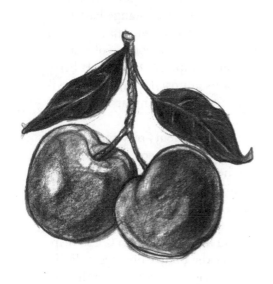

ACEROLA
A BERRY WiTH a HEALTHY PUNCH

HEALiNG POWER
CAN HELP:
Strengthen the immune
system

Speed wound healing

Prevent heart disease

Protect against cancer

Never heard of acerola? That's no sur-
prise. This small, red, cherrylike fruit, which is native to the West Indies and
now grown primarily in Puerto Rico and other Caribbean islands, is harder to
find in the United States than a can of beef stew in a vegetarian's pantry.

That's unfortunate, because acerola happens to be the richest natural
source of vitamin C in the world. This means that this fruit can benefit the body
in a variety of ways, from fortifying the immune system to helping prevent age-
related conditions like heart disease and cancer.

"In Puerto Rico and even the warmer states such as Florida, people grow
acerola in their backyards," says Arturo Cedeño-Maldonado, Ph.D., professor
of plant physiology at the University of Puerto Rico in Mayagüez. One variety of
acerola is quite sweet and can be eaten like grapes. Another variety is lip-smack-
ingly tart but higher in vitamin C. It's often made into jams, jellies, and juices.

A WEALTH OF C

Many of us step up our consumption of orange juice or grapefruit halves
at the first sign of the sniffles. It makes sense because vitamin C, found in abundance in citrus fruits, has been shown to help relieve cold symptoms.

Similarly, people in the Caribbean or West Indies might pop a few fresh

In the Kitchen

Since acerola isn't commercially available in this country, most cooks aren't sure how to use it. But if you're lucky enough to have some growing in your backyard, here are a few tips for getting it ready.

- You can use fresh acerola just as you would other types of berries, in jellies, jams, pies, or other fruit desserts. If you happen to buy the tart variety, however, be prepared to use a lot of sugar to keep your mouth from puckering.
- You can crush dried acerola with a rolling pin, then add it in small amounts to pies, preserves, or fruit butters. It will keep for months when stored in a tightly covered glass jar, as long as you periodically check for and discard berries that are moldy.

acerola berries to head off illness. A single acerola berry provides 80 milligrams of vitamin C, 133 percent of the Daily Value. To put this in perspective, an entire orange has about 70 milligrams. Even guava, one of the richest natural sources of vitamin C, can't compete. One acerola berry contains almost 10 times more vitamin C than a similar amount of guava.

The benefits of vitamin C go beyond relieving cold symptoms. It also helps the body make collagen, a tough, fibrous protein that helps build connective tissue, skin, bones, and teeth and that plays a role in wound healing. Vitamin C also helps protect the body from free radicals, cell-damaging oxygen molecules thought to contribute to the development of cancer, heart disease, and many other conditions.

Getting the Most

Enjoy the sweet taste. Even though the tart varieties of acerola contain more vitamin C than their sweeter kin, it hardly matters. "The sweet fruit also contains a huge amount of vitamin C," says Dr. Cedeño-Maldonado.

Buy it processed. Specialty markets in Puerto Rico carry acerola jams, jellies, and juices. Although they contain somewhat less vitamin C than the fresh berries, they're still very good sources. "These products have been found to retain from 60 to 80 percent of their original vitamin C," says Dr. Cedeño-Maldonado.

Treat the berries gently. Dried and crushed acerola berries can be used to make tea. Unfortunately, boiling or steeping the berries in hot water can reduce the amount of vitamin C by about half. So to get the most vitamin C per cup, you may want to add extra berries.

Aging
Eating Back the Years

When Jeanne Louise Calment was born, Ulysses S. Grant was still president, and Vincent Van Gogh was buying colored pencils in her father's store in France. Calment, who lived to be 122, holds the record as the oldest person on Earth, having beaten the average life expectancy by 45 years.

Most of us can expect to live about 75 years. While that's just a drop in the bucket for the likes of Calment, it's still almost 20 years longer than the average life span just a few generations ago.

Every year, people are living just a little bit longer. This is partly due to our success in battling childhood diseases like polio as well as adult conditions such as heart disease and diabetes. But it's also because scientists are unlocking the secrets of aging itself. We're finding out why our bodies break down and how to put the brakes on our own destruction. In the process we're expanding not only our life spans but also what scientists call our health spans—the number of years that we can expect to live in robust good health.

"Once we can understand and manage the ways in which our bodies generate harmful molecules, which are major factors in biological aging, we will be able to reach out and grasp that 120-year life span," says William Regelson, M.D., professor of medicine at the Virginia Commonwealth University, Medical College of Virginia School of Medicine in Richmond.

The Power of Antioxidants

Researchers have finally identified one of the most important contributors to heart disease, wrinkles, cancer, arthritis, and many of the other problems of aging. "We rust," says Dr. Regelson.

Ironically, the same air that gives us life is what causes iron to rust, fruit to turn brown, and our bodies' cells to break down and age. Through a series of chemical changes, oxygen molecules in our bodies lose electrons, making them unstable. These unstable molecules are called free radicals.

In frantic attempts to stabilize themselves, free radicals pillage electrons from healthy cells throughout your body. Every time they steal an electron, two things happen: A healthy molecule is damaged, and more free radicals are created. Unless this process is stopped, an increasing number of cells is damaged every day, and our health pays the price.

To keep this destructive process under control, nature created an enormous arsenal of antioxidants, which are compounds in foods that can stop free radicals from doing harm. Antioxidants come between free radicals and your body's healthy cells, offering up their own electrons and preventing yours from being pillaged.

Even though the body naturally produces its own antioxidants, studies clearly show that the antioxidants in foods offer superior protection. Three of the strongest antioxidants are beta-carotene and vitamins C and E. Each of these nutrients has been shown to be very effective against age-related illnesses like cancer and heart disease. Although you can get some protection by taking antioxidant supplements, most doctors agree that the antioxidants in foods are a better choice and should be your first line of defense.

"The problem is, if you take too much of one antioxidant, the others shut down," explains Richard Cutler, Ph.D., former research chemist at the Gerontology Research Center of the National Institute on Aging and founder of Genox Corporation, which investigates strategies for stopping free radical damage, both in Baltimore. "It's best to get them through foods like fruits and vegetables, where they exist in the proportions nature intended."

Since so many foods are loaded with antioxidants, you really don't need to take supplements anyway. The quickest way to get vitamin C, for example, is to have a glass of grapefruit juice, an orange, or a half-cup of sweet red peppers, each of which provides more than 100 percent of the Daily Value (DV). For beta-carotene, deep green or bright orange fruits and vegetables are your best picks. One sweet potato or large carrot delivers between 12 and 15 milligrams, slightly more than the 6 to10 milligrams that experts recommend we get.

Unlike vitamin C and beta-carotene, vitamin E is a bit trickier to get from foods because it's found mainly in high-fat foods, such as vegetable oils, that we'd rather avoid. Still, you can get quite a bit of vitamin E in wheat germ, with ¼ cup providing 4 milligrams, 20 percent of the DV. Nuts and seeds are also good sources of vitamin E.

Even though these three are essential antioxidants, they're not the only ones. Fruits and vegetables are loaded with plant compounds called phytonutrients, which also have antioxidant abilities. Some phytonutrients have been shown to disable cancer-causing substances as well.

In a study at the University of Michigan in Ann Arbor, researchers found that people who got the most glutathione, a phytonutrient found in avocados, grapefruit, winter squash, oranges, tomatoes, and potatoes, had lower blood pressures and cholesterol levels and maintained healthier weights than folks who got the least.

"Getting enough of all of these antioxidants won't guarantee that you'll live to be 150," says Dr. Cutler. "But they will help you reach your maximum life span, and with some people only living to 60, adding another 15 years is quite nice."

FUTURE YOUTH

While it's important to eat to prevent aging, you also need to adjust your eating habits *as* you age. As the years pass, your nutritional needs can change dramatically.

"We produce less saliva as we age, so food isn't as easy to digest and swallow," says Susan A. Nitzke, R.D., Ph.D., associate professor in the nutritional sciences department at the University of Wisconsin in Madison. "We experience changes in taste and appetite, so we eat less. We also have less stomach acid, which means that we don't digest foods or absorb nutrients as well as we used to."

In a study of 205 older adults, many of whom had weakened immune systems, researchers in Newfoundland found that almost a third of them were low in iron, zinc, folate, vitamin B_{12}, or protein—or a combination of these nutrients. But the problems were easily corrected. Once the folks began getting the necessary nutrients, they had significant jumps in levels of disease-fighting immune cells.

Doctors don't always think to check for nutritional deficiencies in adults. This is unfortunate because a simple lack of nutrients can easily be mistaken for more serious illnesses, says Dr. Regelson. "I've seen people who thought they were having trouble with senility and who supposedly couldn't take care of themselves anymore. What they really had were nutritional deficiencies," he says.

Zinc, for example, is an essential mineral for maintaining a healthy immune system. It's also one of the nutrients that requires adequate amounts of stomach acid in order to be absorbed. When acid levels decline, getting enough zinc can be a problem, says Dr. Nitzke. This is especially true in people who are taking antacids, she adds.

The easiest way to get all the zinc your body needs is to have a plate of steamed oysters. Just six shelled morsels deliver 77 milligrams of zinc, 513 percent of the DV. Crab is also good, with 3 ounces providing 7 milligrams, 47 percent of the DV.

Many older people have trouble getting enough B vitamins, which are essential for keeping the nerves and brain healthy. "As we age, the lining of the stomach changes, making it harder to absorb these nutrients," says Dr. Regelson. "After age 55, it's particularly easy to be deficient in vitamin B_6."

Potatoes and bananas are your best bets for bringing in the B_6. One potato provides 0.5 milligram, 25 percent of the DV, and a banana has 0.7 milligram, 35 percent of the DV. To get more folate (also a B vitamin), you need to eat greens and beans, particularly pinto and kidney beans. A half-cup of either of these beans provides over 100 milligrams of folate, more than 25 percent of the DV. Spinach is another good source of folate, with 1 cup containing as much as an equal amount of beans. Finally, you can get plenty of vitamin B_{12} in meats and other animal foods. Clams are a top performer: 20 small steamed clams provide an astonishing 89 micrograms of vitamin B_{12}, 1,483 percent of the DV.

As bones get older, it's essential to get extra calcium to prevent them from becoming brittle, says Dr. Nitzke. "Many people believe that they can't eat dairy foods because they're 'lactose intolerant,' but in fact, most people can eat moderate amounts of dairy without trouble," she says.

Low-fat milk and skim-milk cheese and yogurt are your best sources of this bone-building nutrient. One cup of fat-free yogurt contains 415 milligrams of calcium, 41 percent of the DV. Skim milk is also good, with one glass providing 302 milligrams, 30 percent of the DV.

Iron is another mineral that can be tough to get in the correct amounts. Some people don't get enough, while others get too much, says Dr. Nitzke. To be safe, she recommends having your doctor do a blood test for anemia. If it turns out that you do need more iron, you won't have any trouble getting it. Lean meat and seafood contain an abundance of iron, she says. Cream of Wheat and other fortified cereals are also good, with 5 milligrams of iron per serving, 29 percent of the DV.

EAT LESS, LIVE LONGER

Even though we may need to eat more of certain foods in order to live longer, researchers are finding that the opposite can also be true: People who eat a little less sometimes live a little more.

Research has shown that laboratory animals on a restricted-calorie diet have lower blood pressures, higher levels of healthful high-density lipoprotein cholesterol, and lower levels of potentially dangerous blood fats called triglycerides than their all-you-can-eat companions, says George Roth, Ph.D., a scientist at the Gerontology Research Center. In fact, the lean eaters outlive their gluttonous kin by about 30 percent.

"We believe that one of the ways in which calorie restriction works is by shifting animals' metabolisms to a survival mode so that they use the energy they take in most efficiently," says Dr. Roth. "Right now, we are testing calorie-restriction on primates, which will give us a better indication of how well it will work in people." So far, all the signs, such as lower blood pressure and cholesterol levels, are indicating that it will be beneficial, he says.

The research is still preliminary, so it would be a mistake to start cutting calories if you're already at a healthy weight. But it does seem likely that cutting unnecessary calories from your diet will help stretch your life span a little further, says Dr. Roth.

ALZHEIMER'S DISEASE
FOODS FOR LIFELONG THOUGHT

We used to call it senility, and we took it for granted, as if it were natural for people to mentally drift away as they got older. Today, doctors know that "senility" is really Alzheimer's disease, and no one takes it for granted any more.

Doctors aren't sure what causes Alzheimer's disease. What is known is that in people who have this condition, there are declines in the production of certain brain chemicals that allow nerves to send messages back and forth. Further, protein deposits form on their brains, possibly causing the death of brain cells.

Since medications haven't proven very effective, some researchers are turning their attention to nutrition. "I think it's worthwhile to consider diet as a potential factor in Alzheimer's," says James G. Penland, Ph.D., research psychologist at the U.S. Department of Agriculture Human Nutrition Research Center in Grand Forks, North Dakota.

A ROLE FOR ANTIOXIDANTS

The research is very preliminary, but there's some evidence that free radicals, which are harmful oxygen molecules that damage tissues throughout the body, including in the brain, may play a role in causing Alzheimer's disease.

Even though the body produces protective substances called antioxidants that help control free radicals, there aren't always enough of them to stop the onslaught. But you can get more antioxidants into your body simply by eating foods that contain antioxidant substances, such as vitamin E.

Laboratory studies have shown that vitamin E, which is found mainly in wheat germ, cooking oils, and nuts and seeds, can help prevent sticky protein deposits from forming on the brain. In fact, researchers at Columbia University in New York City found that large doses of vitamin E—2,000 international units a day—were as effective as selegiline (Eldepryl), a prescription drug that is used to delay the progression of the disease.

Bs FOR THE BRAIN

Researchers are also investigating B vitamins as a way of treating Alzheimer's disease. The body uses B vitamins to help maintain the protective

7

covering on nerves and to manufacture chemicals that nerves use to communicate. When levels of B vitamins decline, mental performance may suffer, says Dr. Penland.

A study at the University of Toronto has shown, in fact, that in people with Alzheimer's disease, levels of vitamin B_{12} in the spinal fluid are lower than in people without the disease. In addition, the researchers found that giving people with Alzheimer's disease large amounts of thiamin, another B vitamin, can slightly improve mental performance.

Good sources of thiamin include pork, wheat germ, and fresh pasta. For vitamin B_{12}, meats such as turkey, chicken, and liver and seafood such as steamed clams, cooked mussels, and mackerel are all good sources.

ONE TO WATCH

Among some Alzheimer's researchers, interest is brewing in a natural substance called acetyl-L-carnitine, which resembles amino acids found in dairy foods, kidney beans, eggs, and red meats. Research suggests that carnitine, which helps carry fats into brain cells, may help slow the progression of the disease.

In a study at the University of Pittsburgh School of Medicine, researchers found that when people with Alzheimer's were given carnitine for 12 months, damage to the brain appeared to slow down. So far, scientists haven't tried using foods containing carnitine to control Alzheimer's disease, but getting more carnitine in your diet could play at least a small role in slowing it down.

HEAVY METAL

Ever since researchers found small deposits of aluminum in the brains of some people with Alzheimer's, there has been speculation that too much exposure to this metal may play a role in causing the disease.

So far, there's no conclusive evidence that aluminum plays *any* role in Alzheimer's disease. Researchers admit, however, that they really don't know if it does or not. To be on the safe side, you might want to reduce the amount of aluminum you're exposed to. It's not always easy to do, since aluminum is a very common metal in the environment.

Drinking soda from a can, for example, can deliver 4 milligrams of aluminum, which is more than the maximum safe limit of 3 milligrams a day. In addition, foods cooked or stored in aluminum foil or aluminum pots and pans can pick up small amounts of the metal and pass it on to you.

Researchers still don't know how much, if any, of the aluminum we take into our bodies actually makes it to our brains. Being aware of the issue, however, will make it easier for you to at least limit your exposure—by buying sodas in bottles, for example, or using aluminum foil only when it's essential.

ANEMIA
IRONING OUT FATIGUE

In Greek, the word *anemia* means "no blood." But that's an exaggeration. People with anemia have plenty of blood. It's just that the red blood cells are not carrying their usual complement of energy-giving oxygen.

There are many forms of anemia, but the most common is iron-deficiency anemia. When you're not getting enough iron in your diet or you are losing blood—as a result of menstruation, for example—the oxygen-carrying capacity of your blood can drop precipitously. Deprived of oxygen, you wilt. Anemia can make you feel sluggish and weak. Your brain feels fuzzy. You're always cold.

It is estimated that about one-third of U.S. women have low iron stores and are at risk for anemia. Luckily, it's generally an easy condition to correct. And the cure is our favorite thing—food.

IRONING OUT THE PROBLEM

Women of childbearing age need 15 milligrams of iron a day for good health. Women past menopause and men need 10 milligrams. Pregnant women need a much higher amount—30 milligrams a day. It's virtually impossible to get that much iron in the diet, so obstetricians often prescribe supplements.

For the rest of us, how hard is it to get enough iron in food? It's not too tricky if you eat meat, fish, and poultry. These foods contain substantial amounts of iron. For example, 3 ounces of steamed blue mussels has 6 milligrams of iron. A 3-ounce serving of lean, broiled top round steak has 3 milligrams, and the same amount of roasted white turkey meat has 1 milligram.

If you eat little or no meat, though, you'll need to pay more attention to your diet. It's not that vegetables don't have iron. A half-cup of canned pumpkin, for example, has 2 milligrams of iron. Kidney beans and lentils have 3 milligrams in a half-cup serving. As you can see, the total amount of iron isn't the problem with these foods. Something called bioavailability is.

INCREASING ABSORPTION

Bioavailability refers to how well our bodies absorb the nutrients we eat. There are two forms of iron with vastly different levels of bioavailability. The iron found in meat, fish, and shellfish, called heme iron, is readily absorbable. The iron found in plant foods, called nonheme iron, is less so.

Here's an example. Of the 6 milligrams of iron in 3 ounces of mussels, roughly 15 percent will be absorbed by your body. Only 3 percent of the 3 milligrams of iron in a half-cup of lentils, however, will be absorbed, explains Victor Herbert, M.D., professor of medicine at Mount Sinai School of Medicine and Bronx Veterans Affairs Medical Center, both in New York City, and co-editor of *Total Nutrition*.

It's possible to boost the bioavailability of iron with savvy eating. For example, pairing a food that contains vitamin C with a food that contains iron guarantees that you'll get substantially more of the iron into your bloodstream. "Iron is best absorbed in an acidic environment, particularly ascorbic acid—vitamin C," says Carol Fleischman, M.D., assistant professor of medicine at Allegheny University Hospitals in Philadelphia.

Similarly, combining meats and vegetables in the same meal makes it easier to get more iron. The heme iron in meats "potentiates" the iron in vegetables, making it easier to absorb.

"You don't need to spend too much time worrying about the proportion of vitamin C to iron in your food, or the proportion of heme food to nonheme food," adds Dr. Fleischman. "Coordinating it all does give the most benefits, but if a woman is iron-deficient, her absorption of iron will be much more avid. So the more iron she eats, the more she absorbs."

Boosting Your Iron Stores

If you suspect that you have anemia, your doctor will probably want to do a complete checkup to make sure that nothing serious is wrong. When the problem is not getting enough iron in the diet, however, it's almost always easy to correct.

If you like clams, you're in business. A bowl of 20 small steamed clams contains an astonishing 25 milligrams of iron. That's more than three times the amount of iron in a serving of chicken livers.

Meats, legumes, and vegetables are also high in iron. Mixing heme iron from meats with nonheme iron from beans and vegetables will increase absorption of the nonheme iron 10 to 15 percent, "an appreciable amount," says Henry C. Lukaski, Ph.D., supervisory research physiologist at the U.S. Department of Agriculture (USDA) Human Nutrition Research Center in Grand Forks, North Dakota.

To get the most iron from your meals, be sure to have a little vitamin C at the same time. Vitamin C can "double the absorption of nonheme iron," says Janet R. Hunt, R.D., Ph.D., a research nutritionist at the USDA Human Nutrition Resource Center.

There are many ways to include vitamin C with your meals. For example, a tomato has 24 milligrams of vitamin C, 40 percent of the Daily Value (DV). You can also get vitamin C by drinking orange juice, pineapple juice, or other citrus juices.

Another way to mix vitamin C with iron is to eat more potatoes. One baked potato contains 20 milligrams of vitamin C, 33 percent of the DV, as well as 0.6 milligram of iron. Eating the potato with the skin will more than triple the amount of iron it provides.

One nutrient that you don't want to combine with iron is calcium. Especially when you're taking iron supplements, having calcium-rich foods in the same meal may set you back. "They compete for the same receptor sites on your cells," explains Fergus Clydesdale, Ph.D., professor and head of the department of food science at the University of Massachusetts in Amherst. The calcium and iron in foods also compete, but not as much as when you're taking supplements.

Dr. Clydesdale recommends spacing your calcium and iron 3 hours apart. For example, put milk on your cereal in the morning, but wait until later to take your iron supplement.

Really, you only have to remember one thing. If you're concentrating on getting the most iron in this meal, wait until the next one to include calcium-rich foods or supplements.

The same goes for coffee and tea. Both beverages contain tannins, chemicals that have a mild blocking effect on iron supplements, says Dr. Clydesdale. So don't take your pills with your morning coffee, he advises.

One easy way to get more iron in your diet is simply to cook your meals in cast-iron pots, says Dr. Lukaski. "As a rule of thumb, it increases iron by 2 to 5 percent," he says. And at breakfast, don't hesitate to have an old-fashioned meal. Because it's fortified with iron, a half-cup of cooked Cream of Wheat is loaded with 5 milligrams of iron. Instant oatmeal also contains iron, though not as much: about 3 milligrams in a half-cup.

VEGETARIAN DANGERS

Twice as many vegetarians as meat-eaters get anemia, says Dr. Herbert. In this case, the problem is due not only to a lack of iron but also to a lack of vitamin B_{12}. This nutrient, which is needed for cells to divide and mature properly, comes mostly from animal foods, he explains. Consequently, strict vegetarians may get little or no B_{12} in their diets.

The resulting condition, called pernicious anemia, isn't an immediate problem, if only because the body uses vitamin B_{12} sparingly. Most of us have enough in storage to last six years or so—"a grace period," says Dr. Fleischman. Because of this, strict vegetarians may not notice symptoms of B_{12} deficiency, which include fatigue and tingling in the hands and feet, for a very long time.

As with iron-deficiency anemia, being low in B_{12} is easily reversed. "Ve-

THE BEST SOURCES

Your body can't make red blood cells without iron. Reduce the amount of iron in your diet, and you may reduce your number of red blood cells—and with them the amount of oxygen in your bloodstream.

In the table below is a list of the best iron sources you can find, both for absorbable heme iron (found in meat and fish) and less absorbable nonheme iron (found in plants).

Foods Containing Heme Iron

Food	Portion	Iron (mg.)
Clams, steamed	20 small (approx. 3 oz.)	25.2
Chicken livers, simmered	3 oz.	7.2
Mussels, steamed	3 oz.	5.7
Oysters, steamed	6 medium (1 1/2 oz.)	5.0
Quail, whole	1	4.2
Beef, bottom round roast, lean only, braised	3 oz.	2.9
Tuna, light meat, water-packed	3 oz.	2.7
Shrimp, steamed	3 oz.	2.6
Turkey, dark meat, roasted	3 oz.	2.0
Chicken leg, roasted	3 oz.	1.2

Foods Containing Nonheme Iron

Food	Portion	Iron (mg.)
Cream of Wheat cereal, quick-cooking	3/4 cup	7.7
Tofu, regular	1/4 block (approx. 4 oz.)	6.2
Pumpkin seeds, hulled, dried	1 oz.	4.3
Lentils, boiled	1/2 cup	3.3
Potato, baked	7 oz.	2.8
Kidney beans, boiled	1 1/2 cup	2.6
Pinto beans, boiled	1/2 cup	2.2
Black beans, boiled	1/2 cup	1.8
Pumpkin, canned	1/2 cup	1.7
Split peas, boiled	1/2 cup	1.3

gans, strict vegetarians who eat no meats or dairy foods, will probably have to take B$_{12}$ supplements or brewers' yeast," says Dr. Fleischman. "Check with your doctor to see which is best for you."

ANTIOXIDANTS
BODYGUARDS FOR YOUR CELLS

HEALING POWER
CAN HELP:
Reduce the risk
of heart disease

Prevent certain cancers

Reduce the risk
of macular degeneration

Prevent muscle soreness

If you want to know how the antioxidant vitamins work, take yourself back to World War II.

Japan had a fleet of airborne fighters so dedicated to defending their island nation that they would sacrifice themselves, dive-bombing from the sky and crashing into invading ships in the sea below. Antioxidants are to your body what these kamikaze pilots were to 1940s Japan—your bravest, most aggressive servants.

Every day, your body faces about 10,000 attacks from cell-damaging forces known as free radicals, which are unstable oxygen molecules that have lost an electron through exposure to sunlight, pollution, and everyday wear and tear. These volatile molecules cruise around your body trying to stabilize themselves by stealing electrons from other molecules. When they succeed, they create still more free radicals, damaging healthy cells in the process.

Free radical damage is what causes low-density lipoprotein (LDL) cholesterol to adhere to artery walls, leading to hardening of the arteries and heart disease, for example. When free radicals damage DNA inside the cells, the result can be cell mutations that lead to cancer. Free radical assaults on your eyes may lead to cataracts and macular degeneration, the leading cause of vision loss in people over age 50. And many scientists believe that free radicals are the primary force behind aging itself.

Unless something steps in the way, this free radical free-for-all can cause irreparable damage. That's where antioxidants come in. Every time you eat fruits, vegetables, or other antioxidant-rich foods, a flood of these protective compounds enters your bloodstream. They travel throughout your body, stepping between your body's healthy molecules and the pillaging free radicals, offering up their own electrons. This neutralizes the free radicals and keeps your cells out of harm's way.

The Big Three

Just as your body produces free radicals, it also produces antioxidants. Some of these are enzymes created solely to squelch free radicals. Like the kamikaze pilots of yore, however, these defenders can be overwhelmed if you're under serious attack—from car exhaust or cigarette smoke, for example, or even from engaging in strenuous exercise.

That's when you need to call in the reserves—antioxidant compounds. There are literally hundreds of natural food compounds that act as antioxidants in the body. And the nice thing about them is that you never have to run out, because you can just eat more.

Though researchers are investigating new antioxidant compounds every day, most scientific study has focused on three in particular—vitamins C and E and beta-carotene.

"There is no doubt that antioxidants play a crucial role in reducing the risk for all kinds of diseases," says Alfred Ordman, Ph.D., professor of biochemistry at Beloit College in Beloit, Wisconsin. "The scientific evidence is simply overwhelming."

Vitamin C

Like Navy SEALs, molecules of vitamin C (also called ascorbic acid) patrol the waters of your body, capturing free radicals in blood and other fluids, such as lung and eye fluids. Getting lots of vitamin C in your diet can help protect against damage in many of your body's fluid-filled areas, such as the heart, arteries, and eyes.

An important attribute of this aquatic antioxidant, which is found in foods like tropical and citrus fruits, red bell peppers, and broccoli, is that it works so quickly. Vitamin C has been shown to block free radicals before other antioxidant compounds even arrive on the scene.

One of the most exciting findings about vitamin C is that it appears to help curtail the effects of aging. Researchers analyzed a national survey of vitamin C intake and death rate in 11,348 people ages 25 to 74 during a 10-year span. They found that men and women with high intakes of vitamin C—about 300 milligrams a day—from both food and supplements had much lower death rates from heart disease than those with low intakes. Specifically, men had a 42 percent lower death rate from heart disease, and women had a 25 percent lower death rate. Even when vitamin C intakes were less than 50 milligrams a day, women had a 10 percent reduction in death rates from heart disease, while men had a 6 percent reduction.

"Other studies have shown similar results," says James Enstrom, Ph.D., associate research professor at the University of California School of Public Health, Los Angeles.

Like most antioxidants, vitamin C is also widely recognized by researchers for its ability to protect against cancer—particularly against stomach cancer. When comparing vitamin C intake among the populations of seven different countries during a 25-year period, researchers found that the more vitamin C people ate—up to about 150 milligrams a day—the lower their risk of dying from stomach cancer.

"Though the 60 milligram Daily Value (DV) for vitamin C is probably inadequate, you should stay below 1,000 milligrams a day so that the vitamin doesn't interfere with other nutrients in your body," adds Robert R. Jenkins, Ph.D., professor of biology at Ithaca College in New York.

Dr. Ordman recommends taking 500 milligrams of vitamin C twice a day to keep your body's stores at optimum levels. Even better, get as much of that as you can from food, he says.

Maintaining your vitamin C stores is especially important if you're a smoker or you live with one. It takes about 20 milligrams of vitamin C to squelch the free-radical effects of one cigarette.

Vitamin E

While vitamin C is hard at work patrolling the waters of your body, vitamin E (also known as alpha-tocopherol) is delving into denser territories, protecting your fat tissues from free radical invasion.

It's precisely this fat-protecting prowess that makes vitamin E particularly effective in the fight against heart disease. Researchers have found that vitamin E, which dissolves in fat, plays a powerful role in keeping your "bad" LDL cholesterol from oxidizing and sticking to artery walls.

A number of large population studies involving tens of thousands of people have linked high vitamin E intake with a significant decrease in risk for heart disease. In a study of 80,000 nurses, researchers found that women with the highest vitamin E intake—about 200 international units a day—were one-third less likely to suffer from heart disease than their counterparts who were only getting about 3 international units a day.

One of the most promising findings for female health emerged from a study at the University of New York in Buffalo in which researchers examined vitamin E levels in women with a high family risk for breast cancer. They found that women who maintained high levels of vitamin E had significantly lower risks for the disease than women who had low levels. The benefits were most pronounced among younger women, although those past menopause were also protected.

Getting enough vitamin E in the diet—it's found mainly in vegetable cooking oils, wheat germ, and sunflower seeds—is important for men as well. More than 50 percent of men with diabetes, for example, have difficulty achieving erections, often because of free-radical damage to the arteries supplying blood to the penis. Research suggests that getting enough vitamin E in the diet can help keep blood flowing smoothly through those arteries.

While vitamin E is effective in its own right, it works more efficiently when combined with vitamin C, says Dr. Ordman. "It's like vitamin C helps vitamin E get back on its feet again. After vitamin E becomes oxidized by free radicals, vitamin C comes along and regenerates it so that it's ready to work again," he explains.

The DV for vitamin E is 30 international units, but Dr. Ordman recommends shooting for 400 international units in order to get the maximum protection.

BETA-CAROTENE AND FRIENDS

Beta-carotene, a red-yellow food pigment that turns to vitamin A in the body, has been on quite a roller-coaster ride during the past few decades. It enjoyed enormous popularity when scientists linked it with lower rates of heart disease and cancer. The mood changed, however, when researchers discovered that taking beta-carotene supplements seemed to increase the risk for some of these diseases. Now, as medical science learns more about this enigmatic antioxidant, beta-carotene's reputation is ascending again, albeit more cautiously than before.

"We know that beta-carotene has established benefits, but the amounts that people need are well within the range they can get from eating five or more servings of fruits and vegetables a day," explains Dr. Ordman. "So you don't need extraordinary amounts. There are definite risks with supplementation."

Why are food sources of beta-carotene so much better than supplements? Scientists still aren't sure, but they suspect that it may be because beta-carotene has at least 500 siblings, collectively known as carotenoids. It's possible, they say, that it's not just the beta-carotene that's causing the benefits but the combination of beta-carotene plus its less-recognized kin.

Lycopene, a carotenoid found in tomatoes, for instance, may be considerably more potent than beta-carotene in the battle against cancer. When testing the effectiveness of each of these compounds in the laboratory, researchers found lycopene to be more effective than beta-carotene at inhibiting the growth of certain types of cancer cells.

In a study that proves that carrots really are good for your eyes, researchers found that people with the highest levels of carotenoids had one-third to one-half the risk of macular degeneration than those with lower levels.

So the next time you're in the produce aisle, be sure to fill your cart with plenty of carotenoid-rich foods like spinach and other dark green, leafy vegetables, and deep orange fruits and vegetables like pumpkins, sweet potatoes, carrots, and cantaloupe.

THE BEST SOURCES

All fruits and vegetables are great sources of antioxidant compounds. But which are the best? Researchers at Tufts University in Boston have compiled a list of foods that are extremely high in vitamin C and beta-carotene. (It's difficult to get enough vitamin E in foods alone, although cooking oils, nuts, seeds, and wheat germ all are good sources.) Here are some of their favorites.

Food	Portion	Vitamin C (mg.)	Beta-carotene (mg.)
Broccoli, cooked	1/2 cup	37	1.0
Brussels sprouts, cooked	4	36	0.3
Butternut squash, cubed	1/2 cup	15	4.3
Cantaloupe	1/4	56	2.6
Kiwifruit	1	89	0.1
Navel orange	1	80	0.2
Papaya	1/2	94	0.3
Strawberries	1/2 cup	42	—
Sweet potato, baked	1	28	15.0
Sweet red pepper, chopped	1/2 cup	95	1.7
Watermelon, cubed	1/2 cup	8	0.2

WORKING TOGETHER

Even though antioxidants work well on their own, they really aren't solo players. Like a finely tuned orchestra, they perform best when they're performing together.

In one study, researchers from Scotland gave 50 men an antioxidant "cocktail" containing 100 milligrams of vitamin C, 400 international units of vitamin E, and 25 milligrams of beta-carotene. They gave another 50 men inactive pills. After 20 weeks, they found that in the men given antioxidants, disease-fighting white blood cells had sustained only two-thirds as much DNA damage as the white blood cells of men not taking the active pills. This is important, because damage to DNA can lead to the development of cancer.

Moreover, when it comes to keeping your heart ticking, there may be nothing quite as effective as a one-two punch of vitamins C and E, according to a study from the National Institute on Aging in Bethesda, Maryland. In a study of 11,178 people ages 67 to 105, researchers found that those who took vitamins C and E every day cut their risk of dying from heart disease in half.

Although antioxidants certainly have shown their mettle against major

FRUITFUL PROTECTION

The next time your spouse gives you the evil eye for stealing away with a piece of strawberry shortcake, just say that you need it for your fight against free radicals. You may get a skeptical stare, but at least you'll be telling the truth.

Researchers from Tufts University in Boston and other universities evaluated 12 commonly eaten fruits and five fruit juices to determine which had the most free radical–fighting punch. Strawberries won hands down.

For starters, strawberries are a powerhouse of vitamin C, packing more than 70 percent of the Daily Value in a half-cup. They also contain a variety of other antioxidant compounds, such as ellagic acid.

Other fruits that scored particularly high were plums, oranges, red grapes, and kiwifruit.

health threats like heart disease and cancer, they are also useful in preventing lesser ailments. One example is muscle soreness. One study found that folks who are sedentary most of the time and then suddenly exercise intensely may find relief from aching muscles with vitamin E. It appears that vitamin E may reduce free radical damage that can lead to muscle soreness.

THE REST OF THE TROOP

Even though vitamins C and E and beta-carotene are the best-studied of the antioxidants, they're only a small part of a massive army of protective compounds found in foods. For example, the minerals selenium and zinc also act as potent antioxidants. So do the phenolic compounds in green tea and the flavonoids in red wine. "We all agree that everyone should eat at least five servings of fruits and vegetables a day to ensure that they get healthy amounts of all of these antioxidants," explains Dr. Ordman. "But as far as taking extra supplements, you should stick with those that have been studied extensively and proven safe in long-term clinical trials. Those are vitamins C and E. Everything else should come solely from food."

APPENDICITIS
THE FORCE OF FIBER

Researchers have wondered for years why appendicitis is relatively rare in places like Africa and Asia, while in the United States it's extremely common, affecting between 7 and 12 percent of people at some time in their lives.

What are we doing wrong?

"There's always been speculation that high-fiber diets protect against appendicitis," says David G. Addiss, M.D., medical epidemiologist for the division of parasitic diseases at the Centers for Disease Control and Prevention in Atlanta. People in Africa and Asia eat tremendous quantities of fruits, vegetables, whole grains, and other fiber-rich foods. In this country, however, most of us get only 11 to 12 grams of fiber a day. This is less than half of the Daily Value (DV) of 25 grams.

But for a brief time in the 1940s, a curious thing happened. Due to wartime rationing, people started eating less meat and more high-fiber foods, and appendicitis rates started dropping. A coincidence? Some researchers don't think so.

DIGESTION MADE EASY

Appendicitis usually occurs when a firm piece of stool blocks the pea-size opening of the appendix (part of the large intestine), allowing bacteria to flourish inside. Since the fiber found in foods absorbs water, a high-fiber diet causes the stool to become larger, softer, and less likely to break apart. This can help prevent stray particles from blocking the appendix.

Getting more fiber in your diet also causes stool to move more quickly through the digestive tract. "Anything that will decrease the resident time of all the waste products in your large intestine can only help," says Frank G. Moody, M.D., professor of surgery at the University of Texas Medical School in Houston. Even though doctors aren't positive that getting more fiber will prevent appendicitis, it clearly provides some protection.

One of the easiest ways to get more fiber into your diet is to start the day with cereal. Most breakfast cereals, both hot and cold, are wonderful sources of fiber, says Pat Harper, R.D., a nutritional consultant in the Pittsburgh area. Some cereals, in fact, contain 10 or more grams of fiber per serving. That's more than half of the DV, all in one bowl. So the next time you're at the supermarket, be sure to put a few boxes of cereal in your cart. And take a few minutes to read the labels, Harper adds. A cereal should have at least 5 grams of fiber per serving. If it doesn't, you may want to pick another brand. Or if your favorite cereal is fairly low in fiber, you can mix it with a higher-fiber kind to get the extra protection.

Another way to get more fiber is to eat whole-grain foods. Foods like white bread, white rice, and white flour, which are made from processed grains, have been stripped of much of their protective fiber. In fact, you'd have to eat 20 slices of white bread to get just 10 grams of fiber. Foods made from whole grains, however, are loaded with fiber. A slice of whole-wheat bread, for example, has 2 grams of fiber, more than four times the amount in its processed counterpart. A half-cup serving of cooked barley has 3 grams of fiber, while a half-cup of cooked oatmeal has 3 grams. All whole grains are super fiber choices, Harper says.

Legumes are even better sources. A half-cup of cooked split peas, for example, has 8 grams of fiber, nearly a third of the recommended daily amount. The same amount of cooked kidney beans has nearly 6 grams of fiber, and a half-cup of boiled black beans has almost 8 grams.

While fruits and vegetables can't compete with legumes for sheer fiber force, they're still significant sources. A half-cup of broccoli, for example, has 2 grams of fiber. Apples and oranges have about 3 grams of fiber each. And don't forget dried fruits. A half-cup of raisins has 4 grams of fiber, while 10 dried apricot halves have 3 grams.

Even though the juicy flesh of fruits contains some fiber, most of the fiber is found in the peel. So whenever possible, eat fruits (and vegetables, including potatoes) with the skin intact.

Citrus fruits, of course, are an exception to this rule, since you don't eat the skin. Fortunately, though, much of the fiber in oranges, grapefruit, and other citrus fruits is found in the white pith just beneath the skin. To get the most fiber, don't slice citrus fruits. Instead, peel and eat them whole to get the most fiber in each bite.

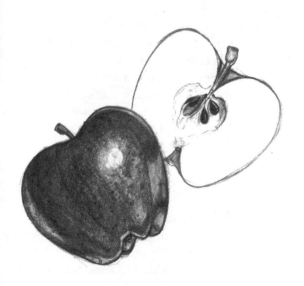

APPLES
THEIR BENEFITS
ARE SKIN-DEEP

HEALING POWER
CAN HELP:
Lower the risk
of heart disease

Prevent constipation

Control diabetes

Prevent cancer

It's really not surprising that apples have long been considered a symbol of good health and vitality. For one thing, you can keep them handy to eat anywhere, anytime, just by dropping one in your briefcase, backpack, or purse. To complete the package, they come ready-wrapped in their own protective but tasty skin, with all their tart sweetness wrapped within. It's almost as if the head designer said, "Apples are good, so I'll make them easy to eat."

Yet apples are more than just a wholesome snack. Studies suggest that eating apples can help reduce the risk of heart disease. In the laboratory, they have been shown to have stopping power against cancer cells. Evidence is still preliminary, but it appears that having an apple or two a day really can help keep the doctor away.

IT'S ALL IN THE SKIN

Even though many people favor the flesh, much of an apple's healing power resides in the skin, which contains large amounts—about 4 milligrams—of a compound called quercetin. Like vitamin C and beta-carotene, this is an antioxidant compound that can help prevent harmful oxygen molecules from damaging individual cells. Over time, this can help prevent changes in the cells

In the Kitchen

There are 2,500 kinds of apples in the United States alone. Even if you can't sample all of the world's apples, you can try some of the more notable varieties. Here are a few to look for.

Braeburn. Ranging in color from greenish gold to almost solid red, Braeburn apples combine sweetness and tartness. A great eating apple.

Fuji. Available year-round, Fuji apples are crisp and sweet, with just a hint of spice. They are wonderful eating apples.

Gala. These apples have distinctive red stripes running down yellow-orange skin. Both crisp and sweet, they are used for munching and also for making applesauce.

Jonagold. Tangy and sweet, Jonagold apples are used both for eating and baking.

Liberty. A favorite of organic growers, Liberty apples are resistant to many diseases and don't require large amounts of pesticides. They're excellent for eating and cooking.

Newtown Pippin. How green grows this apple! The taste is notably tangy, making it a good choice for applesauce and pies.

Northern Spy. Greenish yellow with red stripes, these apples have a tart taste that's wonderful for cooking and baking.

Winesap. Spicy and tart, these are often used for ciders and also for baking and adding to salads.

that can lead to cancer.

Even in the healing world of antioxidants, quercetin is thought to be exceptional. In one study, researchers in Finland compared the amount of various antioxidants in people's diets with their risk of heart disease over a 20-year period. Men who had the highest daily intake of quercetin and other antioxidants (their diets included about a quarter of an apple) had a 20 percent lower risk of heart disease than men who ate the least. The researchers concluded that quercetin was responsible for most of the study's good results.

In a study in the Netherlands, researchers found that men eating an apple a day (along with 2 tablespoons of onions and four cups of tea) had a 32 percent lower risk of heart attack than those who ate fewer apples.

"So eating an apple a day is not a bad idea," says Lawrence H. Kushi, Sc.D., associate professor of public health, nutrition, and epidemiology at the University of Minnesota in Minneapolis.

Heart disease is not the only major malady to feel quercetin's force. The compound has also shown clout against cancer. Laboratory studies show that it can inhibit the growth of tumors and also help prevent cancer cells from spreading.

"When you subject cells to a carcinogen and then put in the quercetin, you prevent mutation from occurring—you prevent the carcinogen from acting," says Dr. Kushi. "Quercetin is one of the things that apples are relatively high in."

FIELDS OF FIBER

Recent discoveries aside, apples are perhaps best known for their fiber. They contain both soluble and insoluble fiber, including pectin. A 5-ounce apple with the skin has about 3 grams of fiber. "They're a good source," says Chang Lee, Ph.D., professor of food science and technology at Cornell University–New York State Agricultural Experimental Station in Geneva.

Insoluble fiber, found mostly in the skin, is the kind that we used to call roughage, which has long been recommended for relieving constipation. More is at stake, though, than just comfort. Studies show that a smoothly operating digestive tract can help prevent diverticulosis, a condition in which small pouches form in the large intestine, and also cancer of the colon. Plus, insoluble fiber is filling, which is why apples are such an excellent weight-control food for people who want to lose weight without being hungry all the time.

The soluble fiber in apples, which is the same kind found in oat bran, acts differently from the insoluble kind. Rather than passing through the digestive tract more or less unchanged, soluble fiber forms a gel-like material in the digestive tract that helps lower cholesterol and, with it, the risk of heart disease and stroke.

It's not just the soluble fiber that's so helpful, but a particular type of soluble fiber called pectin. Pectin, which is the same ingredient used to thicken jellies and jams, appears to reduce the amount of cholesterol produced in the liver, providing double protection. "Plus, pectin's ability to form a gel slows digestion, which slows the rise in blood sugar—so it's good for people with diabetes," says Joan Walsh, R.D., Ph.D., foods and nutritional instructor at San Joaquin Delta College in Stockton, California.

An average-size apple contains 0.7 gram of pectin, more than the amount in strawberries and bananas.

Getting the Most

Look for the brown. "Some varieties of apple, like Granny Smith, are bred to be low in certain protective compounds that make apples brown when you peel them," says Mary Ellen Camire, Ph.D., associate professor and chair of the department of food science and human nutrition at the University of Maine in Orono. Look for varieties that brown easily to reap the most health benefits.

Don't count on apple juice. Although apple juice contains a little iron and potassium, it's no great shakes compared to the whole fruit. By the time apples wind up as juice, they've given up most of their fiber and quercetin.

Of course, if you're choosing between soda and apple juice, by all means choose the juice. But don't use it as a substitute for the real thing.

Apple Crumble with Toasted-Oat Topping

6 medium Jonagold apples

½ cup unsweetened applesauce

¾ cup old-fashioned or quick-cooking rolled oats

3 tablespoons toasted wheat germ

3 tablespoons packed light brown sugar

1 teaspoon ground cinnamon

1 tablespoon canola oil

1 tablespoon unsalted butter, cut into small pieces

Per serving

calories **197**
total fat **5.7 g.**
saturated fat **1.6 g.**
cholesterol **5 mg.**
sodium **3 mg.**
dietary fiber **4.7 g.**

Preheat the oven to 350°F. Coat a 12″ × 8″ baking dish with no-stick spray.

Cut the apples in half lengthwise. Remove the cores and stems and discard. Cut the apples into thin slices.

Place the apples and the applesauce in the prepared baking dish. Toss to coat the apples evenly with the applesauce. Spread out evenly in the baking dish.

In a small bowl, mix the oats, wheat germ, brown sugar, and cinnamon. Drizzle with the oil. Add the butter. Mix with your fingers to work the oil and butter into the dry ingredients.

Sprinkle the oat mixture evenly over the apples. Bake for 30 to 35 minutes, or until the topping is golden and the apples are bubbling. Serve warm.

Makes 6 servings

Cook's Note: Although you can make this recipe with peeled apples, leaving the peels on ensures that you get more fiber as well as the beneficial antioxidant quercetin.

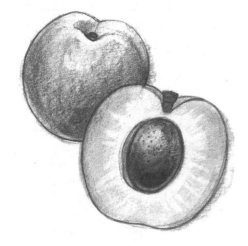

APRICOTS
A BOUNTY
OF BETA-CAROTENE

HEALING POWER
CAN HELP:
Protect the eyes

Prevent heart disease

At one time, Chinese brides nibbled on apricots to increase fertility. It sounds funny today, until you realize that these fruits are, in fact, high in a mineral needed for the production of sex hormones.

These days, of course, few people are likely to rely on apricots to influence family size. Yet this sweet, velvety fruit contains a variety of compounds that research shows can fight infections, blindness, and heart disease.

Most of apricots' health benefits are due to their copious and exceptionally diverse carotenoid content. Carotenoids are the pigments in plants that paint many of our favorite fruits and vegetables red, orange, and yellow and that in humans have a wide range of health-protecting properties. Researchers have identified at least 600 different carotenoids, with some of the most powerful, including beta-carotene, being found in apricots.

"Apricots are one of the best foods to look to for carotenoids," says Ritva Butrum, Ph.D., vice president for research at the American Institute for Cancer Research in Washington, D.C.

FRUIT FOR THE HEART
The apricot's unique mix of healing compounds makes this food a powerful ally in fighting heart disease. Along with beta-carotene, apricots contain

In the Kitchen

Although most of us eat apricots straight from the fruit bin, there are many other ways to prepare—and enjoy—these little golden gems.

Grill them. Grilled apricots take on a smoky, slightly sweet flavor as the sugars caramelize. Simply thread whole or halved fresh apricots on skewers, brush with honey and cook for 7 to 10 minutes, turning frequently.

Broil them. To cook apricots indoors, cut the fruit in half, brush with honey, and broil in the oven, cut side up.

Poach them. Poached apricots are a great way to warm up a cool evening. Put fruit juice and whole cloves or a cinnamon stick in a small saucepan and bring to a simmer. Add whole or halved apricots and cook for 6 to 8 minutes. Remove the apricots and continue cooking the sauce until it thickens. Then use it as topping for the apricots.

lycopene, and both compounds have been shown in studies to fight the process by which the dangerous low-density lipoprotein (LDL) form of cholesterol turns rancid in the bloodstream. This is important because when LDL goes bad, it's more likely to stick to artery walls.

"Lycopene is currently considered one of the strongest antioxidants we know about," says Frederick Khachik, Ph.D., research chemist at the Food Composition Laboratory at the U.S. Department of Agriculture in Beltsville, Maryland.

A 13-year study found that those with the highest intakes of carotenoids had a one-third lower risk of heart disease than those with the lowest intakes. In an 8-year study of 90,000 nurses, those with diets richest in carotenoids had a one-quarter lower risk.

Apricots are a good source of beta-carotene. Three fruits contain 2 milligrams, about 30 percent of the recommended daily amount.

Good for the Eyes

Even if you don't have the spinach-loving personality of Popeye, you can get lots of vitamin A by eating apricots. (The beta-carotene in apricots is converted to vitamin A in the body.) This nutrient helps protect the eyes, and as it turns out, the eyes need all the help they can get.

Every time light passes through the eyes, it triggers the release of tissue-damaging free radicals. Left unchecked, these destructive oxygen molecules attack and damage the lenses of the eyes, possibly setting the stage for cataracts. Free radicals can also attack blood vessels supplying the central portions of the retinas, called the maculas. If the blood supply gets cut off, the result can be macular degeneration, the leading cause of vision loss in older adults.

Vitamin A has been shown in studies to be a powerful antioxidant—that is, it helps block the effects of free radicals. A study of more than 50,000 nurses, for example, found that women who got the most vitamin A in their diets reduced their risk of getting cataracts by more than one-third. Three apricots provide 2,769 international units of vitamin A, 55 percent of the Daily Value (DV).

HELP FROM FIBER

It's almost impossible to exaggerate the benefits of getting enough fiber in your diet. High-fiber foods can help you lose weight, control high blood sugar, and lower cholesterol levels. They're also essential for keeping digestion regular.

So here's another reason to add apricots to your fruit bowl. Three fruits contain 3 grams of fiber, 12 percent of the DV. Better yet, that's at a minimal calorie cost—just 51 calories for all three. When you're eating apricots for fiber, however, be sure to eat the skin, which contains a substantial amount of the fruit's fiber.

Getting the Most

Eat them firm. Even if you enjoy your fruit nice and soft, it's best to eat apricots while they're still slightly firm. Apricots contain the most nutrients when they're at their peak of ripeness; once they start getting soft, these compounds quickly begin to break down.

Shop for color. Unlike most fruits, apricots can be yellow or orange and still be ripe. Both colors are acceptable when you're trying to get the most healing benefits. However, apricots that have green in them were picked early and may never ripen, which means that you lose out on much of their healing goodness.

Store them carefully. It's important to keep apricots cool to prevent them from getting overripe. Unless you're going to eat them within a day or two, it's best to store them in the fruit bin in the refrigerator, where they'll keep for about a week.

Here's another storage tip. Because apricots are such a soft, delicate fruit, they readily pick up flavors—from other fruits they're stored with, for example, or even from refrigerator smells. It's a good idea to store them in a paper or plastic bag.

APRICOT BREAKFAST PARFAITS

1 **cup low-fat granola (without raisins)**

1 **cup nonfat plain yogurt**

8 **large apricots, pitted and thinly sliced**

Ground cinnamon

PER SERVING

calories	**173**
total fat	**2.3 g.**
saturated fat	**0.1 g.**
cholesterol	**1 mg.**
sodium	**75 mg.**
dietary fiber	**2.9 g.**

Place 1 tablespoon of the granola in each of 4 parfait dishes. Add 2 tablespoons of the yogurt per dish, spreading to make an even layer. Divide half of the apricots among the dishes. Sprinkle lightly with the cinnamon. Place 1 more tablespoon of the granola in each dish.

Divide the remaining $1/2$ cup yogurt among the dishes. Top with the remaining apricots and the remaining $1/2$ cup granola, dividing them evenly among the dishes.

Serve immediately, or cover and chill in the refrigerator for up to 2 hours.

Makes 4 servings

Cook's Notes: Use only ripe apricots for this recipe. The fruit is ripe when it yields slightly to a gentle squeeze and is lightly fragrant.

Glass dessert bowls can be used if parfait dishes are unavailable. Spoon the yogurt into 4 bowls, then top with the apricots and granola.

ARTHRITIS
FOODS THAT RELIEVE JOINT PAIN

Here's a traditional Chinese treatment for arthritis. Add 100 dead snakes to 5 liters of red wine and some herbs. Let mellow for three months. Drink the wine three times a day for 6 to 12 weeks.

Admittedly, this concoction is a bit on the strange side, but until recently, most doctors felt that any food-related remedy for arthritis was only slightly less bizarre than this unappetizing brew.

While there isn't a specific food that will help relieve arthritis in all people, doctors today recognize that what you eat—or, in some cases, don't eat—can help ease discomfort and even slow the progression of the disease.

JOINTS OUT OF JOINT

Arthritis, which causes pain, stiffness, and swelling in and around the joints, isn't just one disease, but many. The most common form of arthritis is osteoarthritis, which is caused by wear and tear on cartilage, the shock-absorbing material between the joints. When cartilage wears away, bone grinds against bone, causing pain and stiffness in the fingers, knees, feet, hips, and back.

A more serious form of the disease is rheumatoid arthritis. It occurs when the immune system, instead of protecting the body, begins attacking it. These attacks cause swelling of the membrane that lines the joints, which eventually eats away at the joints' cartilage. It is the form of arthritis most affected by diet.

NUTRITIONAL TRIGGERS

Since there's some evidence that rheumatoid arthritis is triggered by a faulty immune system, and the immune system is affected by what we eat, it makes sense that for some people, diet can make a difference in how they feel.

"Diet is critical in the treatment of this form of arthritis," says Joel Fuhrman, M.D., a specialist in nutritional medicine at the Amwell Health Center in Belle Mead, New Jersey. "In populations that consume natural diets of mostly unprocessed fruits, vegetables, and grains, autoimmune diseases are almost nonexistent. You don't see much crippling rheumatoid arthritis in rural China, for example, because the people there eat differently than we do."

Fast Relief

Although many doctors aren't convinced that fasting will relieve rheumatoid arthritis pain, Joel Fuhrman, M.D., a specialist in nutritional medicine at the Amwell Health Center in Belle Mead, New Jersey, is convinced that it plays a powerful role. "Virtually everyone with rheumatoid arthritis who fasts finds that their pain will temporarily go away," he says.

In many people with rheumatoid arthritis, says Dr. Fuhrman, the immune system works overtime attacking partially digested food particles that the intestine lets escape into the bloodstream. Fasting gives the entire body, including the immune system, time to recover, he says. In addition, if you gradually add foods, one at a time, to your diet after fasting, you can begin figuring out which foods are most likely to trigger flare-ups, he says.

For people who don't like the prospect of total deprivation, even for a few days, it's acceptable to drink fruit juices, vegetable juices, or herbal teas. This modified fast can usually help relieve arthritis pain, while providing the body with extra nutrients.

While fasting is generally safe, Dr. Fuhrman says, it may be dangerous for people on medications. To be safe, always check with your doctor before giving fasting a try.

More is involved than just getting more fruits, vegetables, and grains. Some people are sensitive to certain foods—like wheat, dairy foods, corn, citrus fruits, tomatoes, and eggs—that can switch on the body's inflammatory response. For the most part, food sensitivities are rarely involved in arthritis flare-ups, says David Pisetsky, M.D., Ph.D., co-director of the Duke University Arthritis Center in Durham, North Carolina, and medical adviser to the Arthritis Foundation.

Since there are so many things that can exacerbate the pain of rheumatoid arthritis, knowing which foods, if any, to avoid can be difficult. Dr. Pisetsky recommends starting a food diary so that you can keep track of what you were eating around the time a flare-up occurred. If you discover a pattern—for example, you remember eating tomatoes shortly before an attack—you'll have an idea of what to avoid in the future. Once you've identified a possible culprit, stop eating that food (or foods) for at least five days, he says. Then try the food again and see if your symptoms return.

Vegetarian Relief

Since the proteins found in meats may occasionally play a role in causing arthritis pain, it makes sense that following a vegetarian diet would help relieve it. Research bears this out.

In a study at Norway's University of Oslo, 27 people with rheumatoid arthritis followed a vegetarian diet for one year. (After the first three to five months, they could eat dairy products if they wished.) They also avoided gluten (a protein found in wheat), refined sugar, salt, alcohol, and caffeine. After a month, their joints were less swollen and tender, and they had less morning stiffness and a stronger grip than people who followed their usual diets.

The Fat Connection

These days it's difficult to think of an illness that isn't made worse by a diet high in saturated fats. Arthritis, it appears, is no exception.

In one study, 23 people with rheumatoid arthritis were put on a very low fat (10 percent of calories from fat) diet for 12 weeks. They also walked 30 minutes a day and followed a stress-reduction regimen. People in this group experienced a 20 to 40 percent reduction in joint tenderness and swelling; many of them were able to cut back on arthritis medications. People in a second group who didn't follow the diet showed no such improvement.

"We think that the diet caused most of the improvements in joint swelling and tenderness," says study leader Edwin H. Krick, M.D., associate professor of medicine at Loma Linda University in California.

A diet low in saturated fats reduces the body's production of prostaglandins, hormonelike substances that contribute to inflammation, says Dr. Krick. In addition, a low-fat diet may hinder communications sent by the immune system, thereby interrupting the body's inflammatory response. "Interrupting those chemicals can help the joints get better," he says. "One way to accomplish that is by consuming a low-fat or largely vegetarian diet."

Some doctors recommend limiting dietary fat to no more than 25 percent of total calories, with no more than 7 percent of these calories coming from saturated fats. "There's a very simple way to reduce your intake of saturated fats— just don't add them to food," says Dr. Pisetsky. "When you have a sandwich, for example, use low-fat mayonnaise instead of the real thing."

Replacing butter, sour cream, and cheese with their lower-fat or fat-free counterparts can also lower your intake of saturated fats. Even if you don't cut them out of your diet completely, just cutting back can make a difference.

Fish for Relief

Even though it's generally a good idea to cut back on fats, there is one type of fat that you may want to include in an anti-arthritis diet. The omega-3 fatty acids, found primarily in cold-water fish like mackerel, trout, and salmon, reduce the body's production of prostaglandins and leukotrienes, both substances that contribute to inflammation.

In one study, researchers at Albany Medical College in New York had 37 people with arthritis consume high doses of fish oil. After six months, these people reported having fewer tender joints, less morning stiffness, and better grip strength than those who consumed less or no fish oil.

Although scientific studies often require the use of supplements, you can get similar benefits by eating the fish, according to a study at the University of Washington in Seattle. Researchers found that women who ate one or more servings of baked or broiled fish a week were less likely to get rheumatoid arthritis than women who didn't eat fish.

To get the healing benefits from fish, you need to eat it two or three times a week, says Joanne Curran-Celentano, R.D., Ph.D., associate professor of nutritional sciences at the University of New Hampshire in Durham. Fish rich in omega-3's include salmon, bluefin tuna, rainbow trout, halibut, and pollack. Canned fish such as mackerel, herring, sardines, and tuna are also high in omega-3's.

Help for Wear and Tear

For years, doctors didn't suspect that there could possibly be a link between diet and osteoarthritis. After all, they reasoned, this condition is a "natural" result of wear and tear on the joints. What could diet possibly do?

According to a preliminary study, however, what you eat can make a difference. Researchers at Boston University School of Medicine studied the eating habits of people with osteoarthritis of the knee. They found that those getting the most vitamin C—more than 200 milligrams a day—were three times less likely to have the disease get worse than those who got the least vitamin C (less than 120 milligrams a day).

The researchers aren't sure why vitamin C seemed to make such a difference, says study leader Timothy McAlindon, M.D., assistant professor of medicine at the medical school. Since vitamin C is an antioxidant, it may protect the joints from the damaging effects of free radicals, unstable molecules that can cause joint inflammation. "Vitamin C may also help generate collagen, which enhances the body's ability to repair damage to the cartilage," he says.

Dr. McAlindon recommends that people get at least 120 milligrams of vitamin C a day in their diets, twice the Daily Value. "That's the amount in a couple of oranges," he says. Other fruits and vegetables rich in vitamin C include cantaloupe, broccoli, strawberries, peppers, and cranberry juice.

It's not only what you eat that can affect osteoarthritis but also how much you weigh.

"There's good evidence that people who are overweight are at increased risk for developing osteoarthritis in weight-bearing joints like the knee," says Dr. Pisetsky. Research also suggests that overweight people are at higher risk for developing osteoarthritis in non-weight-bearing joints, such as those in the hands. "Losing weight leads to less pain and improved mobility," he says.

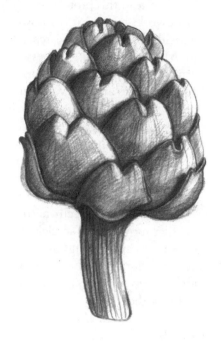

Artichokes
Hearts for Good Health

Healing Power

Can help:
Protect against
skin cancer

Prevent heart
and liver diseases

Prevent birth defects

When Henry II's wife started eating artichokes in France during the Renaissance, the natives deemed it positively scandalous. The artichoke, after all, was rumored to be an aphrodisiac—hardly the food that a lady the likes of Lady Catherine should be eating with abandon.

Four hundred years have passed since then, and there's little evidence that artichokes can fire your libido. But they can do a lot to fuel your health. Research has shown that they contain a compound that can help prevent certain kinds of cancer and even heal a damaged liver.

Green Globes of Protection

Artichokes originated in the scorching Nile Valley and today are grown most prolifically in the sun-baked soil of Castroville, California. So perhaps it's not surprising that the artichoke, which is actually the immature flower of the thistle plant, may provide protection against skin cancer.

In a study at the University Hospitals of Cleveland and Case Western Reserve University School of Medicine, also in Cleveland, researchers found that an ointment made with silymarin, a compound found in artichokes, was able to prevent skin cancer in mice.

In the Kitchen

At first glance, the artichoke is kind of like Rubik's Cube—it looks inviting and intriguing, but you're not sure you want to mess with it.

Appearances can be deceptive. If you follow a few easy tips, preparing and eating artichokes is simple.

- Dirt readily gets lodged beneath their scaly leaves, so it's important to rinse artichokes thoroughly before cooking them.
- Pull off the tough outer, lower petals. With a sharp knife, slice off the stems so that they're level with the bottoms of the artichokes.
- Stand the artichokes in a large saucepan. Cover them halfway with water and simmer, covered, for 30 to 40 minutes. Or place them on a steaming rack and steam for the same amount of time.
- To test for doneness, pull on a center petal. If it comes out easily, the artichoke is done.
- To eat the leaves, hold them by the tip, curved side down, and draw them between your teeth to remove the tender flesh.
- When the leaves are gone, use a fork or spoon to scoop out the hairy layer, called the choke. Discard the hairy choke, then dig into the best part—the tender heart.

You don't have to wear artichokes to reap this protection. "Silymarin works because it is a powerful antioxidant," explains researcher Hasan Mukhtar, Ph.D., professor of dermatology and environmental health sciences at Case Western Reserve University School of Medicine. Antioxidants help prevent cancer in the body by mopping up harmful, cell-damaging molecules known as free radicals before they damage DNA and pave the way for tumors to develop. Free radicals occur naturally, but their formation is accelerated by exposure to such things as sunlight and air pollution. You can't stop free radicals from forming, but artichokes can block their effects.

"It's such an effective antioxidant that silymarin extract is even used medicinally against liver disease in Europe," says Dr. Mukhtar. Studies haven't been done yet to determine how many artichokes you'd have to eat to reap these benefits, he adds. In the meantime, preliminary research suggests that you can't go wrong by including more of these super-healthy—and very tasty—vegetables in your diet.

Hearts for Your Heart

As Americans continue to enjoy the convenience of drive-through, fast-food living, they often come up short on many significant food components, particularly the fiber that only comes from plant foods.

Even though dietary fiber does

not have nutritional value, it's of tremendous importance. By adding bulk to the stool, it causes wastes to be excreted from the body more quickly. This is essential for sweeping toxins and cholesterol from the intestinal tract before they cause problems. In addition, getting enough fiber in your diet (the Daily Value, or DV, is 25 grams) can help prevent high cholesterol, heart disease, high blood pressure, high blood sugar (a precursor of diabetes), and certain kinds of cancer, particularly colon cancer.

Artichokes are an excellent fiber source. One medium cooked artichoke contains more than 6 grams of the rough stuff, providing about a quarter of your daily requirement. Even if you don't eat the leaves, you can get plenty of fiber from the hearts alone. Frozen or fresh, a half-cup serving of artichoke hearts delivers about 5 grams of fiber, 20 percent of the DV.

Artichokes are also a good source of magnesium, a mineral that has been found to be helpful in controlling high blood pressure. Magnesium helps keep muscles running smoothly and lessens the risk of arrhythmia, which is a potentially dangerous variation in the heart's normal rhythm. Studies have shown that 20 to 35 percent of people who have heart failure also have low levels of magnesium.

One medium artichoke delivers 72 milligrams of magnesium, 18 percent of the DV. A half-cup serving of artichoke hearts alone provides 50 milligrams, nearly 13 percent of the DV.

FILLED WITH FOLATE

Pregnant women would be especially wise to sink their teeth into the sweet layers of artichokes because, as researchers have discovered, artichokes are loaded with folate, a B vitamin known for its importance in fetal development.

Even if you're not pregnant, folate is an essential nutrient. It helps the nerves function properly, and studies show that it may be important in protecting against heart disease and certain cancers as well.

Unfortunately, folate deficiency is one of the most common vitamin deficiencies in this country. We simply don't eat enough okra, spinach, and other folate-rich foods to get the 400 micrograms we need each day.

One medium artichoke contains 61 micrograms of folate, 15 percent of the DV. A half-cup of artichoke hearts contains about 43 micrograms, which is 11 percent of the DV.

A BURST OF C

As with most fruits and vegetables grown in the sun-drenched California soils, artichokes are a good source of vitamin C.

Like silymarin, vitamin C is a potent antioxidant, so it squelches free radicals before they do damage. Studies also show that eating plenty of vitamin C helps maintain healthy skin and strong immunity against bacteria and viruses. One medium artichoke contains about 12 milligrams of vitamin C, 20 percent of the DV.

Getting the Most

Enjoy the convenience. The one problem that many people have with artichokes is that they're too much work to eat. An easy alternative is to buy a bag of frozen hearts. They're a snap to prepare, and although they lose some nutrients during processing, they actually have more folate than their fresh counterparts.

For vitamin C, eat it fresh. Vitamin C is easily destroyed during processing. So when you're trying to boost your intake of this important vitamin, fresh artichokes are the way to go.

Go easy on the dip. In their natural state, artichokes are a low-fat food—a benefit that's quickly lost when you dip the leaves in butter. To maintain their low-fat profile while still adding a bit of zest, replace the butter with a dip of low-fat yogurt seasoned with garlic or lemon juice.

Artichoke Gratin

2 **packages (9 ounces each) frozen artichoke hearts**

1 **tablespoon fresh lemon juice**

3 **tablespoons plain dry bread crumbs**

1 **tablespoon grated Parmesan cheese**

1 **teaspoon dried Italian herb seasoning**

1 **clove garlic, minced**

1 **teaspoon olive oil**

Per serving

calories	**95**
total fat	**2.5 g.**
saturated fat	**0.7 g.**
cholesterol	**1 mg.**
sodium	**137 mg.**
dietary fiber	**7 g.**

Preheat the oven to 375°F. Coat a 9" glass pie plate with no-stick spray.

Place the artichokes in a colander and rinse well with cold water to separate. Drain well, then pat dry with paper towels. Place in the prepared pie plate and sprinkle lightly with the lemon juice. Toss to coat.

In a small bowl, combine the bread crumbs, Parmesan, herb seasoning, garlic, and oil. Toss with a fork to mix. Sprinkle the mixture evenly over the artichokes.

Bake for 15 to 20 minutes, or until the topping is golden. Serve warm.

Makes 4 servings

Cook's Notes: Use the artichokes straight from the freezer. There's no need to thaw them.

If Italian herb seasoning is unavailable, substitute 1/2 teaspoon dried oregano, 1/2 teaspoon dried basil, and a pinch of crushed dried rosemary.

Artificial Sweeteners
Sweets without Sin

More than 90 years ago, scientists began looking for substances that would provide the sweetness of sugar without the calories. And soon enough, they found them, to the great joy of cola-drinking, gum-chewing, and snack-eating people who, for the first time, thought they could indulge their cravings for sweets without adding to their waistlines.

Today, artificial sweeteners such as saccharin (Sweet 'N Low), aspartame (NutraSweet), and acesulfame-K (Sunette) are stirred into millions of cups of coffee every year. They're also used commercially in sugar-free gums, candies, and desserts.

What makes artificial sweeteners special is their molecular shape. Even though they tickle the sweet buds on your tongue, they contribute hardly any calories (between 0 and 4, depending on the brand) to your diet. And because artificial sweeteners are chemically different from sugar, they don't cause the same problems, says Stanley Segall, Ph.D., professor of nutrition and food science at Drexel University in Philadelphia.

When you eat sugary foods, for example, bacteria in your mouth quickly multiply, creating acids that can damage the soft enamel on your teeth. Artificial sweeteners, however, don't encourage these bacteria to grow. So if you substitute artificially sweetened foods for those with "natural" sugar, you'll have a much lower risk of tooth decay.

In addition, artificial sweeteners are a real boon for people with diabetes. Unlike sugar, which can cause dangerous swings in blood sugar, artificial sweeteners don't affect it at all. "They're especially helpful when it comes to soft drinks," Dr. Segall says. "Artificial sweeteners allow people with diabetes to enjoy these beverages without paying the sugar penalty."

The Artificial Sweetener Blues

Despite their benefits, though, artificial sweeteners have actually failed in their main mission—to help people enjoy sweets without gaining weight. If anything, people have been getting heavier since the sugar substitutes were first introduced, says Christina M. Stark, R.D., a nutrition specialist in the division of nutritional sciences at Cornell University in Ithaca, New York.

In a landmark study of more than 80,000 nurses, Harvard researchers found that the single best dietary predictor of weight gain was how much saccharin the women ate. A later study revealed that people who used artificial sweeteners were, on average, two pounds heavier than people who did not.

Even though artificial sweeteners add little or no calories, they'll only help you lose weight if you use them *instead* of sugar. "Since artificial sweeteners came out, consumption of both regular sugar and artificial sweeteners has gone up," explains Stark. "We just added them to our sugar consumption, so we're getting more total calories."

Artificial sweeteners can help you lose weight, says Dr. Segall, if you're smart about using them. You can't assume, for example, that "sugar-free" means "calorie-free." A cake made with artificial sweeteners may not contain sugar calories, but it could have a lot of calories from fats or other carbohydrates besides sugar.

One mistake people sometimes make is rewarding themselves for "saving" calories, Dr. Segall adds. If you have a diet cola, for example, you'll save over 100 calories and about 30 grams of sugar over the regular kind. But that won't do you any good if you splurge on a high-calorie drink later on.

FOOD ALERT
ASPARTAME UNDER FIRE

The artificial sweetener aspartame (NutraSweet) is a miracle of food technology. Made from two amino acids, it is 200 times sweeter than sugar, yet delivers almost no calories.

Over the years, however, it has come under fire because of persistent speculation that it may contribute to serious problems such as seizures and attention deficit disorder. While research has shown that aspartame doesn't play a role in either of these conditions, it isn't entirely without risk, at least for a small number of people.

The Centers for Disease Control and Prevention in Atlanta has been tracking problems linked to aspartame. In some people, apparently, it can cause headaches, heart palpitations, or swelling of the face, hands, or feet, among other problems.

More seriously, one small study found that people with a history of depression tended to have more serious symptoms when they consumed as little as 30 milligrams (about one packet) of aspartame a day.

If you're sensitive to aspartame, the only solution is to read food labels carefully and avoid foods that contain it.

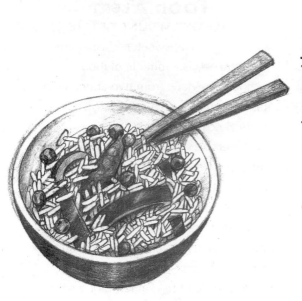

ASIAN DIET
EAST EATS BETTER

HEALING POWER
CAN HELP:
Ease menopausal discomfort

Lower cholesterol

Reduce the risk of cancer
and heart disease

Every year Americans spend more than $884 billion on health care in the quest to stay younger and healthier and live longer. But if we really want to improve our health, perhaps we should take some of that money and get on the next boat to China or Japan. Studies show that people living in Asian countries have lower cholesterol as well as lower rates of heart disease and cancer than people in America.

They're also slimmer. The average 5-foot 4-inch woman in Japan, for example, weighs 126 pounds. That's 24 pounds lighter than her average American counterpart, who weighs about 150.

What's the reason for their good health? Although exercise and close family relationships certainly play a role, the main reason appears to be the traditional Asian diet, which has been called the healthiest in the world.

"I saw people eating a diet similar to the Asian diet when I was a young doctor on a plantation in Hawaii, taking care of Filipinos of all generations," recalls John A. McDougall, M.D., medical director of the McDougall Program at St. Helena Hospital in Napa Valley, California, and author of *The McDougall Program for a Healthy Heart*. "The older, first-generation people never got sick. But their children who adopted American eating habits eventually got fat and got all the diseases we see today."

The Asian diet is surprisingly simple and satisfying. Rice, noodles, breads, and other grains make the foundation, which is topped with generous portions of bok choy, mushrooms, and other fruits and vegetables. The diet also includes beans, seeds, nuts, a smattering of fish, eggs, and poultry, a few sweets, and occasionally some meats.

The term *Asian diet* is typically taken to mean Chinese and Japanese foods, but it also embraces cuisines from Korea, India, Thailand, and Vietnam. In all of these countries, people enjoy a rich array of foods, but the fundamentals of the diet remain the same.

WHERE'S THE BEEF?

While the Asian diet has many important components, perhaps the most healthful element is what it doesn't have—specifically, lots of meat and the accompanying saturated fat and cholesterol.

In China, for instance, people eat an average of 4 pounds of beef a year. In Japan, they eat more, about 23 pounds of beef and veal a year. The average American, in contrast, chows down 94 pounds of beef a year, plus chicken, pork, and other meats. Americans get approximately 35 percent of their calories from fat, while in Japan it's only about 11 percent.

As you would expect, cholesterol levels tend to be much lower in Asian countries, at least among people who eat traditional diets. The benefits can be profound, since lower cholesterol levels reduce not only the risk of heart disease but also the risk of cancer.

THE BENEFITS OF SOY

It's not only the absence of meat and highly processed foods that makes the Asian diet so healthful. People in Asian countries also eat a lot of soy foods—

MAKING THE GOOD BETTER

Although the traditional Asian diet includes many of the foods that we eat every day, there is one notable exception. You won't find a lot of milk, cheese, or other dairy foods. This is one reason that Asian diets are so low in fat. It also may explain why Asian bones aren't as strong as they could be.

Even though you can get a lot of calcium from plant foods like bok choy and broccoli, most scientists agree that dairy foods play a critical role in keeping bones strong. In fact, when researchers compared calcium intake and bone density, they found that women who got their calcium largely from dairy foods had bone densities 20 percent higher than those who got their calcium mainly from plant foods.

"Bone density is a concern in countries like China," explains Robert M. Russell, M.D., of the Jean Mayer USDA Human Nutrition Research Center on Aging at Tufts University in Boston. So even if you find yourself following a traditional Asian diet, be sure to supplement it with low-fat milk, cheese, and other dairy foods, says Dr. Russell.

EATING THE ASIAN WAY

Take a look at almost any loaf of bread, and on the package you'll see the U.S. Department of Agriculture's Food Guide Pyramid, a guide that recommends that everyone eat approximately 15 to 26 servings of fruits, vegetables, beans, grains, and proteins every day. The pyramid is considered the benchmark for healthy eating in this country.

As it turns out, there's also an Asian Pyramid, which is one of the healthiest food plans in the world. Unlike the U.S. pyramid, which includes both milk products and meat as a way of getting enough protein every day, the Asian pyramid replaces those foods with beans, nuts, seeds, and fish. Plus, it includes a fair amount of vegetable oils, as well as moderate amounts of sake, beer, tea, and other beverages. Exercise is also an important part of this plan.

When you follow the Asian plan, be sure to pick most of your foods from the base of the pyramid, leaving those at the top for special occasions. Incidentally, except in India, dairy foods are rarely eaten in Asia.

Meat — Once a month (Or more often in very small amounts)
Sweets
Eggs & poultry — Once a week (Or more often in very small amounts)
Fish & shellfish or dairy — Optional daily
Vegetable oils — Daily
Fruits | Legumes, nuts, and seeds | Vegetables
Regular physical exercise
Moderate alcohol consumption
Rice, rice products, noodles, breads, millet, corn, and other grains (unrefined, if possible)

Adapted from "Traditional Healthy Asian Diet Pyramid"
© 1995 Oldways Production & Exchange Trust

3 to 4 ounces a day of tempeh, tofu, defatted soy flour, and more.

There are several reasons that soy foods are so healthful, says Christopher Gardner, Ph.D., research fellow at the Stanford University Center for Research in Disease Prevention in Palo Alto, California. They're rich in a group of natural compounds called phytoestrogens, which the body converts into hormonelike substances that act like a weak form of estrogen. In premenopausal women, these faux estrogens block the body's estrogen receptors, lowering the amount of estrogen in the body. This can help lower the risk of breast cancer.

Later in life, the phytoestrogens in soy can ease menopausal symptoms such as hot flashes by replacing the estrogen lost during this time. In fact, Asian women rarely experience hot flashes. They're also less likely than American women to have heart disease, because phytoestrogens have a protective effect.

Soy foods are the major source of protein in Asian countries. In China, people get only 11 percent of their protein from meat, while in America, 69 percent of our protein comes from meat. The more protein you eat from animal sources, the more calcium is excreted from the body. This can be a problem for women, who have a higher risk of developing osteoporosis than men do.

Even if you don't follow the Asian diet all that closely, you can't go wrong if you add more soy foods to your diet, Dr. Gardner says.

Natural Goodness

The National Cancer Institute has been preaching "five fruits and vegetables a day," and nutritionists have been begging us to get the Daily Value of 25 grams of fiber instead of the paltry 11 to 12 grams most of us get each day.

The Asian diet, which is packed with fresh fruits, vegetables, and other fiber-rich foods, is on the cutting edge. In China, for example, people get 33 grams of fiber every day. That's serious heart protection, according to researchers at the Harvard School of Public Health, who, in a six-year study of almost 41,000 men, found that those who increased their daily fiber intake by just 10 grams were able to decrease their risk of heart disease by almost 30 percent.

These fruits and vegetables are also rich sources of vitamin C, carotenoids (including beta-carotene), and other antioxidant compounds that help protect the body from disease. Studies show that people who eat the most fruits and vegetables have the lowest rates of heart disease and cancer.

A Cup of Health

Walk into any Asian restaurant and you'll be served a pot of tea. Don't stop with one cup. Research suggests that having four small cups of tea a day can substantially lower your risk of heart disease and stroke. Asians, of course, drink tea by the potful, which may explain their robust good health.

Tea contains potent antioxidant compounds called phenols, which protect the body from disease. In a study of 552 men, researchers in the Netherlands found that those who drank about five cups of black tea a day had about one-third the risk of stroke of those drinking fewer than 2½ cups.

In the world of antioxidants, the phenols in tea are "absolutely exquisite," says Gary Stoner, Ph.D., director of the cancer chemoprevention program at the Ohio State University Comprehensive Cancer Center in Columbus. And green tea, the kind preferred in Eastern countries, has more antioxidant power than black tea.

Fishy Business

Japan is an island, which means that people there eat a lot of fish. For years, researchers believed that the more fish people ate, the healthier they were. Numerous studies show that even small amounts of fish, as little as 3 ounces a week, provide powerful protection. "Fish contains fats that thin the blood and help prevent heart disease," says Dr. McDougall.

But while some fish is good, more isn't necessarily better. A 30-year study of 2,000 men led by researchers at Northwestern University Medical School in Chicago found that those who ate more than 8 ounces of fish a week had higher stroke rates than those who ate less. In fact, stroke and other cerebrovascular diseases are traditionally one of the leading causes of death in Japan.

This doesn't mean that you should stop eating fish, says Dr. McDougall. "It's a delicacy and should be eaten in small amounts," he says. "Don't just replace your chicken with a big slab of fish and think you're eating healthy."

ASIAN NOODLES WITH VEGETABLES

1   **egg, lightly beaten**
9   **ounces dry eggless chow mein noodles or baked ramen noodles**
1   **tablespoon canola oil**
1   **tablespoon minced garlic**
4   **cups thinly sliced bok choy stems and leaves**
1   **medium carrot, shredded**
1   **tablespoon reduced-sodium soy sauce**
1   **teaspoon sugar**
1   **teaspoon dark sesame oil**

PER SERVING

calories	**338**
total fat	**7.2 g.**
saturated fat	**1 g.**
cholesterol	**53 mg.**
sodium	**197 mg.**
dietary fiber	**3.9 g.**

Coat a small no-stick skillet with no-stick spray. Warm over medium heat. Add the egg and swirl the pan so the egg coats the bottom. Cook for about 1 minute, or until almost set. Carefully turn and cook a few seconds until the egg is set on the bottom. Remove from the pan and place on a cutting board to cool slightly. Roll up tightly and cut into strips. Set aside.

Cook the noodles (discard the seasoning packet or reserve for another use) in a pot of boiling water for 3 minutes, or according to the package directions. Drain, rinse with cold water, and drain again. Set aside.

In a large no-stick skillet or wok over medium heat, warm the canola oil. Add the garlic and cook for 30 seconds, or until fragrant. Add the bok choy and carrots. Stir-fry for 1 to 2 minutes, or until the bok choy starts to wilt. Add the noodles, soy sauce, sugar, and sesame oil. Cook, tossing, for 1 to 2 minutes, or until the noodles are heated through. Add the reserved egg strips and toss to combine.

Makes 4 servings

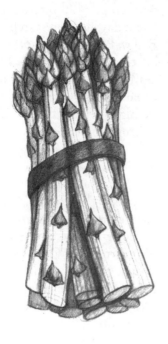

ASPARAGUS
SPEARS
OF PROTECTION

HEALING POWER
CAN HELP:
Prevent birth defects

Reduce the risk
of heart disease
and cancer

Asparagus was extremely popular among the royal households of seventeenth-century France—not just for its fresh taste but also because the tender spears were thought to be a powerful aphrodisiac.

For asparagus aficionados—even those without amour on the brain—there's no more welcome sign of spring than those brilliant green tips poking up from winter's ground. It's a welcome sign for health as well, since asparagus contains compounds that can help fight birth defects, heart disease, and cancer.

FILLED WITH FOLATE

One of the most critical medical breakthroughs of this century was the discovery that the incidence of brain and spinal cord birth defects (called neural tube defects) could be cut in half if women of childbearing age got 400 micrograms of folate a day.

Asparagus is richly endowed with folate, a B vitamin that is essential for helping cells regenerate. Five asparagus spears contain 110 micrograms of folate, about 28 percent of the Daily Value (DV).

If you're pregnant, you may want to take a double serving. While govern-

It's not something that will send you running to the emergency room, but you may have noticed a curious fact about asparagus. After you eat even a small amount, your urine seems to have an unpleasant odor.

It's not your imagination. Asparagus contains an amino acid called aspartic acid. Many people lack the enzyme needed to break aspartic acid down. As a result, it stays in the body and gets converted to a related compound—one with that distinctive sulfurous smell.

While there isn't a "cure" for this telltale aroma, neither is it anything worth worrying about. So have an extra helping of asparagus and ignore the temporary odor.

ment guidelines recommend that women get 400 micrograms of folate a day, folate researcher Lynn B. Bailey, Ph.D., professor of nutrition at the University of Florida in Gainesville, suggests that the optimal level for pregnant women may be higher, "possibly as high as 600 micrograms," she says.

Not only is folate good for women in their childbearing years, it also fights heart disease in everyone. It appears that folate acts as a floodgate, controlling the amount of homocysteine (an amino acid) in the bloodstream. When folate levels drop, homocysteine levels rise, causing damage to the tender arteries supplying blood to the heart and brain.

For preventing heart disease, getting enough folate may be just as important as controlling cholesterol. Indeed, heart researchers say that if Americans would increase their intake of folate to 400 micrograms a day, the number of deaths caused by heart disease would drop by at least 13,500. Currently, only 12 percent of us are getting that much.

PROTECTION AGAINST CANCER

As you've come to expect from all the green vegetables, asparagus offers powerful protection against cancer. It contains a number of compounds that essentially double-team cancer-causing substances before they do harm.

The first of these substances is folate. Studies reveal that people with the most folate in their blood are the ones least likely to develop colon cancer.

The second protective compound in asparagus is glutathione. A small protein, glutathione is a powerful antioxidant. This means that it helps mop up free radicals, high-energy particles that, when left unchecked, ricochet wildly through the body, scarring and punching holes in cells, and doing the types of damage that can lead to cancer. In an analysis of 38 vegetables, freshly cooked asparagus ranked first for its glutathione content.

IN THE KITCHEN

Asparagus is among the easiest vegetables to prepare and cook. What's more, its natural freshness means that you don't need butter or sauces to bring out its flavors. To enjoy great taste with little effort, here's what cooks advise.

Check the tips. When buying asparagus, take a close look at the tips. Fresh asparagus tips are compact and tightly furled. If the tips look loose and frayed, the asparagus is getting old, and you should pass it by.

Remove the stalk. Although you can eat asparagus from top to bottom, the tough, woody stalk is usually discarded. The easiest way to do this is simply to bend the stalk; asparagus naturally snaps off at the point where the tough end stops and the tender top begins.

When the spears are thick, however, the snap method can waste perfectly good flesh. To preserve more of the stalk, use a vegetable peeler to peel the bottom area of each spear. Use a knife to find the point where the flesh turns woody (it will be tough to slice) and cut the bottom off there.

Take the E Train

There's another reason to add more asparagus to your plate. It contains vitamin E, which can be very good for the heart. A study led by researchers at the University of Minnesota School of Public Health in Minneapolis found that getting as little as 10 international units of vitamin E a day can substantially reduce the risk of heart disease in women. Five asparagus spears have 0.4 international unit of vitamin E. That's about 1 percent of the DV.

"This is the first study to examine the effect of vitamin E from food instead of from supplements, and the results surprised even us," says Lawrence H. Kushi, Sc.D., associate professor of public health, nutrition, and epidemiology at the University of Minnesota in Minneapolis and the lead investigator of the study.

Obviously, you'd have to eat a lot of asparagus (119 spears, to be exact) to get the amount of vitamin E that proved most beneficial in the study. In fact, it's difficult to get large amounts of vitamin E from diet alone since it's most abundant in oils and nuts. That's why many doctors recommend taking vitamin E supplements.

Vitamin E does more than protect against heart disease. Research suggests that it may even help prevent Type II, or non-insulin-dependent, diabetes, both by protecting the pancreas (the organ that produces insulin) and by influencing how the body burns sugar. A study of 944 men ages 42 to 60 found that men with low levels of vitamin E had nearly four times the risk of developing this disease.

Getting the Most

Store it carefully. Folate is destroyed by exposure to air, heat, or light, so you need to store asparagus carefully, says Gertrude Armbruster, R.D., Ph.D., director of the dietetic program at Cornell University in Ithaca, New York. She recommends storing it away from light in the back of the refrigerator or in a produce drawer.

Cook it gently. Asparagus is a tender vegetable, and vigorous boiling isn't necessary. "Microwaving asparagus definitely destroys fewer nutrients than does boiling or even steaming," Dr. Armbruster says.

Stand it upright. Since most of asparagus's nutrients are in the tip, it's better to cook it upright in a tall container rather than piling it at the bottom of a baking dish, Dr. Armbruster says. Add a few inches of water to the pot, cover with a lid, and bring to a simmer. Keeping the tips out of the water will not only preserve nutrients but will also help the stalks cook evenly and more quickly.

ASPARAGUS WITH ORANGE-SOY DRESSING

1 **pound asparagus**

1 **tablespoon reduced-sodium soy sauce**

1 **tablespoon fresh orange juice**

½ **teaspoon grated orange rind**

½ **teaspoon grated fresh ginger**

½ **teaspoon dark sesame oil**

2 **shallots or 1 small onion, minced**

Snap any tough bottoms from the asparagus stalks. Rinse the asparagus and place it on a steamer rack in a large saucepan containing 1″ of water. Cover and bring to a boil over high heat. Steam for 5 to 7 minutes, or until crisp-tender.

In a small bowl, combine the soy sauce, orange juice, orange rind, ginger, and oil. Whisk to mix well. Stir in the shallots or onions. Drizzle the mixture over the asparagus and toss gently to coat.

Makes 4 servings

PER SERVING

calories	**40**
total fat	**0.8 g.**
saturated fat	**0.1 g.**
cholesterol	**0 mg.**
sodium	**129 mg.**
dietary fiber	**2.4 g.**

ASTHMA
FOODS FOR EASY BREATHING

If you have asthma, it doesn't take much: A fast walk, a sudden shot of cold air, or even of whiff of pollen can cause airways inside your lungs to narrow suddenly, making each breath seem unbelievably precious.

But asthma can be controlled. A vital part of the strategy is what you eat. "Diet is the key," says Richard N. Firshein, D.O., assistant professor of family medicine at New York College of Osteopathic Medicine, medical director of Paul Sorvino Asthma Foundation in New York City, and author of *Reversing Asthma*.

FIGHTING INFLAMMATION

Much of the battle against asthma is a battle against inflammation. When pollen, pollution, or other airborne irritants enter the lungs, the immune system releases chemicals to "kill" the invaders. Unfortunately, the chemicals that are meant to defend you can actually do a lot of harm. They cause the airways to become inflamed and swollen, which makes breathing difficult. At the same time, the body releases clouds of free radicals, the harmful oxygen molecules that make the inflammation even worse. This is why, in people with asthma, the airways tend to stay inflamed long after the attack is over.

One way to stop asthma is to reduce the inflammation. There's some evidence that foods high in vitamin C and other antioxidants, which block the effects of free radicals, can help the airways return to normal. "We know an asthma attack is an inflammatory thing, and we know it produces a lot of oxygen radicals," says Gary E. Hatch, Ph.D., research toxicologist in the pulmonary toxicology branch of the Environmental Protection Agency. "So antioxidants should help."

The three antioxidants that appear to have the most stopping power against asthma are selenium and vitamins C and E. In addition, there are a number of foods, such as fish, that have been shown to reduce inflammation throughout your body, including in the lungs.

GIVING ASTHMA THE JUICE

As part of nature's plan to control free radicals, vitamin C is naturally concentrated in the lining of the lungs. This is why it's a good idea for people with asthma to eat a diet rich in this antioxidant nutrient.

Two large studies, the National Health and Nutrition Examination surveys, found that people who got the most vitamin C in their diets were much less likely to have respiratory diseases, including asthma, than those who got the least. And it doesn't take a lot of vitamin C to get the benefits, says Dr. Hatch. Research suggests that getting 200 milligrams a day—more than three times the Daily Value (DV) of 60 milligrams—will go a long way toward keeping your lungs strong.

Vitamin C is one of the easiest antioxidants to get a lot of. A 6-ounce glass of freshly squeezed orange juice, for example, delivers 93 milligrams of vitamin C, a third more than the DV. Other super sources include citrus fruits, bell peppers, broccoli, brussels sprouts, and strawberries.

Breathe Deep with E

Research suggests that vitamin E can dramatically lower your risk of asthma. In a large study of 75,000 nurses, for example, Harvard University researchers found that those getting the most vitamin E in their diets were 47 percent less likely to have asthma than those getting the least.

The advantage of vitamin E is that it appears to target free radicals that are caused by air pollution, one of the leading causes of asthma. In addition, vitamin E stimulates the release of chemicals in the body that help relax smooth muscles, including muscles that make up the airways in the lungs.

As with vitamin C, it doesn't take a lot of vitamin E to get the benefits. In the nurses' study, for example, women in the low-asthma group were getting no more than the DV of 30 international units.

Since vitamin E is found mainly in cooking oils, however, it's not always easy to get the necessary amounts. Perhaps the best way to get more of this nutrient in your diet is to put wheat germ on the menu by adding it to other foods, like muffins or meat loaf. One serving of wheat germ has 5 international units. of vitamin E, nearly 17 percent of the DV. You can get smaller amounts of vitamin E in almonds, sunflower seeds, whole-grain cereals, spinach, and kale.

A Nutty Solution

Selenium is one of the trace minerals, which means that you don't need a lot of it. Research suggests, however, that a little selenium goes a long way, especially for people with asthma.

Like vitamins C and E, selenium is an antioxidant that can help protect the lungs from free radicals. What's more, the body uses selenium (in combination with a compound called glutathione) to make vitamins C and E work more effectively.

In a study of 115 people, researchers in New Zealand found that those getting the most selenium in their diets were five times less likely to have asthma than those getting the least.

The DV for selenium is 70 micrograms, which appears to be all you need to keep the risk for asthma low. Meats, chicken, and seafood are good selenium selections, but they can't touch Brazil nuts. One Brazil nut contains 120 micrograms of selenium, 170 percent of the DV.

Restoring the Flow

Even though antioxidants can help control (and prevent) asthma over the long run, they aren't much good when you need fast relief. For that, you might want to sit down to a good meal of halibut, steamed oysters, spinach, and black-eyed peas. Each of these foods is high in magnesium, a mineral that can help you start breathing again.

Magnesium relaxes smooth muscles in the airways, allowing more air to get through. In addition, it reduces the activity of cells in the body that cause inflammation. In hospitals, in fact, doctors often use a form of magnesium—in an injection, unfortunately, not on the half-shell—to provide fast relief from asthma attacks.

In one study, English researchers exposed more than 2,600 people with asthma to an airway-constricting chemical. They found that those getting the least magnesium in their diets were twice as likely to have their airways shut down as those getting the most.

Oysters, halibut, and mackerel are good magnesium finds. Cooked spinach is also good, with a half-cup providing 78 milligrams of magnesium, about 20 percent of the DV.

Catching Your Breath

Finally, you might try fishing for asthma relief at your local fish market. Studies show that the omega-3 fatty acids found in fish can help reduce inflammation in the lungs. What's more, these oils appear to reduce the tissue damage that often follows asthma attacks, says Dr. Firshein.

Salmon, mackerel, and other oily fish, which are high in omega-3's, appear to be the best choices for stopping asthma. In one large survey, Australian researchers found that in families where people ate very little oily fish, almost 16 percent of the children had asthma. In families where these fish were frequently on the menu, however, only 9 percent of the children had asthma. And in families where no fish was served, the rate of asthma in children was 23 percent.

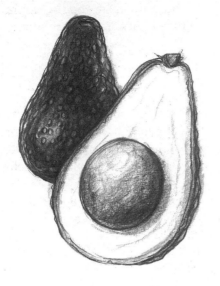

Avocados
No Longer a Forbidden Fruit

Healing Power
Can help:
Control cholesterol

Lower blood pressure

Prevent birth defects

Ounce for ounce, the humble avocado packs more calories than almost any other fruit on the planet: 731. It also has the dubious distinction of being one of the few fruits with a measurable fat content, with up to 30 grams each. That's half the daily recommended amount for an average adult.

You wouldn't think that a food that's so fattening could be good for you. But that's the word from dietitians, who say that adding a little avocado to your diet every day could actually improve your health.

Avocados are great sources of folate and potassium. They also contain high amounts of fiber and monounsaturated fat, both of which are good news for people who are concerned with diabetes or heart health.

Part of a Diabetes Diet

People with diabetes have traditionally been told to eat more carbohydrates and cut back on fat. Overall that's good advice, but it's not necessarily the best advice for everyone.

Doctors have discovered that when some people who have diabetes eat a lot of carbohydrates, they tend to develop high levels of triglycerides, a type of blood fat that may contribute to heart disease. Surprisingly, when people replace some of those carbohydrates with fat, particularly the kind of fat found in avocados, the dangerous fats in the bloodstream tend to decline.

Avocados are a rich source of monounsaturated fats, particularly a kind called oleic acid. "We've found that these monounsaturated fats improve fat levels in the body and help control diabetes," says Abhimanyu Garg, M.D., associate professor of internal medicine and clinical nutrition at the University of Texas Southwestern Medical Center at Dallas.

In one study, scientists in Mexico put 16 women with diabetes on a relatively high-fat diet, with about 40 percent of calories coming from fat. Most of the fat came from avocados. The result was a 20 percent drop in triglycerides. Women on a higher-carbohydrate plan, by contrast, had only a 7 percent drop in triglycerides.

"What's nice about avocados is that they provide a lot of these monounsaturated fats," adds Dr. Garg. Someone on a 2,000-calorie-a-day diet, for example, might be advised to eat 33 grams of monounsaturated fat. "You can get about 20 grams from just one avocado," he points out.

FOOD ALERT
A RISKY COMBINATION

People who are taking warfarin (Coumadin), a heart medication designed to keep blood from clotting, should go easy on the avocados. Though scientists aren't sure why, the natural oil in avocado seems to prevent the drug from working, at least in some people.

In one small study, researchers in Israel found that eating between $1/2$ and one avocado could make the drug work less efficiently. While the effects didn't last long—when people stopped eating avocado, the drug started working again—this could be dangerous for some people. So if you're taking warfarin, check with your doctor before adding avocados to your menu.

HELP FOR HIGH CHOLESTEROL

People with diabetes aren't the only ones who benefit from eating a little more avocado. The oleic acid in avocados can also help people lower their cholesterol.

In a small study from Mexico, where guacamole is considered almost a food group, researchers compared the effects of two low-fat diets. The diets were the same except that one included avocados. While both lowered levels of dangerous, low-density lipoprotein cholesterol, the avocado diet raised levels of healthful high-density lipoprotein cholesterol while slightly lowering triglycerides.

Another way in which avocados help lower cholesterol is by adding healthful amounts of fiber to the diet, adds Dr. Garg. Fiber adds bulk to the

A lot of people have never picked, prepared, or eaten an avocado. But they're very easy to work with.

Here are a few hints for getting started.

Help them ripen. Like bananas, avocados ripen better off the tree, so they are picked and sold unripe. Once you get them home, leave them on the counter for several days or until the fruit is slightly soft.

Make a pit stop. To open an avocado, cut it lengthwise, rotating the knife all the way around the seed. Then twist the halves in opposite directions to separate the halves. To remove the pit, slip the tip of a spoon underneath and pry it free.

Add some lemon. Avocados quickly turn brown once the skin has been removed. Sprinkling the cut surfaces with lemon or lime juice will help the avocado retain its natural color.

stool, causing it, and the cholesterol it contains, to be excreted from the body more quickly. One avocado packs more fiber than a bran muffin—10 grams, 40 percent of the Daily Value (DV).

More Help for Your Heart

Avocados pack a big potassium punch. Half an avocado provides 548 milligrams of potassium, 16 percent of the DV. That's 15 percent more than you'd get in a medium banana.

Studies show that people who eat diets high in potassium-rich foods like avocados have a markedly lower risk of high blood pressure and related diseases like heart attack and stroke.

"You can never get too much potassium," says David B. Young, Ph.D., professor of physiology and biophysics at the University of Mississippi Medical Center in Jackson. Even small additions can make big differences, he says.

A Fortune in Folate

Avocados may be one of the perfect foods when you're eating for two, particularly when it comes to getting enough folate, a nutrient that helps prevent life-threatening birth defects of the brain and spine. Many women don't get enough folate in their diets, but avocados can go a long way toward fixing that. Half an avocado contains 57 micrograms of folate, 14 percent of the DV.

Moms-to-be aren't the only ones who should be dipping their chips in guacamole, though. Everyone needs folate. It's an essential nutrient for keeping nerves functioning properly. It may also help fight heart disease.

Getting the Most

Find fruit from Florida. Even though the monounsaturated fat in avocados is good for cholesterol, it's not so good for your waistline. To get the nutrients from avocado without all the fat, shop for Florida avocados. They have about two-thirds the calories and half the fat of avocados grown in California.

Know when to buy them. Another way to have avocados with a little less fat is to buy those harvested between November and March. They may have one-third the fat of those picked in September or October.

AVOCADO-JICAMA SALAD

2   **cups peeled, matchstick-cut jícama**

¼   **cup fresh orange juice**

2   **tablespoons minced onions**

1   **small serrano pepper, sliced (wear plastic gloves when handling)**

⅛   **teaspoon chili powder**

1   **Florida avocado**

1   **tablespoon chopped fresh cilantro**

PER SERVING

calories	**121**
total fat	**6.9 g.**
saturated fat	**1.4 g.**
cholesterol	**0 mg.**
sodium	**9 mg.**
dietary fiber	**4 g.**

Place the jícama on a serving plate.

In a small bowl, mix the orange juice, onions, peppers, and chili powder. Pour about half of the dressing over the jícama and toss to coat. Spread the jícama out evenly on the plate.

Cut through the avocado lengthwise, then twist gently to separate the halves. Remove the pit and discard it. Peel each half of the avocado, then cut it into thin lengthwise slices. Arrange the slices in spoke fashion on the bed of jícama.

Drizzle with the remaining dressing. With the back of the spoon, spread the dressing gently over the avocado slices to cover thoroughly. Cover and refrigerate for 15 to 30 minutes. Sprinkle with the cilantro.

Makes 4 servings

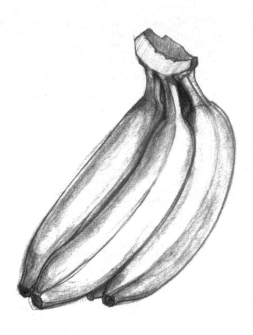

Bananas
A Bunch
of Potassium

Healing Power
Can help:
Decrease risk of stroke

Lower high blood pressure

Relieve heartburn

Prevent ulcers

Speed recovery
from diarrhea

Something about bananas makes people laugh. We talk about "going bananas" and "slipping on banana peels." You would think that these yellow-skinned beauties were made for the comedy club.

But here's something that you'll want to take seriously. Studies have shown that the fruit beneath that slippery skin can do wonders for our health. Bananas may help prevent conditions ranging from heart attack and stroke to high blood pressure and infection. They can even help heal ulcers.

Indeed, despite our lack of reverence, we can eat bananas by the bunches, with every man, woman, and child tossing down about 27 pounds of them each year. After learning more about bananas' remarkable health benefits, you may want to make that 28.

Bananas for the Heart

If the needle on the blood pressure cuff has been inching up in recent years, it may be time for a tropical vacation. If the sun and surf don't bring your pressure down, the bananas sure will.

Bananas are one of nature's best sources of potassium, with each fruit providing about 396 milligrams, 11 percent of the Daily Value (DV) of this essential mineral. Study after study shows that people who eat foods rich in potassium have a significantly lower risk of high blood pressure and related diseases like heart attack and stroke.

Even if you already have high blood pressure, eating plenty of bananas may significantly reduce or even eliminate your need for blood pressure medication, according to scientists at the University of Naples in Italy. Researchers believe that one of the ways that bananas keep blood pressure down is by helping to prevent plaque from sticking to artery walls. They do this by keeping the "bad" low-density lipoprotein cholesterol from oxidizing, a chemical process that makes it more likely to accumulate. That's why bananas may be a good defense against atherosclerosis, or hardening of the arteries, another contributor to high blood pressure, heart attack, and stroke.

And the best part is that you don't have to eat a boatload of bananas to get these benefits, says David B. Young, Ph.D., professor of physiology and biophysics at the University of Mississippi Medical Center in Jackson. Just three to six servings can do the trick.

"Studies show that you can get a significant impact from relatively small changes," says Dr. Young. "My advice would be to think of potassium-rich foods like love and money: You can never get too much."

STOMACH RELIEF

Though more research needs to be done, bananas may replace antacids in your medicine cabinet as an effective way to quell the inner flames of heartburn and indigestion. Although experts don't know why they work, bananas seem to act as a natural antacid.

In addition, bananas may be helpful for preventing and treating ulcers. "There have been a few studies showing that bananas may have a protective effect in ulcer treatment," says William Ruderman, M.D., a gastroenterologist in private practice in Orlando, Florida. "But we need more research before we can know for sure."

Scientists suspect that bananas may guard against stomach damage in two ways. First, a chemical in bananas called protease inhibitor appears to be able to kill off harmful, ulcer-causing bacteria before they do their dirty work. Second, bananas seem to stimulate the production of protective mucus, the layer that helps prevent harsh acids from coming into contact with the tender stomach lining.

RESTORING BALANCE

When you've been run ragged by a case of the runs, it's important that you replenish all the vital fluids and nutrients that diarrhea depletes. And a banana is just the food to do it, says Dr. Ruderman.

"Bananas are a very good source of electrolytes, like potassium, which you lose when you become dehydrated," he explains. Electrolytes are minerals that turn into electrically charged particles in the body, helping to control almost everything that happens inside, from muscle contractions and fluid balance to the beating of the heart.

In addition, bananas contain some pectin, a soluble fiber that acts like a sponge in the digestive tract, absorbing fluids and helping to keep diarrhea in check.

Getting the Most

Broaden your horizons. Even if you're not all that fond of bananas as a snack, there are many other ways to get their healing goodness. In Caribbean countries and Central and South America, for example, people frequently add bananas to everyday recipes—everything from meat loaf to casseroles. Because of their mild, slightly sweet taste, bananas work well in almost any recipe.

Buy a bunch. One reason that people don't eat a lot of bananas is that they tend to get soft and mushy before you get around to eating them. Here's a trick for keeping them fresh. When bananas are getting soft too quickly, put them in the refrigerator. This will quickly stop the ripening process. (Don't be alarmed when the cold turns the skin black—the fruit inside will still be fresh and tasty.)

On the other hand, when you're waiting for that bunch of green bananas to ripen, it's easy to speed up the process. Put them in a brown paper bag at room temperature. The ethylene gas that bananas produce naturally will speed up the ripening.

SAUTÉED BANANAS

4	**large bananas, ripe but firm**
1	**teaspoon unsalted butter**
1	**teaspoon canola oil**
	Ground allspice

PER SERVING

calories	**150**
total fat	**2.8 g.**
saturated fat	**0.9 g.**
cholesterol	**3 mg.**
sodium	**2 mg.**
dietary fiber	**2.9 g.**

Peel the bananas and cut them in half crosswise, then cut the halves lengthwise to make 16 pieces.

In a large no-stick skillet over medium heat, warm the butter and oil. Add the bananas, cut side down, and cook, without moving, for 5 minutes, or until golden. Turn and cook for 1 to 2 minutes, or until lightly golden on the bottom. With a spatula, remove the bananas from the pan and place 4 pieces on each of 4 dessert plates. Season lightly to taste with the allspice. Serve warm.

Makes 4 servings

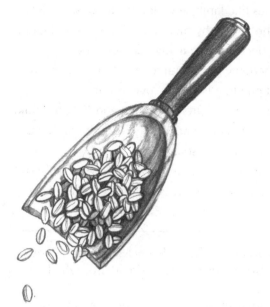

BARLEY
A GREAT GRAIN FOR THE HEART

HEALING POWER
CAN HELP:
Lower cholesterol

Reduce the formation
of blood clots

Improve digestion

Reduce cancer risk

If you're a vitamin E enthusiast, you've probably heard about tocotrienols. Like vitamin E, tocotrienols are antioxidants, meaning that they help reduce damage to the body from dangerous oxygen molecules called free radicals. And barley is one of the richest sources of these compounds.

"Tocotrienols are potentially more powerful antioxidants than other chemical versions of vitamin E," says David J. A. Jenkins, M.D., Sc.D., Ph.D., professor of nutritional sciences and medicine at the University of Toronto. "They have at least 50 percent more free radical–fighting power than other forms." That translates into a lot of heart disease–fighting might.

Tocotrienols fight heart disease in two ways. One, they help stop free radical oxidation, a process that makes low-density lipoprotein (LDL) cholesterol, the dangerous type, more likely to stick to artery walls. And two, they act on the liver to reduce the body's production of cholesterol.

Barley also contains lignans, compounds that have antioxidant ability and thus provide still more protection. According to Lilian Thompson, Ph.D., professor of nutritional sciences at the University of Toronto, lignans can help prevent tiny blood clots from forming, further reducing the risk of heart disease.

Finally, barley is exceptionally high in both selenium and vitamin E. Although research results are mixed, there's mounting evidence that both help pro-

IN THE KITCHEN

Unlike rice and wheat, which are quite mild, barley has a robust, slightly pungent taste that complements highly flavored dishes like lamb stew or mushroom soup. But you prepare it in much the same way as other grains by mixing it with water and letting it simmer, covered, until the kernels are tender. Here are a few additional tips.

Plan for expansion. One cup of dried barley will expand to about four times that amount during cooking, so be sure to use a pan that is slightly oversized.

Give it time to tenderize. Hulled barley can be extremely tough and slow to cook, so it should be soaked overnight before cooking. Pearl barley, on the other hand, has had the tough outer husk removed and doesn't require soaking.

Use it as an add-in. Even properly prepared barley is somewhat chewy, so it's rarely served as a side dish. Most cooks prefer to make barley ahead of time, then add it to soups or stews.

tect against cancer. Indeed, some researchers believe that selenium may work best as an anti-cancer agent when combined with other antioxidants, which, as we've seen, barley has in abundance.

One cup of cooked pearl barley contains 36 micrograms of selenium, more than half the Daily Value (DV), and 5 international units of vitamin E, 17 percent of the DV.

FIBER PROTECTION

Besides helping to reduce damage from dangerous LDL cholesterol, there's another way in which barley helps keep blood vessels healthy. It's loaded with beta-glucan, a type of soluble fiber that forms a gel in the small intestine. Cholesterol in your body binds to this gel, which is then excreted from the body.

Soluble fiber does more than lower cholesterol. It also binds to potential cancer-causing agents in the intestine, keeping them from being absorbed. And because soluble fiber soaks up lots of water in the colon, it helps digestion work more efficiently, thereby preventing constipation.

Getting the Most

Buy it whole. Although pearl barley is the most common form found in American grocery stores, it's been refined no less than five times to scrub off the healthful outer husk and bran layer.

A more nutritious choice is hulled barley. Stripped only of the outer, inedible hull, it's the best source of fiber, minerals, and thiamin. It also has a more distinctive, nuttier flavor than its highly processed counterparts. You can generally find hulled barley at health food stores.

Try it baked. Unless you're extremely fond of cooked barley, it's unlikely that you're ever going to eat 1 cup a day, the amount recommended by Dr. Jenkins to get the most healing power. Here's another way to get more barley into your diet. Add it to baked goods. You can substitute about 1½ cups of barley flour for every 3 cups of regular flour. Or add barley flakes to cookies, muffins, or bread. They will add a distinctly nutty taste while delivering more fiber and nutrients than you'll get from white flour alone.

BARLEY-MUSHROOM SOUP

1 **tablespoon olive oil**

2 **cups chopped onions**

8 **ounces cremini mushrooms, sliced**

1 **medium carrot, finely diced**

1 **cup hulled barley**

2 **cans (16 ounces each) reduced-sodium chicken broth, defatted**

3 **cups water**

2 **teaspoons crushed dried rosemary**

⅛ **teaspoon salt**

In a Dutch oven over medium heat, warm the oil. Add the onions, mushrooms, and carrots. Reduce the heat to medium low and cook, stirring frequently, for 5 minutes, or until the onions soften.

Stir in the barley, broth, water, rosemary, and salt. Bring to a simmer. Reduce the heat to low, partially cover, and cook for 1 to 1½ hours, or until the barley is tender.

Makes 4 main-dish servings

Cook's Note: This soup freezes well and can be kept for several months.

PER SERVING
calories **265**
total fat **6.8 g.**
saturated fat **1.7 g.**
cholesterol **5 mg.**
sodium **185 mg.**
dietary fiber **11 g.**

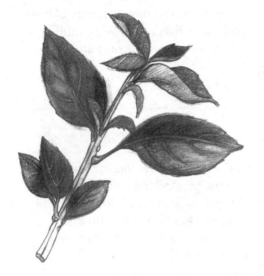

BASIL
LEAVES
FOR GIVING EASE

HEALING POWER
CAN HELP:
Ease digestion

Lower the risk of cancer

Pizza-lovers from Boise to Brooklyn dust their slices with dried basil. Pasta mavens inhale plates of pasta al pesto, redolent with garlic and basil. Gardeners live for the first tomato of the season, drizzled with olive oil and garnished with homegrown, fresh-snipped basil.

Whether it's used dried or fresh, basil's sharp aroma and spicy flavor pleasures the nose as well as the palate. When you treat yourself to basil, you may also be treating yourself to important health benefits. There are substances in this herb that can help calm your stomach and even, researchers believe, play a role in preventing cancer.

KEEPING CELLS HEALTHY

The research is still preliminary, but laboratory studies suggest that compounds found in basil may help disrupt the dangerous chain of events that can lead to the development of cancer.

In one study, researchers in India spiked the food of a group of laboratory animals with basil extract, while animals in a second group were given only their usual diet. After 15 days, animals given the extract had higher levels of enzymes that are known to deactivate cancer-causing substances in the body.

Basil's ability to prevent cancerous changes was linked not to one partic-

IN THE KITCHEN

Your friend with the green thumb hands you a bouquet of fresh basil, still warm from the sun. It smells heavenly—but how do you use it? Here are a few suggestions.

Treat it gently. Basil is a delicate herb, and rough handling will cause the leaves to droop. To keep it looking fresh, gently remove the stems and flowers. Then spray the leaves with cool (not cold) water and pat dry with a paper towel. Let the leaves air-dry on another paper towel before storing.

Wrap it well. When storing fresh basil, place the leaves in a plastic bag. Remove as much of the air from the bag as you can, then seal it well and store it in the refrigerator. When properly stored, basil will keep for about four days.

Save it for later. One way to ensure that you always have fresh basil in the house is to freeze it. Pour a small amount of olive oil in a blender or food processor, add fresh basil leaves and process until the mixture has a pastelike consistency. Then freeze the mixture in ice cube trays and store the frozen cubes in a freezer bag. That way you'll always have small portions of fresh-tasting basil for all your favorite recipes.

ular compound in the herb but instead to several compounds working together, the researchers speculate. While it's too soon to say whether basil will have the same beneficial effects in humans, it's certainly not too soon to put more of this flavorful herb on your menu.

A Digestive Aid

The next time your stomach sends out a postprandial SOS, try sipping a cup of basil tea. This herb has a reputation for easing a variety of digestive disorders, especially gas.

No one's sure exactly why basil appears to soothe stomach upsets. One possible explanation is a compound called eugenol. This compound, which is found in basil, has been shown to help ease muscle spasms. This could explain why basil appears to help ease gas and stomach cramps.

To make a soothing basil tea, pour ½ cup of boiling water over 1 to 2 teaspoons of dried basil. Let the brew steep for 15 minutes, then strain and serve. People who frequently have gas may benefit by drinking 2 to 3 cups a day between meals.

Getting the Most

Mix it up. While many fresh foods are more nutritious than their dried counterparts, basil is good both ways. One teaspoon of ground dried basil contains more essential minerals, like calcium, iron, magnesium, and potassium, than 1 tablespoon of fresh-snipped leaves. On the other hand, ground basil has a larger surface area exposed to the environment, which can accelerate the natural breakdown of its beneficial compounds. Your best bet, researchers say, is to make liberal use of both forms of the herb.

Store it carefully. Exposing dried basil to heat, light, or air for long periods will cause many of the protective compounds to break down. To extract the most healing power, it's important to store basil in a cool, dark place, preferably in a glass or metal container.

PASTA WITH PESTO AND TOMATOES

¼ cup blanched almonds

2 cups loosely packed fresh basil leaves

2 cloves garlic

2 tablespoons extra-virgin olive oil

2 tablespoons grated Parmesan cheese

¼ teaspoon salt

¼ teaspoon ground black pepper

   Pinch of ground nutmeg

3 tablespoons defatted reduced-sodium chicken broth

8 ounces penne or rotini

2 ripe medium tomatoes, cut into thin wedges

Place the almonds in a food processor and process with on/off turns until finely chopped. Pour into a small bowl.

Add the basil and garlic to the food processor. Process until coarsely chopped. Add the oil, Parmesan, salt, pepper, nutmeg, and the broth. Process until finely minced. Add the reserved almonds. If the mixture is very dry, add 1 tablespoon broth and process to mix.

Cook the pasta in a large pot of boiling water according to the package directions. Drain and place in a large bowl. Pour the pesto over the pasta. Add the tomatoes and toss to coat.

Makes 4 servings

PER SERVING

calories	**398**
total fat	**12.4 g.**
saturated fat	**2 g.**
cholesterol	**3 mg.**
sodium	**211 mg.**
dietary fiber	**10.4 g.**

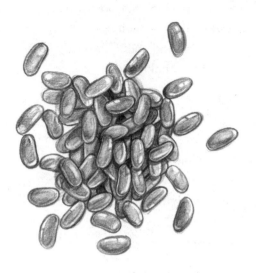

Beans
Small but Mighty

Healing Power
Can help:
Lower cholesterol

Stabilize blood sugar
levels

Reduce the risk of breast
and prostate cancers

Prevent heart disease
in people with diabetes

A generation ago, beans were culinary outcasts. Dusty sacks of pinto and navy beans as well as chickpeas languished on supermarket shelves. Crocks of kidney beans, usually untouched, sat next to cling peaches at steakhouse salad bars. And the three-bean salad at the annual family picnic drew more flies than raves.

Not anymore. Our consumption of beans rose from 5.5 pounds per person in 1974 to 7.3 pounds in 1994. There's a good reason for this surge in popularity. Beans, are the ultimate power food—low in fat and high in protein, fiber, and a variety of vitamins and minerals.

"Beans are actually little chemical factories with lots of biologically active substances in them, and there's good evidence that eating them may protect against cancer," says Leonard A. Cohen, Ph.D., head of the experimental breast cancer program at the American Health Foundation in Valhalla, New York.

Sending Cholesterol South

While beans aren't the only food that can help lower cholesterol, they're certainly one of the best. Beans are packed with soluble fiber, the same gummy stuff found in apples, barley, and oat bran. In the digestive tract, soluble fiber traps cholesterol-containing bile, removing it from the body before it's absorbed.

IN THE KITCHEN

If you roll right by the dried beans at the supermarket because you don't have time for all the soaking and boiling and waiting around, put on the brakes. Cooking beans from scratch doesn't have to be a daylong project, says Patti Bazel Geil, R.D., diabetes nutrition educator at the University of Kentucky in Lexington and author of *Magic Beans*. With the quick-soaking method, you can shave hours off the cooking time.

1. Rinse the beans in a colander, put them in a large pot, and cover with 2 inches of water. Bring to a boil, reduce the heat to medium, and boil for 10 minutes.

2. Drain the beans and cover with 2 inches of fresh water. ("Discarding the water that the beans were cooked in gets rid of most of their gas-producing sugars," Geil explains.)

3. Soak for 30 minutes. Then rinse, drain, and cover with fresh water again. Simmer for 2 hours or until the beans are tender.

"Eating a cup of cooked beans a day can lower total cholesterol about 10 percent in six weeks," says Patti Bazel Geil, R.D., diabetes nutrition educator at the University of Kentucky in Lexington and author of *Magic Beans*. While 10 percent may not seem like much, keep in mind that every 1 percent reduction in total cholesterol means a 2 percent decrease in your risk for heart disease.

Beans can lower cholesterol in just about anyone, but the higher your cholesterol, the better they work. In a study at the University of Kentucky, 20 men with high cholesterol (over 260 milligrams per deciliter of blood) were given about ¾ cup of pinto and navy beans a day. The men's total cholesterol dropped an average of 19 percent in three weeks, possibly reducing their heart attack risk by almost 40 percent. Better yet, the dangerous low-density lipoprotein cholesterol—that's the artery-plugging stuff—plunged by 24 percent.

It appears that all beans can help lower cholesterol, even canned baked beans. In another University of Kentucky study, 24 men with high cholesterol ate 1 cup of beans in tomato sauce every day for three weeks. Their total cholesterol dropped 10.4 percent, and their triglycerides (another blood fat that contributes to heart disease) fell 10.8 percent.

Beans play another, less direct role in keeping cholesterol levels down. They're extremely filling, so when you eat beans, you'll have less appetite for other, fattier foods. And eating less fat is critical for keeping cholesterol levels low.

"Beans are a high-fiber food, and high-fiber foods make you feel fuller," says Geil. In fact, one small study found that people who ate a bean puree felt more satisfied for a longer time than those who ate a similar puree made from potatoes.

KEEPING BLOOD SUGAR STEADY

Keeping blood sugar levels steady is the key to keeping diabetes under control. "Many people don't realize how good beans are for people with diabetes," says Geil. In fact, eating between ½ and ¾ cup of beans a day has been shown to significantly improve blood sugar control.

Beans are rich in complex carbohydrates. Unlike sugary foods, which dump sugar (glucose) into the bloodstream all at once, complex carbohydrates are digested more slowly. This means that glucose enters your bloodstream a little at a time, helping to keep blood sugar levels steady, says Geil.

In addition, beans are high in soluble fiber. Studies have shown that a diet high in soluble fiber causes the body to produce more insulin receptor sites—tiny "docks" that insulin molecules latch on to. More insulin gets into individual cells where it's needed, and less is present in the bloodstream, where it can cause problems.

In an English study, people were given either about 1¾ ounces of a variety of beans—including butter beans, kidney beans, black-eyed peas, chickpeas, and lentils—or other high-carbohydrate foods, like bread, pasta, cereals, and grains. After 30 minutes, blood sugar levels in the bean-eaters were almost half that of those who ate other high-carbohydrate foods.

Beans provide another benefit, says Geil. "People with diabetes are four to six times more likely to develop heart disease," she says. "Eating more beans will help keep their cholesterol low, thereby reducing their risk."

CANCER-LICKING LEGUMES

Studies suggest that low-fat, fiber-rich beans are some of the best cancer-fighting foods. Beans contain compounds—lignans, isoflavones, saponins, phytic acid, and protease inhibitors—that have been shown to inhibit cancer cell growth. These compounds appear to keep normal cells from turning cancerous and prevent cancer cells from growing, says Dr. Cohen.

These compounds are as protective to a plant as they are to a human, says Dr. Cohen. "Basically, they're natural insect repellents—they're ways in which plants protect themselves from insects and other predators," he explains. "If beans can block the growth and invasion of insects, molds, and bacteria, it's not surprising that they might also be able to do the same with a cancer cell."

Soybeans (unlike other legumes) are also rich in genistein and daidzein, two compounds that some experts speculate may play a role in preventing cancer. Known as phytoestrogens, these are weaker versions of the estrogen that we produce naturally. Experts believe that these compounds may help reduce the risk of breast and prostate cancer by blocking the activity of testosterone and estrogen, male and female sex hormones that, over time, can spur the growth of cancerous tumors.

Experts know that Hispanic women have about half the risk of getting breast cancer that White women face. Studies suggest that beans, which are eaten almost daily in many Hispanic households, may be responsible, says Dr. Cohen.

In one study, Dr. Cohen and his colleagues looked at the diets of 214 White, African-American, and Hispanic women. They found that the Hispanic women ate significantly more beans—7.4 servings per week, compared to 4.6 servings per week for the African-American women and less than 3 servings a week for the White women.

"Beans were a major source of fiber for the Hispanic women," says Dr. Cohen. In fact, the Hispanic women consumed nearly 25 percent of their dietary fiber from beans—twice the national average, noted the researchers.

THE HEALTHY MAN'S MEAT

Beans used to be called the poor man's meat. But a more accurate name would be the healthy man's meat. Like red meat, beans are loaded with protein. Unlike meat, they're light in fat, particularly dangerous, artery-clogging saturated fat.

For example, a cup of black beans contains less than 1 gram of fat. Less than 1 percent of that comes from saturated fat. Three ounces of lean, broiled ground beef, on the other hand, has 15 grams of fat, 22 percent of which is the saturated kind.

Beans are also a great source of essential vitamins and minerals. A half-cup of black beans contains 128 micrograms, or 32 percent of the Daily Value (DV) for folate, a B vitamin that may lower risk of heart disease and fight birth defects. That same cup has 2 milligrams of iron, 11 percent of the DV, and 305 milligrams of potassium, or 9 percent of the DV. Potassium is a mineral that has been shown to help control blood pressure naturally.

Getting the Most

Go for the fiber. While virtually all dried beans are good sources of fiber, some varieties stand out from the pack. Black beans, for example, contain 6 grams of fiber in a half-cup serving. Chickpeas, kidney beans, and lima beans all weigh in at about 7 grams of fiber, and black-eyed peas are among the best, with about 8 grams of fiber.

Enjoy them canned. Don't have time to soak and cook dried beans? No problem. Canned beans are just as good for you as the dried kind, says Geil. They're higher in sodium, however, so drain and rinse canned beans well before using them.

Use gas-deflating spices. Has the fear of uncomfortable and embarrassing gas kept you from reaping beans' nutritional benefits? Try spicing them with a pinch of summer savory or a teaspoon of ground ginger. According to some university studies, these spices may help reduce beans' gas-producing effects.

BLACK BEAN CONFETTI SALAD

2 **cans (15 ounces each) black beans, rinsed and drained**

1 **small sweet red pepper, finely diced**

4 **scallions, thinly sliced**

2 **tablespoons chopped fresh cilantro**

2 **tablespoons white-wine vinegar**

1 **tablespoon extra-virgin olive oil**

In a large glass bowl, combine the beans, peppers, scallions, cilantro, vinegar, and oil. Stir well to combine. Let stand for 15 minutes to allow the flavors to blend.

Makes 4 main-dish servings

Cook's Note: You can prepare this salad up to a day in advance. Cover and refrigerate. Bring to room temperature before serving.

PER SERVING

calories	**207**
total fat	**4.1 g.**
saturated fat	**0.6 g.**
cholesterol	**0 mg.**
sodium	**179 mg.**
dietary fiber	**11.7 g.**

MIXED-BEAN SOUP

2 **cups mixed dried beans**

1 **teaspoon olive oil**

2 **cups chopped onions**

4 **cloves garlic, minced**

7 **cups water**

1 **can (14 ounces) vegetable broth**

2 **teaspoons dried summer savory leaves**

  Ground black pepper

Place the beans in a colander and rinse with cold water. Transfer to a Dutch oven and cover with 2" of cold water Bring to a boil over high heat, then reduce the heat to medium and boil for 10 minutes.

Drain the beans, return them to the pot, and cover with 2" of cold water. Set aside to soak for 30 minutes. Drain in a colander, rinse with cold water, and drain again. Set aside.

Wipe the Dutch oven dry. Add the oil and warm over medium heat. Add the onions and garlic. Cook, stirring occasionally, for 6 to 8 minutes, or until softened.

(continued)

MIXED-BEAN SOUP—*Continued*

PER SERVING

calories	**247**
total fat	**2 g.**
saturated fat	**0.1 g.**
cholesterol	**0 mg.**
sodium	**418 mg.**
dietary fiber	**17 g.**

Stir in the water, broth, and savory. Bring to a boil over high heat. Add the beans and stir to combine. Reduce the heat to low. Partially cover and cook for 2 hours, or until the beans are tender. Season to taste with the pepper.

Makes 6 servings

Cook's Notes: If you buy a multibean soup mix that contains a flavoring packet, reserve the seasoning blend for another use.

If dried summer savory is unavailable, substitute 1 teaspoon dried sage and 1 teaspoon dried marjoram.

GINGERED LENTILS

1¼   **cups brown lentils**

2   **teaspoons canola oil**

2   **tablespoons grated fresh ginger**

2   **cloves garlic, minced**

1¼   **teaspoons curry powder**

¼   **teaspoon salt**

1   **lemon, halved**

PER SERVING

calories	**208**
total fat	**3 g.**
saturated fat	**0.3 g.**
cholesterol	**0 mg.**
sodium	**137 mg.**
dietary fiber	**7.4 g.**

Place the lentils in a colander and rinse with cold water, then drain. Transfer the lentils to a large saucepan and add 4 cups water. Bring to a boil over high heat. Reduce the heat to low. Partially cover and cook for 30 to 35 minutes, or until the lentils are tender but not mushy.

Drain the lentils and set aside. Wipe the pan dry. Add the oil and warm over medium heat. Add the ginger, garlic, curry powder, and salt. Stir for a few seconds, until fragrant. Add the lentils and stir well to reheat. Remove from the heat.

Squeeze the juice from 1 half of the lemon and stir it into the lentils. Cut the remaining half into 4 wedges. Serve the lentils with the lemon wedges.

Makes 4 main-dish servings

Cook's Note: This makes a great meatless meal. Serve it with bread or rice and a steamed vegetable.

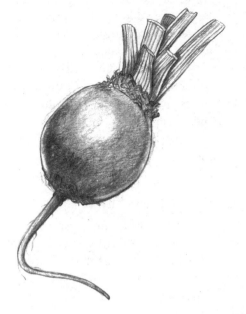

BEETS
BETTER LIVING THROUGH BORSCHT

HEALING POWER
CAN HELP:
Protect against cancer

Prevent birth defects

When you think of healthy cuisine, foods from the Great Bear—Russia—don't come immediately to mind.

It's little wonder, really. We don't usually think of such things as butter-laden cabbage and potatoes, washed down with a slug of vodka, as haute cuisine—or healthy cuisine.

Yet there's one traditional Russian dish that deserves a second look: borscht. Served hot or cold, this sweet crimson soup is made from fresh beets, and that means that it's brimming with nutrients that can fight birth defects and perhaps even stave off cancer.

GIVING CANCER THE RED FLAG

Folk medicine is full of stories about using beets and beet juice for fighting cancer. Though much more research needs to be done, some scientists suspect that the compound that gives beets their rich, crimson color—betacyanin—is also a powerful tumor-fighting agent.

"Beet juice is used in Europe for the treatment of cancer," says Eleonore Blaurock-Busch, Ph.D., president of Trace Minerals International in Boulder, Colorado. "The pigment found in beets may have anti-cancer properties."

In one study on beets' effectiveness against cancer, researchers tested beet

Seeing Red

You've been grating beets on your salads, eating them sliced, and nibbling them from jars. Much to your alarm, this beet feat has you seeing red—in what seems to be the worst possible place.

Don't panic when your urine runs red. Many people who eat beets will experience a condition called beeturia, or the passage of pink or red urine.

When you don't know what's happening, this condition is certainly alarming. But it's harmless, say experts, and will usually pass the same day, unless, of course, you keep eating beets.

juice, along with the juices of other vegetables and fruits, against some common cancer-causing chemicals. Beet juice ranked close to the top in preventing cell mutations that commonly lead to cancer.

"Beets aren't as well-studied as other vegetables, like broccoli," notes Dr. Blaurock-Busch. "But there's certainly enough evidence to warrant including them in your diet."

A Font of Folate

If there's one nutrient that women often don't get enough of, it's the B vitamin folate. They just don't eat enough lentils, spinach, or other folate-rich foods to get the 400 micrograms of folate that they need each day.

Meeting the daily requirement for folate is essential for normal tissue growth and perhaps for protecting against heart disease and certain cancers. Plus, doctors have found that folate is a pregnant woman's best friend because it helps protect against birth defects.

In the Kitchen

Beets aren't the easiest vegetable to work with. They have a strong flavor, they're often tough, and they bleed red. Indeed, cooking with beets is like throwing a pair of red socks into a load of whites—you know that something's going to turn pink.

Here are a few ways to keep this unruly vegetable under control.

Control the color. To keep "beet bleeding" to a minimum, chefs advise washing fresh beets gently during preparation, taking care not to tear the skin, since the tougher outer skin layer keeps most of the pigments inside the vegetable. For the same reason, don't peel beets or remove the root ends or stems until they're cooked and in a separate bowl.

Buy them small. For the best results, choose small- or medium-size beets. They're tender enough at that age that you may not have to peel them at all.

A half-cup of boiled, sliced beets contains 45 micrograms of folate, nearly 11 percent of the Daily Value.

INCREASING IRON STORES

For providing iron, beets can't match such mineral powerhouses as lean beef. But if you're among the millions of Americans who are cutting back on meat or giving it up entirely, then boning up on beets is one way to go.

Getting the Most

Cook them lightly. Studies show that the anti-tumor power of beets is diminished by heat. So cook them lightly to get the most effectiveness.

Try the canned kind. One of the neat things about beets is that they're nearly as nutritious out of a can as they are fresh from the ground. So you can enjoy their health benefits in and out of season.

CHILLED BEET SOUP

2 **cans (15 ounces each) reduced-sodium beets**

2 **tablespoons red-wine vinegar**

1 **teaspoon packed light brown sugar**

½ **cup diced cucumbers**

4 **tablespoons nonfat sour cream**

1 **tablespoon chopped fresh dill**

PER SERVING

calories	**89**
total fat	**0.3 g.**
saturated fat	**0.1 g.**
cholesterol	**0 mg.**
sodium	**116 mg.**
dietary fiber	**3.9 g.**

Drain the beets, reserving 1½ cups of the liquid. Dice the beets and set aside ½ cup.

Place the remaining beets in a blender or food processor. Add the vinegar, sugar, and the reserved beet liquid. Process for 1 to 2 minutes, or until the mixture is a chunky puree. If desired, chill for up to 12 hours.

Serve sprinkled with the cucumbers and the reserved diced beets. Top each serving with 1 tablespoon of the sour cream and a sprinkle of dill.

Makes 4 servings

Cook's Notes: If you use regular canned beets, the sodium will increase 305 milligrams per serving.

For variety, you could replace 1 cup of the beet liquid with apple juice.

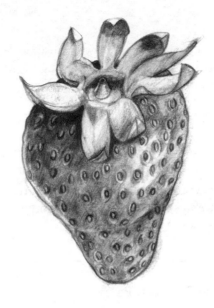

BERRIES
MORE THAN JUST DESSERT

HEALING POWER
CAN HELP:
Prevent cataracts

Ward off cancer

Prevent constipation

Reduce the risk
of infection

The Romans believed that strawberries could cure everything from loose teeth to gastritis. Raspberries, according to folklore, had the ability to soothe inflamed tonsils.

While the benefits of berries have been somewhat exaggerated, their reputation for healing is on the mark. Berries contain a number of substances that show promise for preventing such serious problems as cataracts and cancer.

A HEALING ACID

What makes berries so special is a compound called ellagic acid, which is believed to help prevent cellular changes that can lead to cancer. All berries contain some ellagic acid, with strawberries and blackberries having the most. "Ellagic acid is a good friend to us, helping fight the cancer process," says Hasan Mukhtar, Ph.D., professor of dermatology and environmental health sciences at Case Western Reserve University School of Medicine in Cleveland.

Berries—and the ellagic acid they contain—may help fight cancer on several fronts, says Gary D. Stoner, Ph.D., director of the cancer chemoprevention program at the Ohio State University Comprehensive Cancer Center in Columbus. Ellagic acid is a powerful antioxidant, meaning that it can reduce damage caused by free radicals, harmful oxygen molecules that can literally punch holes in healthy cells and kick off the cancerous process. "It also detoxifies carcinogens," Dr. Stoner says.

In one study, animals exposed to a cancer-causing substance and given a purified extract of ellagic acid were far less likely to develop esophageal cancer than those given the carcinogen alone. Other experiments have found that animals are 70 percent less likely to develop liver tumors when they're given ellagic acid along with the harmful substance.

It's not yet known how much ellagic acid humans might need to get the same benefits, says Dr. Stoner. "While in early experiments laboratory animals were fed purified ellagic acid, in some later experiments they were fed dried strawberries," he explains. "Although the amount of ellagic acid from strawberries was just one-third the amount given in purified form, the animals were still able to fight off chemically induced esophageal cancer. That tells us that there may be some benefit in giving the ellagic acid as nature intended it—in the real food."

FOOD ALERT
DANGEROUS PICKINGS

Even though elderberries are a treasure trove of nutrients, you don't want to pick them in the wild. Before they get ripe, they may contain compounds called cyanogenic glycosides, which can be poisonous, says Ara DerMarderosian, Ph.D., professor of pharmacognosy and medicinal chemistry at Philadelphia College of Pharmacy and Science.

It's not only the berries that are dangerous, he adds. The leaves and bark of the tree also contain the poisonous compounds. In fact, there have been a number of cases of poisoning in children who carved elderberry branches, used them as peashooters, and didn't even eat the berries.

You don't have to avoid elderberries to be safe, however. Just treat them as you would wild mushrooms—a tasty food that's best picked at your favorite fruit stand instead of in the woods. It's also a good idea to cook the berries, because heat destroys the dangerous compounds, Dr. DerMarderosian adds.

Help for the Eyes and More

Ellagic acid isn't the only compound in berries that fights free radicals. Berries are also very high in vitamin C, which is one of the most powerful antioxidants. Getting a lot of vitamin C in your diet may help reduce the risk of heart disease, cancer, and infections. Vitamin C seems particularly important in preventing cataracts, which are thought to be caused by the oxidation of the protein that forms the lenses of the eyes.

All berries contain large amounts of vitamin C. A half-cup of strawberries,

Fresh berries are highly perishable, and need special handling to maintain peak freshness.

Look for leakage. Berries that are leaking from the bottom of the package are either old or have been crushed and are giving up their juice. Look for a fresher, drier batch.

Give them room. When storing berries at home, don't crowd them together, which will cause them to deteriorate rapidly. It's best to store them, unwashed and uncovered, in a large bowl in the refrigerator or spread out on a platter.

Plan ahead. Berries freeze well, so you can enjoy their fresh taste all year long.

for example, has 42 milligrams, 70 percent of the Daily Value (DV). (That's more vitamin C than you'll get in a similar amount of grapefruit.) A half-cup of elderberries has 26 milligrams of vitamin C, 43 percent of the DV, and a half-cup of blackberries has 15 milligrams, 25 percent of the DV.

Berry Full of Fiber

One of the sweeter things about berries is their ability to help prevent a distinctly unsweet problem: constipation. Berries contain large amounts of insoluble fiber, which is incredibly absorbent. It draws rivers of water into the intestine, which makes stools heavier. Heavy stools travel through the intestine faster, which means that you're less likely to become constipated.

The fiber in berries is helpful in yet another way. It helps prevent bile acid (a chemical that the body uses for digestion) from being transformed into a more dangerous, potentially cancer-causing form.

Elderberries are an incredible source of fiber, with a half-cup containing 5 grams. A half-cup of blackberries has more than 3 grams of fiber, while a half-cup of raspberries has 4 grams.

Getting the Most

Shop by color. To get the most nutrients in each bite, it's important to buy (or pick) berries that are at their peak of freshness. Perhaps the easiest way to tell is by checking the color. Blackberries should be jet black; raspberries should be black, golden, or red; blueberries, a powdery blue; and strawberries, a bold red.

Eat them fresh. Cooking destroys large amounts of vitamin C. In fact, even slicing strawberries can cause vitamin C levels to decline because it causes the release of an enzyme that quickly destroys the vitamin. So to get the most vitamin C, it's best to buy strawberries that are still wearing their little green caps and slice them just before serving.

DOUBLE-BERRY SUNDAES

½ pint raspberries

12 ounces blueberries

2 tablespoons fresh orange juice

1 tablespoon honey

1 teaspoon vanilla

¼ teaspoon almond extract

1 pint nonfat vanilla frozen yogurt

PER SERVING

calories **170**
total fat **0.6 g.**
saturated fat **0 g.**
cholesterol **0 mg.**
sodium **45 mg.**
dietary fiber **4 g.**

Place half of the raspberries in a medium glass bowl. Mash lightly with a fork. Add the blueberries, orange juice, honey, vanilla, almond extract, and the remaining raspberries. Stir well to mix. Cover and let stand for at least 30 minutes to allow the flavors to blend.

Scoop the frozen yogurt into 4 dessert dishes. Stir the berry mixture and spoon over the yogurt.

Makes 4 servings

STRAWBERRY TART WITH OAT-CINNAMON CRUST

Crust

⅔ cup old-fashioned or quick-cooking rolled oats

½ cup unbleached all-purpose flour

1 tablespoon sugar

1 teaspoon ground cinnamon

¼ teaspoon baking soda

2 tablespoons canola oil

2–3 tablespoons nonfat plain yogurt

Strawberry Filling

1½ pints strawberries

¼ cup all-fruit strawberry spread

½ teaspoon vanilla

To make the crust: Preheat the oven to 375°F. Coat a baking sheet with no-stick spray.

In a medium bowl, combine the oats, flour, sugar, cinnamon, and baking soda. Mix with a fork until blended. Stir in the oil and 2 tablespoons of yogurt to make a soft, slightly sticky dough. If the dough is too stiff, add the remaining 1 tablespoon yogurt.

Place the dough on the prepared baking sheet and pat evenly into a 10" circle. If the dough sticks to your hands, coat them lightly with no-stick spray. Place a 9" cake pan on the dough and trace around it with a sharp knife. With your fingers,

(continued)

Strawberry Tart
with Oat-Cinnamon Crust—*Continued*

PER SERVING

calories	**161**
total fat	**5.5 g.**
saturated fat	**0.5 g.**
cholesterol	**0 mg.**
sodium	**73 mg.**
dietary fiber	**2.6 g.**

push up and pinch the dough around the outside of the circle to make a 9″ circle with a rim $\frac{1}{4}$″ high.

Bake for 15 minutes, or until firm and golden. Remove from the oven and set aside to cool. With a pancake turner, gently ease the crust onto a large, flat serving plate.

To make the strawberry filling: Wash the strawberries and pat dry with paper towels. Slice off the stem ends and discard.

In a small microwaveable bowl, combine the strawberry spread and vanilla. Microwave on high power for 10 to 15 seconds, or until melted.

Brush or dab a generous tablespoon evenly over the crust. Arrange the strawberries, cut side down, evenly over the crust. Brush or dab the remaining spread evenly over the strawberries, making sure that you get some of the spread between the strawberries to secure them.

Refrigerate for at least 30 minutes, or until the spread has jelled. Cut into wedges.

Makes 6 servings

Cook's Note: You can serve the tart with a scoop of nonfat vanilla frozen yogurt on the side.

Birth Defects
Focus on Folate

Women who are preparing to have babies have long known the importance of eating a healthful diet, with lots of fruits, vegetables, legumes, and whole grains. Even more important, researchers say, is getting more foods high in folate, a B vitamin that has been shown to reduce the risk of birth defects.

For a long time, folate was on the nutritional B-list. Doctors knew that we needed it, but it wasn't considered to be all that important. Then, in the early 1990s, studies proved just how important it is. A study of more than 3,600 mothers found that those who got the Daily Value (DV) of 400 micrograms of folic acid (the supplement form of folate) a day were 60 percent less likely to have children with neural tube defects, in which the skull or spinal cord doesn't fuse properly, than those who got less.

It's not only women planning to have babies who should be getting more folate, adds J. David Erickson, D.D.S., Ph.D., chief of the birth defects and genetic diseases branch of the Centers for Disease Control and Prevention in Atlanta. Since many birth defects occur very early in pregnancy—often before a woman knows she's pregnant—getting enough folate is important for all women of childbearing age, he says.

To get more folate into your diet, some of the dark green, leafy vegetables are good choices, says Patricia A. Baird, M.D., professor of medical genetics at the University of British Columbia in Vancouver. One cup of spinach, for example, has 110 micrograms of folate, 28 percent of the DV. Lima beans are also a good source, with a half-cup providing 140 micrograms, 35 percent of the DV. In addition, packaged foods such as flour, pasta, and rice are fortified with this essential nutrient.

If you are planning to become pregnant, the National Health and Medical Research Council recommends making a special effort to get more folate-rich foods beginning one month before pregnancy begins and continuing for three months afterward.

Incidentally, to get the most folate from the foods you eat, it's important not to overcook them. Boiling or overcooking foods can destroy up to 90 percent of the folate. To get the most of this nutrient, either munch foods raw or cook them gently, using the microwave or a steamer.

Off the A-list

In order to get more folate, many women do the easy thing and take a multivitamin. But if you don't read the label carefully, you could be taking some chances, since some multivitamins contain large amounts of vitamin A, which can increase the risk of birth defects, says Dr. Erickson.

In a study of 22,748 women, for example, researchers found that those getting more than 10,000 international units of vitamin A a day were almost five times more likely to have children with certain head birth defects than those getting less than the DV of 5,000 international units.

You don't have to worry about the vitamin A you get from foods, Dr. Erickson adds. But if you are taking a multivitamin that contains vitamin A, check with your doctor to make sure it's a safe amount.

Dangerous Spirits

The ancient Greeks didn't have microscopes or maternal-care units, but they knew that pregnancy and alcohol don't mix. In fact, they had laws prohibiting newly married couples from drinking.

The Greeks were ahead of their time. Studies have shown that drinking alcohol—not just hard liquor but also beer and wine—during pregnancy can cause problems. In fact, one study found that drinking can double the risk of certain birth defects.

Doctors don't know for sure how much alcohol it takes to cause problems, says Dr. Erickson. Since everyone absorbs alcohol differently, the best advice is for women to avoid alcohol completely until after their babies are born.

Blood Pressure Control
Getting the Numbers Down

It's called the silent killer, but nobody really dies from high blood pressure. Stroke, heart attack, and heart failure are the diseases that kill, yet each one can be caused, at least in part, by high blood pressure.

The scary thing about high blood pressure is that you can have it for years without symptoms. You don't feel it. You can't see it. And you can only detect it with a sphygmomanometer, which you can't even pronounce, except as "blood pressure cuff."

But while high blood pressure works quietly, it's frequently deadly. "High blood pressure is just a reflection of a cardiovascular system that's about to burst internally," says John A. McDougall, M.D., medical director of the McDougall Program at Saint Helena Hospital in Napa Valley, California, and author of *The McDougall Program for a Healthy Heart*. "But if you eat a good diet—lots of fruits and vegetables and starch-based foods versus rich foods—you can help change all that," he says.

The How of Hypertension

How does high blood pressure commit so much mayhem? It sends blood whooshing through the arteries with damaging force. It weakens the arteries, overworks the heart, stirs up blood clots, and tosses them about. Experts can't explain the exact cause of high blood pressure, but the factors that may lead to it are well-known: high cholesterol, hardening of the arteries, kidney disease, and for those who are sensitive to sodium, too much salt in the diet.

High blood pressure is extremely common, affecting up to one in four adults, or up to 50 million Americans. Most high blood pressure, about 80 percent, is classified as mild, or Stage 1. If, when you have your blood pressure taken, your reading ranges from 140 to 159 over 90 to 99, you have mild high blood pressure. (The top figure measures systolic pressure, or how hard your heart works pumping blood through your arteries. The bottom number, the diastolic reading, measures the pressure of blood on artery walls between beats.) Normal blood pressure is less than 130 over 85.

Mild high blood pressure responds well to a variety of nondrug therapies. If you feed and exercise your body well, you may be able to avoid blood pressure drugs (and their often-troublesome side effects) and calm your rushing blood. Don't be misled by the "mild" label, though. "Most heart attacks and strokes that occur do so in people with Stage 1 high blood pressure," says Norman Kaplan, M.D., professor of internal medicine and chief of the hypertension division at the University of Texas Southwestern Medical Center at Dallas.

Researchers at the University of British Columbia in Vancouver examined 166 studies that looked at both drug and nondrug treatments for high blood pressure to compare their effectiveness. They found that weight loss (with exercise) worked as well as drugs to reduce blood pressure. Reducing sodium and alcohol consumption and increasing potassium in the diet were also effective. Scientists in the United States have begun studying the potential of fiber and two other minerals, magnesium and calcium, to reduce blood pressure, too. Here's a summary of what they've found so far.

GIVING YOUR HEART A BREAK

Experts are unanimous that losing weight is the first task to tackle when you're trying to lower blood pressure. In fact, people who are 30 percent overweight are the folks most likely to develop high blood pressure. There's good news about weight loss, though. Dropping just 5 to 10 pounds can have a beneficial effect on blood pressure.

What's the connection? The more tissue you have in your body, the harder your heart has to pump to feed it. And that work exerts more pressure on artery walls.

Everybody knows that losing weight is no piece of cake. But exercise makes it easier. And the best weight-loss diet is the same as the best diet for controlling blood pressure: low-fat foods, including lots of fruits and vegetables.

"We really emphasize following a low-fat, high-fruit-and-vegetable diet. It's almost certain to lower your blood pressure because it lowers sodium and increases all the good stuff that's hypothesized to lower blood pressure—fiber, calcium, and potassium—and it's an effective avenue to weight loss," says Pao-Hwa Lin, Ph.D., director of the clinical nutrition research unit at the Sarah W. Stedman Center for Nutritional Studies at Duke University Medical Center in Durham, North Carolina, and co-author of *Eating Well, Living Well with Hypertension.*

A diet low in fat won't include large amounts of red meat, which is packed with saturated fat. Nor will it include many processed foods, because they're high-fat mine fields. Processed foods are also high in salt and low in potassium, so when you get rid of them, you wipe out three bad birds with one dietary stone.

THE STORY OF SALT

Many experts believe that about half of the people with high blood pressure are salt "responders," meaning that their blood pressure levels depend on the amount of salt they eat. "But there is some controversy about the issue," says Lawrence Appel, M.D., associate professor of medicine and epidemiology at Johns Hopkins University School of Medicine in Baltimore. "I believe most people are salt responders, but some have a greater response than others," he says. "Older people tend to be more sensitive to salt, too, as do African-Americans."

Here's what happens. When you eat the typical American's ration of sodium—3,000 to 6,000 milligrams or more a day, compared to the recommended 2,400-milligram limit—your blood pressure rises. If you're sensitive to salt, the sodium it contains makes your body attract water like a sponge. You soak it up and your blood vessels expand with it, producing higher pressure.

SALT MINES

If you're sodium-savvy and watching your blood pressure, you already know to say no thanks to foods such as chips and salty pickles. Yet sodium appears in many foods in which you might not expect it. Baking soda and baking powder, for instance are both sodium bicarbonate. Dried fruit contains sodium sulfite, and ice cream often has sodium caseinate and sodium alginate.

Even a sharp-eyed sodium detective can miss a few salt mines. Here are some to watch out for.

Instant chocolate-flavored pudding. A half-cup contains 470 milligrams of sodium, more than the amount in two slices of bacon.

Ketchup. One tablespoon contains 156 milligrams of sodium.

Pastries. A fruit Danish has 333 milligrams of sodium, while a cheese Danish has 319. Scones and baking-powder biscuits also tend to be high in sodium.

Cheese. Most types are high in sodium. This includes cottage cheese, which has 425 milligrams in a half-cup serving.

Sodium may also damage the walls of blood vessels, causing scarring and increasing clogging.

"If you have high blood pressure, your sodium needs to be reduced by half," says Dr. Kaplan. " Don't put salt on the table or in the food you cook. Avoid most processed foods, which is where 80 percent of the sodium in American diets comes from. If that doesn't bring your blood pressure down, then sodium isn't the culprit," he says.

Cutting sodium intake by half will lead to a drop of 5 points (or more) in blood pressure in about half the people with high blood pressure, according to Dr. Kaplan.

MINING FOR MINERALS

Potassium and calcium are two minerals that act like massage on a tense body. They help the blood vessels relax. When arteries relax, they dilate, or open up, and give blood the room it needs to move calmly. No sweat. No pressure.

"You can think of potassium as the opposite of sodium," says Harvey B. Simon, M.D., associate professor of medicine at Harvard Medical School. Potassium helps the body excrete sodium, so the more potassium you get in your diet, the more sodium you get rid of. In fact, the landmark INTERSALT study looked at more than 10,000 people from 32 countries and found that people with the highest amounts of potassium in their blood had the lowest blood pressures, and those with the lowest amounts had the highest.

"Fruits and vegetables are naturally low in sodium and high in potassium," says Dr. Lin. "A diet high in vegetables and fruits almost mimics a vegetarian diet, which is known to be linked to lower blood pressure," she says. Foods that are especially rich in potassium include beans, potatoes, avocados, steamed clams, lima beans, bananas, and dried fruits such as apricots and raisins.

Calcium has shown similar ties to blood pressure in studies. Some have found that low intake is actually a risk factor for developing high blood pressure. The landmark Framingham Heart Study looked at the calcium intakes of 432 men. Those who ate the most (between 322 and 1,118 milligrams a day) had a 20 percent lower risk of developing high blood pressure than those who ate the least (8 to 109 milligrams a day).

To put those amounts in perspective, a cup of nonfat yogurt contains about 415 milligrams of calcium and a glass of skim milk has about 352. Besides low-fat and nonfat dairy products, your best sources of calcium include tofu, calcium-fortified orange juice, kale, broccoli, and collard greens.

EATING RIGHT

For starters, you should practice what Dr. Appel calls active shopping. In other words, read the labels. Whenever you buy any food with a nutrition label, glance at the sodium content. One 8-ounce can of stewed tomatoes can contain over 800 milligrams of sodium, while another can might have only 70. "You often have to look hard for low-sodium cereals," Dr. Appel adds. "Shredded wheat is one of the low-salt ones."

Sodium-free is a good phrase to look for on a label. So is *low-sodium*. The word *light*, however, is not as conclusive. Light soy sauce, for instance, can still have 605 milligrams of sodium per tablespoon.

While bread is often a nutritious, wholesome food, occasionally it's high in salt. If you buy it fresh at a bakery where it isn't labeled, don't be shy about asking how much salt is in each loaf. "The amount is variable, and it can be almost nothing or as high as 2 tablespoons for a 2-pound loaf," says Brian Johnson, a graduate of Cordon Bleu, London, who is pastry chef for Metropolitan Bakery in Philadelphia.

When you're buying canned foods, salt can be a real problem. In most cases, however, rinsing the food will eliminate a good percentage of the salt. If you don't have a can of beans that states it's low-sodium, for example, you can rinse off at least half the salt the food was packed in, says Neva Cochran, R.D., a nutrition consultant in Dallas and spokeswoman for the American Dietetic Association. To get the best results, rinse foods such as beans or tuna under running water twice.

Since produce is the cornerstone of a diet for healthy blood pressure, you should always be looking for ways to get more fruits and vegetables. Here are a few of Dr. Lin's suggestions.

- Roast vegetables, lightly drizzled with light olive oil, in the oven.
- Buy prewashed or even precut salads for busy days.
- Order a fruit plate as an appetizer before your meal in a restaurant.
- Eat two vegetarian dinners a week.

When you're picking up produce, be sure to grab some apples, pears, and oranges. These three fruits are fiber queens. And heart researchers are starting to find that not only does fiber decrease dangerous cholesterol, it may also lower blood pressure. Fruit fiber made a strong showing in a study at Harvard Medical School, where scientists tracked more than 30,000 men. The men in the study who ate less than 12 grams of fruit fiber a day (about four oranges or three apples or pears) were 60 percent more likely to develop high blood pressure.

Finally, it's essential to reduce the amount of fat in your diet. You don't have to be fanatical, however. Instead of cutting out fat with a cleaver, start by slicing it off with a scalpel, bit by bit. Dr. Lin recommends making small, gradual changes that will cut the total amount of fat you use in half. Buy butter substitutes and lower-fat versions of margarine. For sautéing, use spray oil instead of liquid oils or butter. Use mustard instead of mayonnaise and snack on low-salt pretzels instead of potato chips.

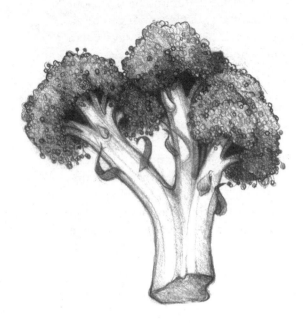

BROCCOLI
KING OF THE CRUCIFERS

HEALING POWER
CAN HELP:
Protect against
heart disease

Fight off cancer

Boost immunity

Ask researchers to name the one vegetable that they buy specifically for cancer prevention, and they'll say that broccoli is the one.

It's difficult to overestimate broccoli's healing powers. This crisp, delicious member of the cruciferous family has been shown to fend off a host of serious conditions, including heart disease and cancer.

DOUBLE CANCER PROTECTION

Broccoli's impressive power as a cancer fighter is due in part to its two-pronged attack. It contains not just one but two separate compounds—indole-3-carbinol (or I3C, for short) and sulforaphane—that help sweep up cancer-causing substances before they have a chance to do harm.

The compound I3C, which is also found in cabbage and brussels sprouts, is particularly effective against breast cancer. In laboratory studies, I3C has been found to lower levels of harmful estrogens that can promote tumor growth in hormone-sensitive cells, like breast cells.

While I3C is working against hormone-induced cancers, sulforaphane is offering protection on another front, by boosting the production of cancer-blocking enzymes, says Thomas Kensler, Ph.D., professor in the department of environmental health sciences in the School of Public Health at Johns Hopkins University in Baltimore.

In one pioneering study, Dr. Kensler and his colleagues at Johns Hopkins University exposed 145 laboratory animals to a powerful cancer-causing agent. Twenty-five of the animals had not received any special treatment, while the rest were fed high doses of sulforaphane. After 50 days, 68 percent of the unprotected animals had breast tumors, compared with only 26 percent of those given the sulforaphane.

It is no wonder that researchers put broccoli at the top of their lists of nutritional superstars. "We know that people who eat lots of cruciferous vegetables, like broccoli, are protected from every kind of cancer," says Jon Michnovicz, M.D., Ph.D., president of the Foundation for Preventive Oncology and the Institute for Hormone Research, both in New York City. Broccoli and other crucifers are particularly helpful when it comes to preventing cancers of the colon, breast, and prostate gland, he adds.

A Boost from Beta-Carotene

While much recent research has focused on "exotic" compounds like sulforaphane, broccoli is also chock-full of more common, but still powerful, compounds like beta-carotene. This nutrient, which the body converts to vitamin A, is one of the antioxidants. That is, it helps prevent disease by sweeping up harmful, cell-damaging oxygen molecules that naturally accumulate in the body. High levels of beta-carotene have been linked to lower rates of heart attack, certain cancers, and cataracts.

Broccoli is an excellent source of beta-carotene, providing about 0.7 milligram in a half-cup cooked serving. This provides 7 to 12 percent of the recommended daily amount.

Supporting Players

Broccoli isn't called the king of the crucifers for nothing. Besides beta-carotene, sulforaphane, and I3C, broccoli contains a variety of other nutrients, each of which can help fend off a host of conditions, from heart disease to osteoporosis.

For example, just a half-cup of chopped, cooked broccoli contains almost 100 percent of the Daily Value for vitamin C. This antioxidant vitamin has been proven in studies to help boost immunity and fight diseases like heart disease and cancer.

Broccoli also ranks up there with diamonds as a woman's best friend. It's one of the best vegetable sources of calcium, packing in 72 milligrams per cooked cup—about a quarter of the amount in an 8-ounce glass of skim milk. Calcium is well-documented as the single most important nutrient that women

IN THE KITCHEN

One of the problems with cooking broccoli is consistency—or, more specifically, a lack thereof. Broccoli consists of both tough stalks and tender florets, the result being that it often ends up with some parts either overdone or underdone.

To help ensure even cooking, it's helpful to cut broccoli into little spears. First, cut off and discard the thick, woody part of the stalk, generally from the bottom up to where the broccoli florets begin to branch. Then cut any large florets and stems in half lengthwise.

If you find that the stems are still too tough for eating, either trim them farther up from the bottom or peel them before cooking.

need to keep osteoporosis (the breaking down of bones) at bay.

Broccoli is also rich in folate, a nutrient that's essential for normal tissue growth and that studies show may protect against cancer, heart disease, and birth defects. Women, especially those who take birth control pills, are often low in this vital nutrient.

Finally, if you're looking to keep your digestive system running smoothly, make broccoli your fuel of choice, experts advise. A half-cup provides 2 grams of fiber, which is a proven protector against constipation, hemorrhoids, colon cancer, diabetes, high cholesterol, heart disease, and obesity.

Experts aren't yet sure how much broccoli you need to maximize its healing potential. Dr. Kensler advises eating at least five servings of fruits and vegetables a day, while reaching for this crunchy crucifer whenever you can.

Getting the Most

Heat it—but just a little. While gently cooking broccoli helps release some of its protective compounds, overheating it can destroy others. "Carotenoids like beta-carotene are preserved by heat, but the indoles, like I3C, don't withstand a lot of heat," explains Dr. Michnovicz. "Light steaming is a great way to cook broccoli. And microwaving is okay, too."

Buy it purple. You'll notice at the supermarket that broccoli is sometimes so dark that it's almost purple. That's good. The dark color means that it has more beta-carotene, experts say. If it's yellowish, on the other hand, skip it. That means that it's old, and its nutritional clock is running down.

Look for the sprouts. Studies at Johns Hopkins University in Baltimore found that three-day-old broccoli sprouts contain 20 to 50 times the amount of protective substances in the mature vegetable. Broccoli sprouts aren't widely available yet. Ask your grocer when you'll be able to find them at your supermarket.

Broccoli Salad

4 cups broccoli florets

¼ cup finely diced red onions

3 tablespoons raisins

2 tablespoons dry-roasted sunflower seeds

¼ cup nonfat plain yogurt

2 tablespoons fresh orange juice

1 tablespoon reduced-fat mayonnaise

Per serving

calories	**100**
total fat	**3.7 g.**
saturated fat	**0.5 g.**
cholesterol	**2 mg.**
sodium	**68 mg.**
dietary fiber	**3.5 g.**

In a large bowl, combine the broccoli, onions, raisins, and sunflower seeds.

In a small bowl, whisk the yogurt, orange juice, and mayonnaise until blended. Pour over the broccoli mixture and toss to coat.

Makes 4 servings

Broccoli in Hoisin Sauce

1 teaspoon canola oil

2 teaspoons grated fresh ginger

3 cloves garlic, minced

4 cups broccoli florets

1½ tablespoons hoisin sauce

Per serving

calories	**52**
total fat	**1.7 g.**
saturated fat	**0.1 g.**
cholesterol	**0 mg.**
sodium	**118 mg.**
dietary fiber	**2.7 g.**

In a large skillet or wok, warm the oil over medium-high heat. Add the ginger and garlic and stir for 10 seconds, or until fragrant. Add the broccoli and 2 tablespoons water. Cook, tossing, for 1 to 2 minutes, or until the broccoli is crisp-tender and the water is absorbed. Stir in the hoisin sauce and toss to coat.

Makes 4 servings

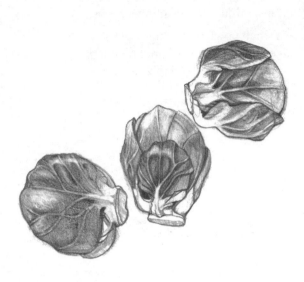

Brussels Sprouts
Good Things in Small Packages

Healing Power

Can help:
Reduce the risk
of breast, prostate,
and colon cancers

Lower cholesterol

Prevent constipation

Lower the risk
of heart disease

If any one food has the reputation for being "the thing on your plate you'd most like to slip to your dog," it might be brussels sprouts. Just say the name and people start crinkling their noses.

Well, believe it or not, brussels sprouts have gotten a lot tastier during the past decade. What's more, scientists have found that they're even better for you than they ever imagined.

New Taste in the Marketplace

Brussels sprouts are miniature members of the cabbage family. And while the brussels sprouts of yore were often strong and bitter, the taste has literally changed, says Steve Bontadelli, a brussels sprouts grower in Santa Cruz, California.

The taste problem originally began when brussels sprouts growers started using machines instead of harvesting sprouts by hand. To make machine harvesting easier, they developed a new strain of sprouts. Unfortunately, these "new and improved" plants yielded some really bitter sprouts, recalls Bontadelli.

"It wasn't until the past 10 years or so that brussels sprouts growers started changing the hybrids to make them taste better," he says. "Today they are much sweeter and milder."

So now you'll be smacking your lips instead of holding your nose when you spoon these health-saving leafy nuggets onto your plate. Taste aside, brussels sprouts are packed with plant chemicals that provide protection against major league diseases like cancer and heart disease.

BELGIUM'S BURLY CANCER-BEATERS

Like other cruciferous vegetables, brussels sprouts are chock-full of natural plant compounds called phytonutrients, which may help protect against cancer. These compounds may be particularly effective against common cancers like those of the breast and colon.

One of the key protective compounds in brussels sprouts is sulforaphane. Sulforaphane triggers the release of enzymes that help rid your body's cells of toxic wastes and reduce your risk for cancer, says Jon Michnovicz, M.D., Ph.D., president of the Foundation for Preventive Oncology and the Institute for Hormone Research, both in New York City.

In a groundbreaking study at Johns Hopkins University in Baltimore, scientists exposed 145 laboratory animals to a powerful cancer-causing agent called DMBA. Twenty-five of the animals had not received any special treatment, while the rest had been fed high doses of sulforaphane. Fifty days later, 68 percent of the unprotected animals had breast tumors, compared with only 26 percent of those that received the sulforaphane.

Brussels sprouts contain another protective phytonutrient called indole-3-carbinol, or I3C. This compound works as an anti-estrogen, meaning it helps sweep up your body's harmful estrogens before they contribute to the growth of cancer cells. It also helps boost the production of certain enzymes that help clear cancer-causing toxins from the body. "Indoles are probably very useful against colon, breast, and prostate cancers," explains Dr. Michnovicz. "And population studies show that they probably protect against other cancers as well."

In one small study, researchers in the Netherlands found that people who ate more than 10 ounces of brussels sprouts (about 14 sprouts) a day for one week had levels of protective cancer-fighting enzymes in their colon that were, on average, 23 percent higher than people who did not eat brussels sprouts.

In another study, five people ate more than 10 ounces of brussels sprouts a day for three weeks, while another five avoided the sprouts and other similar vegetables. At the end of the study, the sprout-eating group had 28 percent less wear and tear to their DNA. It's a promising find, say experts, because the healthier you keep your DNA, the healthier you stay.

In the Kitchen

For such tiny vegetables, brussels sprouts sure cause some large culinary conundrums. Not only is it challenging to cook them just so, but it's also likely that you'll smell up the house while you do it.

It doesn't have to be this way. If you follow these tips, you'll get the health benefits of brussels sprouts without the hassles.

Mark the spot. To allow the tough stems to cook as quickly as the leaves, make an "X" on the bottom of each stem, using a sharp knife. Then steam them for 7 to 14 minutes, until they're just tender enough to poke with a fork.

Quell the smell. The big sulfur smell thrown off by these little cabbages discourages some people from taking advantage of their healing power. Try tossing a stalk of celery in the cooking water. It will help neutralize the smell.

Use them fast. Although brussels sprouts will keep for a week or more in the refrigerator, they start getting bitter after about three days, which may discourage you and your family from eating them and reaping their benefits. Buy only as many as you'll use in the next few days.

Brussels for Your Bowels

Aside from all the "science-y" compounds in brussels sprouts, there are also plenty of good old-fashioned vitamins, minerals, and other substances that can help fight off cancer, heart disease, high cholesterol, and a host of other health problems.

Topping this list is fiber. Brussels sprouts are a good source of fiber, with about 3 grams in a half-cup serving. You'd have to eat more than two slices of whole-grain bread to get the amount of fiber in a half-cup of these little green gems.

Eating your daily fill of brussels sprouts can help you avoid all the conditions that a diet rich in fiber is known to prevent, like constipation, hemorrhoids, and other digestive complaints.

A half-cup of brussels sprouts provides 48 milligrams of immunity-building vitamin C, more than 80 percent of the Daily Value (DV). It also provides 47 micrograms of folate, about 12 percent of the DV. Folate is essential for normal tissue growth, and studies show that it may protect against cancer, heart disease, and birth defects. Women, especially those on birth control pills, often have low levels of this important vitamin.

Getting the Most

Steam them. Though you'll lose some nutrients during the cooking process, raw brussels sprouts just don't go down well. Gently steaming brussels sprouts will help release some of their healing compounds. But don't steam them too long; cooking sprouts until they're mushy makes them lose too much vitamin C, along with other valuable phytonutrients. Plus, overcooking gives them a bitter kick, says Dr. Michnovicz.

GLAZED BRUSSELS SPROUTS

1 **pound small brussels sprouts**

1 **teaspoon unsalted butter**

2 **tablespoons all-fruit apricot spread**

¼ **teaspoon salt**

¼ **teaspoon dry mustard**

PER SERVING

calories	**83**
total fat	**1.7 g.**
saturated fat	**0.7 g.**
cholesterol	**3 mg.**
sodium	**164 mg.**
dietary fiber	**5.7 g.**

Trim the bottoms of the brussels sprouts and cut them in half lengthwise. Place in a large saucepan and add 2 tablespoons water. Bring to a boil over high heat, then cover and reduce the heat to medium-high. Cook, stirring once, for 5 to 7 minutes, or until the sprouts are crisp-tender. If the sprouts start to dry out, add another 1 to 2 tablespoons water.

If any water remains in the pan, drain the sprouts in a colander. Transfer to a medium bowl.

Add the butter to the pan and melt over medium heat. Stir in the apricot spread, salt, and mustard. Cook for 30 seconds, or until bubbly and hot. Add the brussels sprouts to the pan and toss to coat with the glaze.

Makes 4 servings

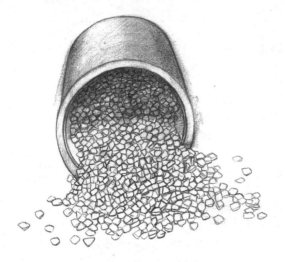

BUCKWHEAT
HOMEGROWN PROTECTION

HEALING POWER

CAN HELP:
Prevent cancer
and heart disease

Control diabetes

Modern epicures generally regard Paris as *the* city for fabulous food. For Mark Twain, however, who toured Europe in 1878, the City of Lights was a disappointment. He couldn't find the one American staple his homesick taste buds hankered for most: buckwheat pancakes.

Even though buckwheat, or kasha, as the roasted form of the grain is called, is as American as corn, it's not very popular in this country anymore, says buckwheat researcher Michael Eskin, Ph.D., professor of food chemistry at the University of Manitoba in Winnipeg. But it is popular in Japan—and some researchers suspect that this may partially explain that country's remarkably low cancer rates, says Dr. Eskin.

TWO-PRONGED PROTECTION

Buckwheat contains a variety of compounds called flavonoids that have been shown in studies to help block the spread of cancer. Two compounds in particular, quercetin and rutin, are especially promising because they appear to thwart cancer in two ways.

These substances make it difficult for cancer-promoting hormones to attach to healthy cells. They can literally stop cancers before they start. Should cancer-causing substances get into cells, these compounds may be able to reduce damage to DNA, the body's chemical blueprint for normal cell division.

KEEPING BLOOD FLOWING

The rutin in buckwheat plays yet another protective role. Working in concert with other compounds, it helps prevent platelets—the components in blood that assist in clotting—from clumping together. By helping to keep blood fluid, buckwheat can play an important part in any heart-protection plan.

There's another way in which the rutin in buckwheat can help keep blood flowing. It appears to shrink particles of the dangerous low-density lipoprotein (LDL) cholesterol. This makes them less likely to stick to artery walls, further reducing the risk of heart attack or stroke.

This could explain why the Yi people of China, who consume a high-buckwheat diet from an early age, have exceptionally low levels of total cholesterol. Better yet, their levels of LDL cholesterol are quite low, while levels of the good high-density lipoprotein (HDL) cholesterol remain high.

Rutin has also been reported to stabilize blood vessels and check excessive fluid accumulation in the body. This may help lower blood pressure and with it the risk of heart disease.

Research suggests that when flavonoids are combined with vitamin E, which is also found in buckwheat, the benefits are even more pronounced. Fat-soluble vitamin E can neutralize dangerous free radicals, harmful oxygen molecules that can damage cells, in the fatty portions of cells. Flavonoids, on the other hand, are water soluble; they attack free radicals in the watery parts of cells. "That puts an antioxidant in both the watery and fatty portions of cells," says Timothy Johns, Ph.D., associate professor in the School of Dietetics and Human Nutrition at McGill University in Montreal.

PROTEIN POWER

Here's great news for vegetarians and others trying to cut back on meat. Buckwheat is the best known grain source of high-quality protein. We need protein for everything from healing wounds to producing brainpower. Yet buckwheat protein does more. It helps lower cholesterol as well.

In laboratory experiments, animals that were fed extracts of buckwheat protein had significantly lower cholesterol levels than their non-buckwheat-eating companions. Levels in the buckwheat-fed animals, in fact, were even lower than in animals given soy protein extract, one of the most powerful cholesterol-busting foods.

In addition, buckwheat is an excellent source of essential nutrients. "It's rich in several minerals, most especially magnesium and manganese but also zinc and copper," says Dr. Eskin.

HELP FOR DIGESTION

One of the most valuable aspects of buckwheat is its ability to help control blood sugar levels in people with adult-onset diabetes, the most common form of the disease.

The carbohydrates in buckwheat, amylose and amylopectin, are digested more slowly than other types of carbohydrates. This causes blood sugar levels to rise more evenly. While this is good for everyone, it's especially important for those with diabetes, whose blood sugar levels tend to rise steeply and stay high too long. Keeping blood sugar under control has been shown to reduce or prevent many of the serious complications of diabetes, including kidney damage.

Even if you don't have diabetes, buckwheat can help. Because it's absorbed more slowly than other grains, it leaves you feeling full longer. This makes it easier to eat less and help control your weight.

And don't forget buckwheat if you or someone you know has celiac disease. This is a potentially serious intestinal problem that occurs in people sensitive to gluten, a protein found in wheat and other grains. Because buckwheat is free of gluten, you can eat as much as you want.

Getting the Most

Fire up the oven. Even though buckwheat is often served as a side dish, you can use the flour to make breads, muffins, and pancakes. It's important, however, to use "light" buckwheat flour, since it actually contains more nutrients that the healthier-sounding "whole" flour.

Whole buckwheat flour is made by grinding the buckwheat hull and adding it to the mix. This adds a robust, dark color but virtually no nutrients, says Clifford Orr, director of the Buckwheat Institute in Penn Yan, New York. In fact, this process "dilutes" the more-nutritious light flour, giving less bang for the buck—8 percent less, to be exact. "Everyone associates the whole version with being healthier, but in this case, it's just not true," Orr says.

Kasha Pilaf

2	teaspoons canola oil
³/₄	cup chopped onions
³/₄	cup kasha (toasted buckwheat groats)
¹/₂	cup shredded carrots
1	egg white, lightly beaten
1¹/₂	cups defatted reduced-sodium chicken broth
1	teaspoon dried marjoram
¹/₄	teaspoon ground black pepper
¹/₈	teaspoon salt (optional)
1	tablespoon minced fresh parsley

In a large skillet over medium heat, warm the oil. Add the onions and cook, stirring occasionally, for 5 minutes, or until softened. Transfer the onions to a plate and set aside.

Add the kasha to the skillet. Reduce the heat to low. Cook, stirring, for 30 seconds. Add the carrots and stir to combine. Add the egg white, stirring constantly with a fork so that it adheres to the kasha and carrots. Cook, stirring to break up large clumps, for 1 minute, or until the egg white is set and the kasha looks dry and crumbly.

Gradually stir in the broth, marjoram, and the reserved onions. Partially cover and cook for 10 to 12 minutes, or until the kasha absorbs the liquid. Add the pepper and salt (if using). Stir to combine. Sprinkle with the parsley.

Makes 4 side-dish servings

Per serving

calories	**175**
total fat	**3.2 g.**
saturated fat	**0.4 g.**
cholesterol	**0 mg.**
sodium	**80 mg.**
dietary fiber	**4 g.**

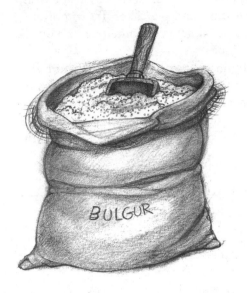

BULGUR
A WHOLE-GRAIN HEALER

HEALING POWER
CAN HELP:
Prevent constipation

Prevent colon
and breast cancers

Reduce the risk
of diabetes
and heart disease

Despite its unfamiliar name, bulgur is simply wheat in its whole form. And as you would expect, this wholesome grain is one of the healthiest foods you can eat.

Research shows that bulgur may play a role in preventing colon and breast cancers and diabetes. In addition, it's extremely high in fiber, which means it can help prevent and treat a variety of digestive problems, including constipation and diverticular disease.

CHEMICAL REPAIR

No matter how carefully you watch your diet, you're probably being exposed to dangerous chemicals nearly every day. Two of the most common are nitrates and nitrites. Nitrates occur naturally in lots of vegetables, including beets, celery, and lettuce. Nitrites are common ingredients in processed foods such as cured fish, poultry, and meat.

These compounds themselves aren't harmful. But when you get them from food, your body transforms them into related compounds called nitrosamines, which have been linked to cancer.

While it's difficult to avoid nitrates and nitrites, a diet high in bulgur can help reduce the potentially dangerous effects. Bulgur contains a compound

In the Kitchen

Even if you've never cooked bulgur, don't let the exotic name put you off. It's extremely easy to prepare. Here's how.

Choose the right kind. Bulgur comes in three grinds, each of which is recommended for different types of recipes.

- The **coarse grind,** which has a consistency similar to rice, is recommended for making pilaf or when using bulgur in any rice recipe.
- Use the **medium grind** when making breakfast cereal or bulgur filling.
- The **fine grind** is usually used for making tabbouleh.

Start it hot. You don't have to cook—and cook and cook—bulgur the way you do other grains. Just cover it with about 2 cups of boiling water for each cup of bulgur. Then let it stand, covered, for about a half-hour, or until the grains are tender.

called ferulic acid, which helps prevent these compounds from making the troublesome conversion into nitrosamines.

Bulgur protects against cancer in yet another way because it contains lignans. "Lignans are potent cancer warriors, especially against colon and breast cancer," says Lilian Thompson, Ph.D., professor of nutritional sciences at the University of Toronto.

Lignans have antioxidant properties, which means that they gobble up dangerous oxygen molecules (free radicals) before they damage individual cells. "Lignans also subdue cancerous changes once they've occurred, rendering them less likely to race out of control," Dr. Thompson says.

Help for the Heart

We've seen that free radicals can contribute to cancer. The same pernicious molecules can also damage blood vessels, setting the stage for heart disease.

Somewhat paradoxically, the lignans in bulgur can help protect the heart by protecting cholesterol. Why would you want to protect a bad guy? Because when cholesterol is damaged by free radical molecules, it is more likely to stick to artery walls, contributing to the development of heart disease.

Bulgur can help in yet another way. This grain has a low glycemic index, meaning that the sugars it contains are released relatively slowly into the bloodstream, says David Jenkins, M.D., Sc.D., Ph.D., professor of nutritional sciences and medicine at the University of Toronto. Not only does this help keep blood sugar levels stable, which is important for people with diabetes, it also may play a role in reducing the risk of heart disease.

Rich in Fiber

Getting more fiber in your diet helps lower cholesterol, reduces cancer and diabetes risk, and helps treat or prevent many digestive complaints, from constipation to hemorrhoids. Bulgur is a good fiber source, with 1 cup of cooked bulgur providing over 8 grams, almost a third of the Daily Value (DV). Compare that to a cup of cooked oatmeal, which has 4 grams of fiber, or a cup of cooked white rice, which has a measly 0.8 gram.

Many of bulgur's benefits come from insoluble fiber. This type of fiber doesn't break down in the body. Instead, it stays in the intestine, soaking up large amounts of water. This makes wastes heavier, so they move through the digestive system faster. Potential cancer-causing substances are ushered out of the body more quickly, giving them less time to create problems.

In a four-year study at the New York Hospital–Cornell Medical Center in New York City, researchers studied 58 men and women with histories of intestinal polyps. (While polyps themselves aren't dangerous, over time they may become cancerous.) In the study, those given bran cereal containing 22 grams of insoluble fiber were more likely to have their polyps shrink or disappear entirely than were those who were given a low-fiber lookalike.

Insoluble fiber has also been shown to prevent (and relieve) constipation. This isn't just a matter of comfort. Moving wastes more quickly through the digestive tract reduces the time that harmful substances are in contact with the intestine. In addition, preventing constipation also helps relieve conditions such as hemorrhoids and diverticular disease.

Minerals for Health

Finally, bulgur is a virtual metal warehouse, rich in minerals essential to health. In addition to iron, phosphorus, and zinc, 1 cup of cooked bulgur contains the following minerals.

- 1 milligram of manganese, about half of the DV. Manganese is needed to ensure healthy bones, nerves, and reproduction.
- 15 micrograms of selenium, 22 percent of the DV. Selenium is needed to help protect the heart and immune system.
- 58 milligrams of magnesium, 15 percent of the DV. Magnesium helps keep your heart beating, nerves functioning, muscles contracting, and bones forming.

Getting the Most

Have it with hot dogs. Since bulgur can help block the process that converts the nitrites in processed foods into cancer-causing substances, it's a good idea to combine it with these foods whenever possible. Tabbouleh, which is made from cooked bulgur mixed with chopped tomatoes, onions, parsley, and mint and flavored with olive oil and lemon juice, makes a wonderfully fresh salad that goes well with any meal.

Buy it in bulk. Unlike many whole grains, which can be extremely slow-cooking, bulgur is steamed, dried, and crushed before it gets to the store. Essentially it's precooked, meaning that it's ready to go in about 15 minutes. If you always have it on hand, you'll find out how easy it is to get more of this healthful grain into your diet.

Keep it cold. Since bulgur is cracked open during processing, the fatty portion of the germ is exposed to air and tends to go rancid. To keep bulgur fresh and ready to eat, be sure to keep it refrigerated until you're ready to use it.

BULGUR SALAD WITH CURRANTS

1	cup fine bulgur
3	cups cold water
¼	cup minced fresh parsley
¼	cup chopped scallions or onions
¼	cup dried currants
2	tablespoons freshly squeezed lemon juice
1	tablespoon extra-virgin olive oil
⅛	teaspoon salt (optional)

PER SERVING
calories	**180**
total fat	**3.9 g.**
saturated fat	**0.5 g.**
cholesterol	**0 mg.**
sodium	**77 mg.**
dietary fiber	**7.4 g.**

In a medium bowl, combine the bulgur and water; stir to mix. Let stand for 30 minutes, or until the bulgur has absorbed the water. If the bulgur is tender but has not completely absorbed the water, drain through a fine sieve and return to the bowl.

Add the parsley, scallions or onions, currants, lemon juice, oil, and salt (if using). Toss to combine. Serve at room temperature.

Makes 4 servings

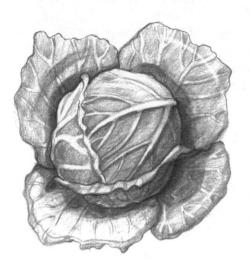

CABBAGE FAMILY
A HEAD ABOVE THE REST

HEALING POWER

CAN HELP:
Prevent breast, prostate, and colon cancers

Lower the risk of cataracts

Prevent heart disease and birth defects

Ancient Roman healers thought that they could cure breast cancer by rubbing on pastes made from cabbage. A few years ago, modern scientists would have dismissed that practice as so much folklore. Now they're not so sure.

"Studies have shown that if you make cabbage into a paste and rub it on the backs of laboratory animals, you can prevent tumors from developing," says Jon Michnovicz, M.D., Ph.D., president of the Foundation for Preventive Oncology and the Institute for Hormone Research, both in New York City.

Of course, the best way to absorb the healing properties of cabbage is simply to eat it. Cabbage not only fights off a variety of cancers but also contains a wealth of nutrients that can ward off heart disease, digestive problems, and other conditions, according to research.

CABBAGE AGAINST CANCER

Like other members of the cruciferous vegetable family, cabbage contains several compounds that studies show can help prevent cancers from occurring. It's particularly effective in preventing cancers of the breast, prostate gland, and colon.

There are two compounds in particular that scientists believe make cabbage a particularly potent cancer-fighting food. The first of these, indole-3-carbinol, or I3C, is especially effective against breast cancer, research shows. The compound acts as an anti-estrogen, meaning that it sweeps up harmful estrogens that have been linked to breast cancer.

In one study, researchers gave a group of Israeli women about a third of a head of cabbage a day for three months. After five days of eating the cabbage-fortified diet, the women's levels of harmful hormones dropped significantly.

"There was no doubt that if we gave women pure I3C, it would work," says Dr. Michnovicz. "But this study showed that for the average person, eating cabbage or a cabbagelike vegetable, like broccoli, would have the same effect."

For even more protection, try replacing your usual cabbage with bok choy, or Chinese cabbage. Laboratory research has found that a compound in bok choy called brassinin may help prevent breast tumors.

Cabbage contains another compound, sulforaphane, which has been shown to block cancer by stepping up the production of tumor-preventing enzymes in the body.

In a pioneering study at Johns Hopkins University in Baltimore, scientists exposed 145 laboratory animals to a powerful cancer-causing chemical. Twenty-five of the animals had not received any special treatment, while the rest had been fed high doses of sulforaphane. Fifty days later, 68 percent of the unprotected animals had breast tumors, compared with only 26 percent of those given high doses of sulforaphane.

Sulforaphane makes cabbage a particularly prized fighter in the battle against colon cancer, adds Dr. Michnovicz, because it stimulates levels of an enzyme called glutathione in the colon, which researchers believe sweeps toxins out of the body before they have a chance to damage the delicate cells lining the intestinal wall.

Eating any kind of cabbage on a regular basis will probably lower your risk for cancer. To get the best possible protection, however, you can't do better than savoy cabbage, say researchers. Savoy contains not only I3C and sulforaphane but also four other tongue-twisting phytonutrients—beta-sitosterol, pheophytin-a, nonacosane, and nonacosanone—that studies show are powerful contenders against potential cancer-causing agents.

ANTIOXIDANT PROTECTION

You've heard a lot about antioxidants such as vitamins C and E and beta-carotene, which help ward off disease by mopping up harmful oxygen molecules called free radicals that naturally accumulate in the body. Free radicals damage healthy tissues throughout the body, causing changes that can lead to heart disease, cancer, and other serious conditions.

As produce goes, cabbage is a cook's best friend. It's versatile, inexpensive, readily available, and easy to prepare. Sure, there's that cabbage-y smell, but that's easily remedied.

The next time you're cooking cabbage, add a celery stalk or whole English walnut (in the shell) to the pot. This will help neutralize the powerful odor. Or simply cook the cabbage more quickly, using the microwave or wok rather than a slow-cooking pot. Long cooking times release more of the strong-smelling sulfur compounds.

Members of the cabbage family are packed with these nutritious compounds. Particularly good are cabbages like bok choy and savoy, which are super sources of beta-carotene, a nutrient that other cabbages don't have in abundance. High blood levels of beta-carotene are related to lower incidences of heart attacks, certain types of cancers, and cataracts.

Not only are these cabbages high in beta-carotene; they're also a good source of vitamin C, which has been shown to boost immunity as well as reduce blood pressure and fight heart disease. A half-cup serving of raw bok choy provides 16 milligrams of vitamin C, 27 percent of the Daily Value (DV), while the same amount of raw savoy cabbage supplies 11 milligrams, 18 percent of the DV.

Both bok choy and savoy cabbage are also decent sources of folate, with a half-cup of either providing about 35 micrograms, or 9 percent of the DV. Your body uses folate for normal tissue growth. Studies show that folate also may protect against cancer, heart disease, and birth defects. Research shows that women are at high risk for folate deficiency, especially if they take birth control pills.

Getting the Most

Keep a cool head. Boiling cabbage removes about half the valuable indoles, experts say. To preserve these compounds at maximum levels, experts advise eating cabbage raw—mixed in with a green salad, for example, or concentrated in coleslaw.

Enjoy the variety. To get the healing benefits of cabbage several times a week without getting bored, explore the different varieties. Green, red, and savoy cabbages, along with bok choy, all are high in protective compounds. They can be eaten raw in coleslaw, slow-cooked in soup, or wrapped around your favorite filling.

Stock up. We often avoid stocking up on fresh produce because it can go bad so quickly. Never fear with cabbage. A head of cabbage will keep for up to 10 days in the crisper drawer, making it easy to eat a little bit each day without worrying about it spoiling.

Bok Choy with Mushrooms

1   pound bok choy
4   large shiitake mushrooms
1   teaspoon canola oil
2   teaspoons reduced-sodium soy sauce
2   teaspoons packed light brown sugar
½   teaspoon dark sesame oil

Per serving

calories **46**
total fat **1.9 g.**
saturated fat **0.2 g.**
cholesterol **0 mg.**
sodium **123 mg.**
dietary fiber **2.2 g.**

Trim the bok choy and cut the leaves from the stems. Thinly slice both the stems and leaves.

Remove and discard the mushroom stems. Cut the caps into narrow slices.

In a wok or large skillet over medium heat, warm the canola oil. Add the mushrooms and stir-fry for 2 to 3 minutes, or until they soften. Add the bok choy stems and stir-fry for 1 minute. Add the bok choy leaves and stir-fry for 20 seconds. Add the soy sauce, brown sugar, and sesame oil. Stir-fry for 1 to 2 minutes, or just until the bok choy is wilted.

Makes 4 servings

Red Cabbage and Kohlrabi Slaw

3   cups shredded red cabbage
1   medium kohlrabi, peeled and cut into matchstick pieces
¼   cup cider vinegar
1   tablespoon honey
1   tablespoon brown mustard seeds
⅛   teaspoon salt

Per serving

calories **41**
total fat **0.4 g.**
saturated fat **0.1 g.**
cholesterol **0 mg.**
sodium **126 mg.**
dietary fiber **2.3 g.**

In a medium bowl, combine the cabbage and kohlrabi. Toss to mix.

In a small bowl, whisk together the vinegar, honey, mustard seeds, and salt. Pour over the cabbage and kohlrabi. Toss to combine. Let stand, tossing once or twice, for 30 minutes to allow the flavors to blend. Or refrigerate for up to 8 hours. Toss just before serving.

Makes 4 servings

CANCER
FOODS AS ULTIMATE PROTECTOR

When it comes to cancer prevention, food is powerful medicine. Study after study shows that a healthful diet—eating less fat and getting more fruits, vegetables, whole grains, and legumes—can vastly reduce the risk of cancer. In fact, research indicates that if we all ate more of the right foods and less of the wrong ones, the incidence of all cancers would be reduced at least 30 percent.

"Food goes beyond being crude fuel, as we once believed," says Keith Block, M.D., medical director of the Cancer Institute at Edgewater Hospital in Chicago. "Our experience over the past two decades indicates that diet plays an important role when dealing with cancer. We're discovering that there are compounds in foods that can actually both prevent and help fight cancer at the cellular level."

PROTECTION FROM THE GARDEN

Researchers have known for a long time that people who eat the most fruits, vegetables, and other plant foods are less likely to get cancer than those who fill up on other, less wholesome foods. But it's only recently that they've discovered the reason. Certain substances found only in plant foods and known collectively as phytonutrients (phyto is a Greek word meaning "plant") have the ability to stop cancer.

Research has shown, for example, that broccoli contains phytonutrients called isothiocyanates, which literally prevent cells from becoming cancerous. In a study at Johns Hopkins University in Baltimore, laboratory animals given a small amount of sulforaphane (one type of isothiocyanate) were about half as likely to develop breast tumors as animals that didn't get the compound.

Phytonutrients are also abundant in foods made from soybeans, like tofu, tempeh, and soy milk. Specifically, soy foods contain a compound called genistein, which inhibits the growth of tumors by preventing blood vessels from growing nearby. This may explain why Japanese women, who eat a lot of soy foods, have a lower rate of breast cancer than their American counterparts. Also, preliminary research suggests that soy foods may help reduce the risk of prostate cancer in men.

As you might expect, garlic, which has a long tradition as a healing food, is also very rich in phytonutrients. Some of the most impressive are called allyl sulfides, which appear to help destroy cancer-causing substances in the body. In a study of nearly 42,000 women, researchers at the University of Minnesota School of Public Health in Minneapolis found that those who ate more than one serving of garlic—either one fresh clove or a shake of powder—a week were 35 percent less likely to get colon cancer than those who ate none.

The Power of Antioxidants

Every day your body is attacked, again and again, by a barrage of harmful molecules called free radicals. These are oxygen molecules that have lost an electron, and they careen around your body looking for replacements. In the process of pilfering electrons, they damage healthy cells, possibly kicking off the cancer process.

Nature anticipated this threat by packing fruits, vegetables, and other foods with antioxidants, protective compounds that either stop the formation of free radicals or disable them before they do harm.

There are many compounds in foods that act as antioxidants in the body, but three of the best-studied and most-powerful are beta-carotene and vitamins C and E.

Beta-carotene is the pigment that gives many fruits and vegetables their lush, deep orange to red hues. It's more than nature's palette, however. Beta-carotene has been shown to stimulate the release of natural killer cells, which hunt down and destroy cancer cells before they have a chance to cause damage.

Literally dozens of studies have shown that people who get a lot of beta-carotene in their diets can reduce their risks of certain cancers, especially those of the lungs, intestinal tract, mouth, and gums.

It doesn't take a lot of beta-carotene to get the benefits. Evidence suggests that getting 15 to 30 milligrams a day—the amount provided by one to two large carrots—is probably all it takes. Cantaloupes, sweet potatoes, spinach, and bok choy all are excellent sources of beta-carotene.

Another powerful antioxidant is vitamin C, which has been shown to help prevent cancer-causing compounds from forming in the digestive tract. In one large study, Gladys Block, Ph.D., professor of epidemiology and director of the public health nutrition program at the University of California, Berkeley, analyzed dozens of smaller studies that looked at the relationship between vitamin C and cancer. Of the 46 studies she examined, 33 showed that those who consumed the most vitamin C had the lowest risk of cancer.

The Daily Value (DV) for vitamin C is 60 milligrams, an amount that's very easy to get in foods. One green pepper, for example, contains 66 milligrams of vitamin C, while a half-cup of broccoli has 41 milligrams.

Perhaps the most versatile antioxidant for fighting cancer is vitamin E. It not only blocks free radicals, it also fends off cancer by stimulating the immune system. In addition, it actually prevents the formation of cancer-causing compounds in the body.

Vitamin E is particularly important for women with a family history of breast cancer. Researchers at the State University of New York at Buffalo found that women who got the most vitamin E were 80 percent less likely to get breast cancer than those getting the least. Even in women without a family history of breast cancer, those getting the most vitamin E were 40 percent less likely to get the disease.

The one problem with vitamin E is that it's difficult to get from foods. Some cooking oils contain a lot, but they're also extremely high in fat. A leaner way to get more vitamin E in your diet is with wheat germ. A little less than 2 tablespoons of wheat germ contains about 4 international units of vitamin E, 13 percent of the DV. Whole grains, legumes, nuts, and seeds are also good sources of vitamin E.

THE FACTS ABOUT FAT

There's no longer any doubt that a diet filled with potato chips, pizza, cheeseburgers, and doughnuts—that is to say, a fatty diet—is one of the greatest risk factors for developing cancer.

"There is enormous evidence linking dietary fat to a variety of cancers, particularly of the breast, colon, and prostate gland," says Daniel W. Nixon, M.D., associate director of cancer prevention and control at the Hollings Cancer Center in Charleston, South Carolina, and author of *The Cancer Recovery Eating Plan.*

A high-fat diet steps up the body's production of free radicals, which not only damage healthy cells but also increase damage to the body's genetic material, says Dr. Keith Block.

In addition, a high-fat diet increases the amount of bile acid, which the body uses to digest fats, that flows into the intestine. Since bile acid may be transformed in the body into cancer-causing compounds, getting too much fat can dramatically increase the risk for colon cancer.

Finally, high-fat diets increase the body's production of estrogen and testosterone, which in large amounts can trigger the growth of tumors in the breasts and prostate gland.

A study of women in 21 countries, for example, found that those who ate high-fat diets (45 percent of calories coming from fat) had more than five times the risk of breast cancer of women who got only 15 percent of calories from fat.

Reducing fat in your diet even slightly can have large benefits. In one study, researchers found that women who got just 10 fewer grams of fat a day were able to cut their risk of ovarian cancer by 20 percent.

As part of an anti-cancer plan, the National Cancer Institute recommends that you get no more than 30 percent of your calories from fat. "I advise getting even less, between 20 and 25 percent," says Dr. Nixon.

Perhaps the easiest way to reduce fat without changing your diet entirely is to cut back on meats, dairy foods, and processed foods, which are typically very high in fat. Once you cut back on these foods, you'll automatically find yourself eating more low-fat foods, like vegetables, whole grains, and legumes, says Dr. Nixon. If you do this consistently, the amounts of fat in your diet will naturally drop to lower levels.

THE FIBER SOLUTION

For a long time, no one took dietary fiber seriously. It's not a nutrient. It isn't absorbed by the body. In fact, it doesn't seem to do much of anything.

As it turns out, fiber does more than anyone ever imagined. "Consuming a high-fiber diet is essential for reducing the risk of certain types of cancer, particularly colon cancer," says Dr. Nixon.

Fiber works against cancer in several ways, he explains. Since fiber is absorbent, it soaks up water as it moves through the digestive tract. This makes stools larger, which causes the intestine to move them along more quickly. And the more quickly stools move, the less time there is for any harmful substances they contain to harm the cells lining the intestine.

In addition, fiber helps trap cancer-causing substances in the colon. And since the fiber itself isn't absorbed, it exits the body in the stool, taking the harmful substances with it.

According to doctors at the National Cancer Institute, you need between 20 and 35 grams of fiber a day to keep your risk of cancer low. That may sound like a lot, and it would be if you ate it all at once. But since many foods contain at least some fiber, it's fairly easy to get enough if you pick the right foods.

Simply make it a point to eat more fruits and vegetables—raw, when possible, and with their skins rather than peeled—than you're currently eating. If you do this regularly, you'll soon find that you're getting most of the fiber you need, says Dr. Keith Block.

Beans, vegetables, and whole grains are among the best sources of fiber you can find. Eating one of them a few times a day will automatically bring your fiber intake into the comfort zone. A half-cup of kidney beans, for example, contains 7 grams of fiber, while the same amount of chickpeas contains 5 grams. As for greens, a half-cup of cooked okra contains 3 grams of fiber, while the same amount of brussels sprouts has 3 grams.

Whether you're eating whole-wheat toast (2 grams of fiber per slice) for breakfast or a bowl of kasha (about 3 grams per half-cup, cooked), whole grains are also great sources of fiber. If you can, get 6 to 11 servings of whole grains a day. A sandwich, incidentally, counts as two servings. Each slice of bread is one serving.

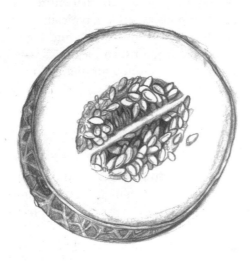

CANTALOUPE
SWEET FRUIT FOR CIRCULATION

HEALING POWER

CAN HELP:
Lower high blood
pressure and cholesterol

Reduce the risk
of heart disease

Reduce the risk of cancer

Prevent cataracts

The show: Meal of Fortune. The question: "For $10,000 and a brand-new car, name the difference between a cantaloupe and a muskmelon."

You smile and hit the buzzer. "Nothing," you say.

Then you jump up and down because you know what the other contestants don't. A cantaloupe is a type of muskmelon. And you also know that cantaloupe—or muskmelon, whichever you prefer—is filled with healing substances that can help control blood pressure, lower cholesterol, keep the blood running smoothly, and protect against cancer.

"Cantaloupe is one of the few fruits or vegetables rich in both vitamin C and beta-carotene," says John Erdman, Ph.D., director of the division of nutritional sciences at the University of Illinois in Urbana. Both of these antioxidant compounds have been shown to protect against cancer, heart disease, and other age-related health conditions, such as cataracts.

POTASSIUM PROTECTION

When you think of cantaloupe, you probably imagine a shimmering wedge of pale orange fruit next to a bowl of cereal. But if your blood pressure is rising, you may find yourself wanting cantaloupe away from the breakfast table, too.

Cantaloupe is great source of potassium, a mineral that can help lower blood pressure, says George Webb, Ph.D., associate professor of physiology and biophysics at the University of Vermont College of Medicine in Burlington.

Half a cantaloupe contains 825 milligrams of potassium, or 24 percent of the Daily Value (DV). "You get more potassium by eating half a cantaloupe than you do by eating a banana," says Dr. Webb.

The body uses potassium to help eliminate excess sodium, which in large amounts can cause blood pressure to rise, says Dr. Webb. The more potassium you eat, the more sodium you lose—and the lower your blood pressure is likely to be. This is particularly true in people who are sensitive to salt, he says.

In a large international study of more than 10,000 people, researchers found that those with the highest levels of potassium had the lowest blood pressures. Those with the least potassium, on the other hand, were more likely to have higher blood pressures.

In addition, studies show that potassium may help keep the body's low-density lipoprotein (LDL) cholesterol—the dangerous kind—from undergoing chemical changes that cause it to stick to artery walls. "There's evidence that a high-potassium diet tends to lower LDL cholesterol and raise 'good' HDL (high-density lipoprotein) cholesterol," says Dr. Webb. Potassium may also help thwart hardening of the arteries (atherosclerosis) and the formation of blood clots that can trigger heart attack and stroke.

IN THE KITCHEN

Few foods are as sweetly aromatic as a perfectly ripe cantaloupe (which may explain its nickname, muskmelon). On the other hand, a cantaloupe that hasn't reached its peak of freshness will leave you underwhelmed. To pick the best, here's what you need to do.

Trust your nose. While thumping melons is the traditional way of testing for ripeness, your sense of smell is a superior judge. A ripe cantaloupe should have a strong, sweet fragrance. If you can't smell it, pass it by.

Check the stem. There shouldn't be one. Mature cantaloupes will only have a smooth, symmetrical basin where the stem once was and flesh that yields slightly to pressure.

THE DYNAMIC DUO

As we mentioned earlier, cantaloupe is a rich source of two potent antioxidants, vitamin C and beta-carotene. Antioxidants are compounds that neutralize free radicals—cell-damaging molecules that occur naturally and that are thought to cause cellular changes that can lead to heart disease, cancer, and cataracts.

Like potassium, vitamin C helps keep the arteries clear and blood moving smoothly by preventing LDL cholesterol from oxidizing and gumming up the artery walls. The body also uses vitamin C for producing collagen, a protein that makes up skin and connective tissue. Cantaloupe is an excellent source of vitamin C, with 1 cup containing 68 milligrams, 113 percent of the DV.

Cantaloupe is also a good source of beta-carotene, which fights heart disease and cancer. Half a cantaloupe provides 5 milligrams of beta-carotene—about half of the daily amount recommended by most experts.

Getting the Most

Buy them ripe. The riper the cantaloupe, the more beta-carotene it contains, says Dr. Erdman. To check for ripeness in the store, put cantaloupes to the "heft-and-sniff test." Heft the fruit to make sure that it's heavy for its size. Then smell it to make sure that it exudes a sweet, musky perfume. If there's no smell, put it down and try another.

Eat it quickly. Vitamin C degrades quickly when exposed to air, so it's important to eat cantaloupe fairly soon after cutting, says Dr. Erdman. This is especially true when the fruit is cut into small pieces, which substantially increases the amount of air to which it's exposed.

ZESTY CANTALOUPE SALAD

1 **medium cantaloupe**

1 **small jalapeño pepper, seeded and finely minced (wear plastic gloves when handling)**

2 **tablespoons fresh lime juice**

1 **tablespoon minced fresh mint**

1/8 **teaspoon salt**

Cut the cantaloupe in half. Scoop out and discard the seeds. Cut each half into 6 wedges. Peel and cut into 1/2" dice. Place in a medium bowl.

Add the peppers, lime juice, mint, and salt. Stir to mix.

Makes 4 servings

Cook's Note: Serve as a side dish for grilled chicken, grilled fish, or vegetarian burgers.

PER SERVING

calories	**56**
total fat	**0.4 g.**
saturated fat	**0.1 g.**
cholesterol	**0 mg.**
sodium	**83 mg.**
dietary fiber	**1.4 g.**

CAROTENOIDS
More Than
Pretty Colors

All great chefs know that the eyes eat first. That's why they put so much effort into presentation, livening up the plate with vivid vegetables.

For a long time, in fact, nature's colorful bounty—an emerald bed of lettuce, shiny scarlet tomato wedges, or bright orange slivers of carrots—was used mainly as a bit of colorful warmth to fill up the empty spaces between the meat and potatoes.

Now we know that there's a better reason to serve vegetables. The pigments that give fruits and vegetables their cheery hues, called carotenoids, are more than pretty colors. They could save your life.

Researchers have found that people who eat the most carotenoid-rich yellow, orange, and red vegetables, like pumpkins, sweet potatoes, watermelons, and sweet red peppers, have significantly lower risks of dying from heart disease and cancer. The same is true of the dark green, leafy vegetables, like spinach and kale. (The chlorophyll they contain masks the lighter carotenoid hues.)

How can a simple food coloring be so good for you? The reason, as is often true with nutrition, comes down to chemistry. Our bodies are constantly under attack by free radicals—oxygen molecules that have lost an electron and zip through the body trying to steal replacement electrons from healthy cells. In time, this process causes internal damage to tissues throughout the body, possibly causing heart disease, cancer, and many other serious conditions. The carotenoids in vegetables neutralize free radicals by offering up their own electrons. This effectively stops the destructive process, helping prevent your cells from being damaged.

"Carotenoids certainly seem to be important in disease prevention," says Dexter L. Morris, M.D., Ph.D., vice chairman and associate professor in the department of emergency medicine at the University of North Carolina School of

The 24-Carat Carotenoids

All rich yellow, orange, and red vegetables contain generous amounts of carotenoids. So do the deep green, leafy vegetables, like spinach and kale. To get the most of these healing compounds into your diet, here are some of the best food sources.

Cantaloupe
Carrots
Kale
Leafy greens
Oranges
Peaches
Pumpkin
Spinach
Sweet potatoes
Tomatoes

Medicine at Chapel Hill. "The best way to get them is by eating five to nine servings of fruits and vegetables every day. That way you're sure to get a wide variety of these compounds in the amounts that nature intended."

There are more than 500 carotenoids, although only 50 to 60 of them are found in common foods. The key carotenoids identified so far are alpha-carotene, beta-carotene, gamma-carotene, beta-cryptoxanthin, lutein, lycopene, and zeaxanthin, although scientists continue to investigate others.

Carotenoids for your Heart

People have been fighting the cholesterol war since doctors first uttered the words "hardening of the arteries." Along with avoiding high-fat foods, you can make progress in winning this war by eating carotenoid-rich fruits and vegetables, like sweet potatoes, spinach, and cantaloupe, every day.

Carotenoids contribute to heart health by helping prevent the dangerous low-density lipoprotein (LDL) cholesterol from oxidizing—the process that causes it to stick to artery walls. Studies show that people with high levels of carotenoids have significantly lower risks for heart disease than those who don't.

Researchers at Johns Hopkins University in Baltimore found that smokers who already had one heart attack were less likely to have a second if they had high blood levels of four important carotenoids—beta-carotene, lutein, lycopene, and zeaxanthin.

Keeping Cancer in Check

The same process by which carotenoids protect against heart disease also seems to protect against cancer. Researchers believe that these compounds, by neutralizing free radicals, can prevent damage to DNA, the genetic material that controls how cells behave.

In one study, researchers at the University of Arizona in Tucson found that high doses of beta-carotene—about 30 milligrams—have the ability to shrink precancerous lesions in the mouth, in some cases by about 50 percent.

"There are several studies now yielding the same results," says Harinder Garewal, M.D., Ph.D., assistant director of cancer prevention and control at the Department of Veterans' Affairs Hospital and a cancer specialist at the University of Arizona Cancer Center in Tucson. "These findings are important because they suggest that you can do something to reverse the onset of cancer."

Another carotenoid that seems to be a crusader against cancer is lycopene—the pigment that gives tomatoes their rosy glow and that is also found in watermelons, guavas, and pink grapefruit. Researchers from the Harvard School of Public Health found that people who ate 10 or more servings per week of tomato-based foods had a 45 percent decrease in their risk for prostate cancer. Those who only ate four to seven servings a week—less than one a day—still came out ahead, with a 20 percent reduction in risk. It wasn't only whole tomatoes that provided the benefits either. Pizza, tomato juice, and other tomato-based foods also were protective.

Although evidence clearly shows that people who get the most carotenoids in their diets tend to get less cancer, the case for taking supplements isn't quite so clear.

For example, when researchers tested the effectiveness of beta-carotene supplements, they found that this compound wasn't effective in preventing cancer. In fact, some studies have shown that taking beta-carotene supplements may accelerate the disease.

"There is very clear evidence that we know less than we thought we did," says Walter Willett, M.D., Dr. P.H., professor of epidemiology and nutrition and chair of the department of nutrition at the Harvard School of Public Health. It's possible that beta-carotene supplements cause problems because high doses interfere with the body's absorption of other protective carotenoids.

For now, the best strategy for preventing cancer is to get carotenoids from food rather than supplements. "Our hope is that with more research we'll be able to pinpoint which compounds are most beneficial and which fruits and vegetables people should emphasize in their diets," says Dr. Willett.

Good for the Eyes

As his name suggests, Popeye has his share of vision problems. But according to research on his favorite leafy elixir, he won't likely have problems with macular degeneration—the leading cause of irreversible vision loss in older adults.

People who eat spinach, collard greens, and other dark green, leafy vegetables five or six times a week have about a 43 percent lower risk for macular degeneration than those who eat it less than once a month, according to a large study in Massachusetts.

The carotenoids that seem to be responsible, zeaxanthin and lutein, are believed to block the effects of free radicals in the outer retina, preventing them from damaging healthy eye tissue.

BUTTERNUT SQUASH, KALE, AND TOMATO STEW

1 **small butternut squash**

1 **tablespoon olive oil**

1 **tablespoon minced garlic**

1 **can (16 ounces) whole tomatoes (with juice)**

½ **cup water**

8 **ounces kale**

1 **tablespoon chopped fresh sage**

1 **tablespoon chopped fresh basil**

PER SERVING

calories	**134**
total fat	**4.1 g.**
saturated fat	**0.6 g.**
cholesterol	**0 mg.**
sodium	**207 mg.**
dietary fiber	**6.2 g.**

With a sharp knife, pierce the squash in 3 or 4 places. Microwave on high power, turning once, for 2 to 3 minutes, or just until the squash starts to soften under the skin. To test, press with your thumb. Carefully cut the squash into quarters. Scoop out and discard the seeds. Cut off and discard the peel. Cut the squash into 1″ chunks.

In a large saucepan over medium heat, warm the oil. Add the garlic and cook for 20 seconds, or until fragrant. Add the squash, tomatoes (with juice), and water.

Cover and reduce the heat to medium low. Cook for 25 to 30 minutes, or until the squash is tender but not mushy. Test for doneness by inserting the tip of a sharp knife in a piece of squash. Add more water if necessary to keep the squash from sticking. With the back of a large spoon, break the tomatoes into smaller pieces.

Rinse the kale and strip the leaves from the coarse stems. Coarsely chop the leaves and add to the saucepan. Add the sage and basil. Cook for 3 to 4 minutes, or until the kale softens.

Makes 4 main-dish servings

Cook's Note: Serve over hot cooked brown rice or quinoa.

Carpal Tunnel Syndrome
More Flex with Flax

Just as highways go through tunnels in order to get around (or under) obstacles, some structures in your body, such as nerves and ligaments, also use tunnels to get where they're going. One of the busiest tunnels is the carpal tunnel, which allows a nerve, blood vessels, and ligaments to pass through the wrist and into the fingers.

There's usually a lot of room inside the carpal tunnel. But when you use your hands and wrists a lot while typing, sewing, or doing other repetitive motions, tissues inside the tunnel may become inflamed and swollen, causing them to press against the nerve. This can cause pain in the wrist as well as tingling or numbness in the fingers, says James L. Napier Jr., M.D., assistant clinical professor of neurology at Case Western Reserve University School of Medicine in Cleveland. Doctors call this condition carpal tunnel syndrome.

One of the best remedies for carpal tunnel syndrome is simply to give your wrists a rest. In addition, there's some evidence that eating flaxseed may help reduce inflammation in the body, including in the wrists, says Jack Carter, Ph.D., professor emeritus of plant science at North Dakota State University in Fargo and president of the Flax Institute.

Flaxseed contains a compound called alpha-linolenic acid, which has been shown to reduce levels of prostaglandins, chemicals in the body that contribute to inflammation, says Dr. Carter. It also contains other compounds called lignans, which have antioxidant properties that can block the effects of harmful oxygen molecules called free radicals. This is important because free radicals are produced in large amounts whenever there's inflammation, and unless they're stopped, they make the inflammation even worse.

So far, researchers haven't put flaxseed to the test against carpal tunnel syndrome, so there's no way to know for sure how much you might need to get the benefits, says Dr. Carter. Some evidence suggests, however, that getting 25 to 30 grams (about 3 tablespoons) of ground flaxseed or 1 to 3 tablespoons of flaxseed oil might be enough to help ease the symptoms.

Since the body can't digest whole flaxseed, be sure to buy flaxseed that's been ground, or grind it yourself. (Look for it at health food stores.) You can add the ground seed to hot cereals or mix it into flour when you bake.

A Weighty Problem

While you're thinking about ways to get more flaxseed into your diet, you should probably also be thinking about how to get extra calories out. There's scientific evidence that people who are overweight are more likely to get carpal tunnel syndrome than those who are lean, says Peter A. Nathan, M.D., hand surgeon and carpal tunnel researcher at the Portland Hand Surgery and Rehabilitation Center in Oregon. In fact, research by Dr. Nathan suggests that people who are overweight have greater risks of getting carpal tunnel syndrome than typists, cashiers, or other folks whose use their hands and wrists a lot on the job.

"Heavy people have a tendency to accumulate more fluid in the soft tissues, including in the wrist," Dr. Nathan explains. As fluids accumulate, they may begin putting pressure on the nerve inside the carpal tunnel, while also reducing the amount of oxygen it receives.

Losing weight isn't necessarily a "cure" for carpal tunnel syndrome, Dr. Nathan adds. But if you are overweight and having problems, losing even a few pounds might take some pressure off this vulnerable nerve.

Too Much of a Good Thing

Since the 1970s, some doctors have tried to treat carpal tunnel syndrome with large doses of vitamin B_6, a nutrient that the body uses to form myelin, the fatty tissue that coats nerve fibers. The problem is that the amounts of vitamin B_6 that are frequently recommended—usually between 150 and 300 milligrams, which is 70 to 150 times the Daily Value (DV)—may be dangerous. "Such hefty doses of vitamin B_6 may actually cause nerve problems," says Alfred Franzblau, M.D., associate professor of occupational medicine in the department of environmental and industrial health sciences at the University of Michigan in Ann Arbor.

There's little evidence that extra vitamin B_6 is helpful for carpal tunnel pain. Dr. Franzblau studied 125 employees of two auto parts factories, 71 of whom had symptoms of carpal tunnel syndrome. He found no evidence linking low levels of vitamin B_6 with this condition.

Even though supplements don't appear to be the answer, it's certainly important for nerve health to get enough of this nutrient in your diet. A serving of skinless chicken breast, an excellent source, has 0.5 milligram, 26 percent of the DV, and a serving of pork tenderloin has 0.4 milligram, 18 percent of the DV. Orange roughy is a good source, with a 3-ounce serving containing 0.3 milligram, 15 percent of the DV.

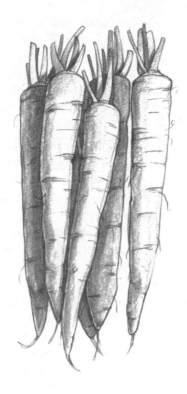

CARROTS
GOOD FOR THE EYES—AND MORE

HEALING POWER
CAN HELP:
Improve night vision

Reduce the risk
of cancer and heart disease

As kids, we all heard how good carrots are for our eyes. But nowadays, researchers are seeing carrots in a whole new light.

The healing potential of carrots goes far beyond their ability to help our vision. They contain a variety of compounds that may help prevent certain cancers, lower cholesterol, and prevent heart attacks.

CAROTENE'S NAMESAKE

The same substance that gives carrots their brash orange color is also responsible for providing many of their health benefits. Carrots are rich in beta-carotene, an antioxidant compound that fights free radicals, the unstable molecules in the body that contribute to conditions ranging from heart disease and cancer to macular degeneration, the leading cause of vision loss in older adults.

Research suggests that the more antioxidants we get in our diets, the less likely we are to die of cancer. In a study of 1,556 middle-age men, researchers from the University of Texas School of Public Health in Houston and Rush–Presbyterian–St. Luke's Medical Center and Northwestern University Medical School, both in Chicago, found that those with the highest levels of beta-carotene and vitamin C in their diets had a 37 percent lower risk of death from cancer than the men with the lowest levels.

Even when vitamin C isn't added to the mix, beta-carotene has powerful effects. Large population studies have shown that having low levels of beta-carotene leaves people more open to developing certain cancers, especially those of the lungs and stomach.

What's good for your body's cells is also very good for your heart. Evidence shows that eating large amounts of carrots and other fruits and vegetables rich in beta-carotene and related compounds may reduce the risk of heart disease. "A half-cup serving of cooked carrots contains 12 milligrams of beta-carotene, about twice the amount you need to get the benefits," says Paul Lachance, Ph.D., professor of nutrition and chairman of the department of food science at Rutgers University in New Brunswick, New Jersey.

It's not only beta-carotene that gives carrots their protective edge. They contain another antioxidant, alpha-carotene, that also appears to help fight cancer. In one study, researchers at the National Cancer Institute found that lung cancer occurred more often in men with low intakes of alpha-carotene than in men who got more.

BETTER VISION

The beta-carotene in carrots does double duty. It converts to vitamin A in the body and helps improve vision. This eye appeal is so well-known that researchers in World War II cultivated carrots that were high in beta-carotene to help pilots see better at night.

Vitamin A helps vision by forming a purple pigment that the eye needs in order to be able to see in dim light. This pigment, called rhodopsin, is located in the light-sensitive area of the retina. The more vitamin A you get, the more rhodopsin your body is able to produce. Conversely, people with low levels of vitamin A may suffer from night blindness, which can make it difficult to drive after dark or to find your seat in a dark theater.

FOOD ALERT
THE COLOR OF INDULGENCE

Orange and yellow are attractive colors for autumn leaves, but not at all pleasing when it's your own skin that's making the change.

People who enjoy their carrots a bit too much may experience a colorful condition called carotenosis, in which the skin turns a faint orange hue. Doctors tell stories of frantic parents rushing to the hospital because they think their children are jaundiced, when in fact they just ate a lot of baby-food carrots.

"Children are particularly prone to it because parents will give them pureed carrots or squash or sweet potatoes, usually in a number of servings," says John Erdman, Ph.D., director of the division of nutritional sciences at the University of Illinois in Urbana.

Carotenosis is harmless, Dr. Erdman says. It's also easy to remedy. Stop eating carrots, and within a day or two your skin color should return to normal.

Getting the Most

Add a little fat. Beta-carotene needs a small amount of fat to make the trip through your intestinal wall and into your body, says John Erdman, Ph.D., director of the division of nutritional sciences at the University of Illinois in Urbana. So the next time you're serving carrot sticks, you may want to accompany them with a small amount of a dip such as ranch dressing.

Eat them cooked. While many foods are more nutritious raw than cooked, carrots benefit from a little cooking. The reason is that carrots have a lot of dietary fiber—over 2 grams in one carrot—which traps the beta-carotene, says Dr. Erdman. Cooking carrots helps free beta-carotene from the fiber cells, making it easier for your body to absorb.

Save the nutrients. One problem with cooking carrots is that some of the nutrients escape into the cooking water, says Carol Boushey, R.D., Ph.D., assistant professor of food and nutrition at Southern Illinois University in Carbondale. To get nutrients into your body instead of pouring them down the sink, try reusing the cooking water—in a sauce, for example, or for moistening mashed potatoes.

Enjoy some juice. Another way to release more of the beta-carotene from carrots is to make a carrot cocktail. Processing carrots in a blender breaks apart the fibers, allowing the beta-carotene to get out, says Dr. Erdman.

Trim them well. When you buy carrots with the greenery still on them, it's important to trim it off before storing them. Otherwise, those pretty, leafy tops will act like nutrient vampires, sucking out the vitamins and moisture before you eat the carrots.

Carrot Slaw with Lime Dressing

4   large carrots

6   tablespoons nonfat plain yogurt

1½   tablespoons fresh lime juice

1½   tablespoons honey

⅛   teaspoon salt

Per serving

calories   **77**
total fat   **0.2 g.**
saturated fat   **0 g.**
cholesterol   **0 mg.**
sodium   **116 mg.**
dietary fiber   **2.4 g.**

Shred the carrots and place them in a medium bowl.

In a small bowl, whisk together the yogurt, lime juice, honey, and salt. Pour over the carrots and toss to coat.

Makes 4 servings

Cinnamon Carrot Coins

3   cups thinly sliced carrots

6   tablespoons fresh orange juice

1½   teaspoons unsalted butter

¾   teaspoon ground cinnamon

Ground black pepper

Per serving

calories   **75**
total fat   **1.7 g.**
saturated fat   **1 g.**
cholesterol   **4 mg.**
sodium   **78 mg.**
dietary fiber   **3.2 g.**

In a medium saucepan, combine the carrots and orange juice. Cover and cook over medium-low heat, stirring once or twice, for 6 to 8 minutes, or until the carrots are crisp-tender.

Add the butter and cinnamon. Cook for 1 minute, stirring to coat. Season to taste with the pepper.

Makes 4 servings

CATARACTS
SET YOUR SIGHT ON ANTIOXIDANTS

It seems as if, with every year that goes by, we have to hold the newspaper a little farther away to read the headlines. Traffic signs get harder to see, and as for reading the menu in a dim restaurant, well, forget it.

It's natural for the eyes to undergo slight changes over time. But for people with cataracts—proteins that accumulate inside the lenses of the eyes—the loss of vision can be profound. Wearing sunglasses and not smoking may reduce the risk of cataracts, but an even better strategy is to eat more fruits and vegetables, says Allen Taylor, Ph.D., director of the Laboratory for Nutrition and Vision Research at the Jean Mayer USDA Human Nutrition Research Center on Aging at Tufts University in Boston. These foods contain a variety of protective compounds that can stop damage to the eyes before cataracts have a chance to form.

The eyes are constantly being bombarded by free radicals, harmful oxygen molecules that are missing electrons and spend their lives looking for replacements. They grab extra electrons wherever they can, damaging healthy cells every time they strike. One way to help stop this damage is by filling your body with antioxidants like beta-carotene and vitamins C and E. Each of these compounds blocks the effects of free radicals, says Dr. Taylor.

SEEING COLORS

Popeye used spinach to build strong muscles, but it works just as well for strengthening the eyes. In fact, studies show that spinach might be one of your best defenses against cataracts.

In a 12-year study of more than 50,000 nurses, Harvard researchers found that those who got the most carotenoids, which are natural plant pigments such as beta-carotene, in their diets were 39 percent less likely to develop serious cataracts than women who got the least. And when the researchers looked at specific foods that contained carotenoids, they found that spinach appeared to be the most protective.

Spinach (along with kale, broccoli, and other dark green, leafy vegetables) contains more than just beta-carotene. It also contains two other carotenoids, lutein and zeaxanthin, which concentrate in the fluids of the eyes. This means that you're getting the most protection right where you need it most.

Here's another reason to eat more fruits and vegetables. They often contain large amounts of vitamin C, which appears to be a key player in keeping the eyes clear. A number of large studies have found that people who get the most vitamin C in their diets are much less likely to get cataracts than those getting the least.

Even though the Daily Value (DV) for vitamin C is 60 milligrams, Dr. Taylor recommends boosting that amount to 250 milligrams for maximum eye protection. It's easy to get that much vitamin C in your diet, he adds. A half-cup of broccoli, for example, has about 30 milligrams of vitamin C, and a large glass of fresh-squeezed orange juice has about 90 milligrams. You can also get lots of vitamin C from citrus fruits, brussels sprouts, green and red peppers, tomatoes, and melons.

OILING UP YOUR EYES

Vitamin E is yet another antioxidant that spends much of its life swimming in the lenses of your eyes. Here's the payoff. In a study of over 15,000 male physicians, researchers at Harvard University found that those whose eyes contained the most vitamin E were less likely to develop cataracts than those who had smaller amounts.

The one problem with vitamin E is that it's hard to get the necessary amounts without taking supplements. This is because vitamin E is found mainly in high-fat foods, such as corn, cottonseed, and peanut oils. But it is possible to get vitamin E without the fat by eating more wheat germ. A quarter-cup of wheat germ has more than 7 international units of vitamin E, about 27 percent of the DV. Almonds, mangoes, and whole-grain cereals are also good sources of vitamin E.

MAKING THE MOST OF MILK

You wouldn't think to toast your eyes with a glass of Bessie's best, but milk, along with chicken and yogurt, provides some of the best eye protection that you can find.

All of these foods contain large amounts of riboflavin, a B vitamin that appears to help prevent cataracts from forming. In a study of more than 1,000 people, researchers at State University of New York at Stony Brook found that those getting the most riboflavin were much less likely to have cataracts than those getting smaller amounts.

The connection, once again, appears to be antioxidants. The body uses riboflavin to manufacture glutathione, a powerful compound that battles free radicals. When you don't get enough riboflavin, glutathione levels fall, and that gives free radicals more time to damage the eyes.

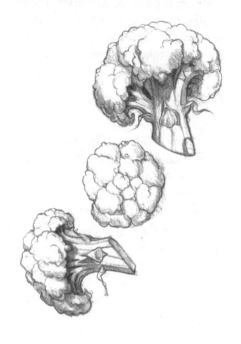

CAULIFLOWER
A White Knight against Cancer

Healing Power
Can help:
Inhibit tumor growth

Boost the immune system

Mark Twain once called cauliflower "a cabbage with a college education"—a bit more refined, perhaps, but essentially the same plain-Jane vegetable.

What Twain didn't know is just how valuable cauliflower is in our quest for good health. (If he had, Huckleberry Finn and Jim might have spent their days eating raw cauliflower instead of greasy catfish fillets.) Like other members of the cruciferous family, cauliflower is loaded with nutrients that seem to wage war against a host of diseases, including cancer. It's also an excellent source of vitamins and minerals that are essential for keeping the immune system strong.

Formidable Florets

Although cauliflower's darker-hued brother, broccoli, has gotten most of the attention for its healing potential, cauliflower is also generously endowed with cancer-preventing powers, says Jon Michnovicz, M.D., Ph.D., president of the Foundation for Preventive Oncology and the Institute for Hormone Research, both in New York City. In fact, cauliflower is one of the most powerful healing foods you can buy.

Researchers have found two potent munitions in cauliflower's cancer-fighting arsenal: the phytonutrients sulforaphane and indole-3-carbinol, or I3C.

Michelangelo, Leonardo da Vinci, and Henry VIII all had one thing in common. They should have stayed away from cauliflower.

If you have gout, like they did, you should, too.

Cauliflower contains amino acids called purines that break down into uric acid in the body. The uric acid crystals can trigger a painful case of gout—a form of arthritis that occurs when the sharp-edged crystals jab into the joints, causing pain and swelling.

If you have gout and can't eat cauliflower, you can still get the same cancer-fighting benefits from its cruciferous siblings like broccoli, cabbage, and brussels sprouts, which contain lower concentrations of purines.

These compounds, which are found in all cruciferous vegetables, may be the reason that studies consistently show that folks who make a habit of crunching crucifers are less likely to get cancer.

In one study, scientists at Johns Hopkins University in Baltimore exposed 145 laboratory animals to high doses of an extremely powerful cancer-causing agent. Of those, 120 were given high levels of protective sulforaphane. Fifty days later, 68 percent of the unprotected animals had breast tumors, compared with only 26 percent of those that received the sulforaphane.

Sulforaphane works by stepping up the production of enzymes in your body that sweep toxins out the door before they can damage your body's cells, making them cancerous, explains Dr. Michnovicz.

Cauliflower's other tumor-squelching compound, I3C, works as an anti-estrogen, explains Dr. Michnovicz. In other words, it reduces levels of harmful estrogens that can foster tumor growth in hormone-sensitive cells, like those in the breasts and prostate gland.

"That's why, although studies show that people who eat cruciferous vegetables are protected from all kinds of cancers, these foods are probably most useful for fighting cancers of the colon, breast, and prostate," says Dr. Michnovicz.

IMMUNE POWER

Cauliflower does more than protect against cancer. It's also packed with vitamin C and folate, two nutrients that are well-known for keeping your immune system in peak condition.

Just three uncooked florets of this crisp crucifer supply 67 percent of the Daily Value (DV) for vitamin C—more than the amount in a tangerine or a white grapefruit. By upping your level of vitamin C, along with other antioxi-

A Crucifer Combo

Maybe you don't like the cabbage-y flavor of cauliflower. Or the way those stringy broccoli florets get stuck between your teeth. Is there a way to combine the benefits of crucifers with a taste and texture you enjoy?

Look for that nitro-green vegetable in the produce section—the one that looks like cauliflower on Saint Patrick's Day: broccoflower.

A California-born hybrid that combines the best of broccoli and cauliflower, broccoflower is sweeter, milder, and easier to chew than either of its parents. Plus it has more nutrients: a half-cup serving has as much as 125 percent of the Daily Value for vitamin C. It's also rich in tumor-squelching phytonutrients like sulforaphane and indoles, experts say.

dant vitamins like vitamin E and beta-carotene, you can keep your immune system strong while staving off a host of conditions, among them heart disease, cancer, and cataracts.

Cauliflower also contains folate, which is important because too little folate is perhaps the country's most common nutritional deficiency. Three uncooked florets of cauliflower provide 9 percent of the DV for folate.

Since folate can help blood work more efficiently, it's often recommended for preventing anemia. In addition, research has shown that folate is essential for normal tissue growth. Not getting enough folate over the long term could set the stage for diseases like cancer and heart disease down the road, say researchers.

Folate is particularly important for women of childbearing age because it plays an important role in preventing birth defects of the brain and spinal column.

Getting the Most

Look for a clear complexion. Unless you're lucky enough to live near a farmer's market, it's not always easy to find cauliflower that's truly at its nutritional prime. But wherever you shop, always avoid cauliflower if it has brown spots on its ivory (or purple) florets. That means that it's already past its nutritional peak.

Enjoy it raw. To keep cauliflower's cancer-fighting indoles intact, keep it out of the heat, advises Dr. Michnovicz. Your best bet is either eating it raw or cooking it quickly in a steamer, wok, or microwave, he says. Boiling is the worst way to cook this crucifer. Submerging cauliflower in the hot, roily water will cause it to lose about half of its valuable indoles, he says.

CAULIFLOWER MEDITERRANEAN-STYLE

4 cups cauliflower florets

5 black olives, pitted and minced

1 tablespoon minced fresh parsley

1 teaspoon red-wine vinegar

1/8 teaspoon crushed red-pepper flakes

In a medium saucepan, combine the cauliflower and 1/4 cup water. Cover and cook over medium heat for 4 to 5 minutes, or until the cauliflower just starts to soften. Stir in the olives, parsley, vinegar, and red-pepper flakes. Cook for 1 minute, or until heated through.

Makes 4 servings

PER SERVING
calories	**42**
total fat	**1.5 g.**
saturated fat	**0.1 g.**
cholesterol	**0 mg.**
sodium	**99 mg.**
dietary fiber	**2.2 g.**

CAULIFLOWER WITH SPICY PEANUT DIP

1/2 cup crumbled firm regular tofu

1 1/2 tablespoons reduced-fat peanut butter, at room temperature

1 tablespoon honey

1 tablespoon rice vinegar or white-wine vinegar

1 teaspoon grated fresh ginger

1 clove garlic, minced

1/8 teaspoon ground red pepper

4 cups cauliflower florets

In a blender or food processor, combine the tofu, peanut butter, honey, vinegar, ginger, garlic, and pepper. Transfer to a small bowl. Serve immediately with the cauliflower or cover and refrigerate for several hours.

Makes 8 servings

PER SERVING
calories	**48**
total fat	**2 g.**
saturated fat	**0.4 g.**
cholesterol	**0 mg.**
sodium	**30 mg.**
dietary fiber	**1.4 g.**

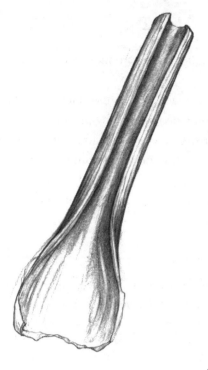

CELERY
STALKS OF PROTECTION

HEALING POWER
CAN HELP:
Reduce high blood pressure

Lower the risk of cancer

The ancient Romans, notorious party animals that they were, wore wreaths of celery to protect them from hangovers, which may explain the practice of putting celery sticks in Bloody Marys.

While there's no evidence that donning a celery chapeau will save you from the consequences of having one too many, celery does have other healing properties. This member of the parsley family contains compounds that may help lower blood pressure and perhaps help prevent cancer. Celery is also a good source of insoluble fiber as well as a number of essential nutrients, including potassium, vitamin C, and calcium.

CHOMP DOWN ON BLOOD PRESSURE

Celery has been used for centuries in Asia as a folk remedy for high blood pressure. In the United States, it took one man with high blood pressure and persistence to persuade researchers at the University of Chicago Medical Center to put this remedy to the scientific test.

The story began when a man named Mr. Le was diagnosed with mild high blood pressure. Rather than cutting back on salt as his doctor advised, he began eating a quarter-pound (about four stalks) of celery per day. Within a week his blood pressure had dropped from 158/96 to 118/82.

William J. Elliott, M.D., Ph.D., who was then assistant professor of medicine and pharmacological and physiological science at the University of Chicago, decided to put celery to the test. Researchers injected test animals with a small amount of 3-n-butyl phthalide, a chemical compound that is found in celery. Within a week, the animals' blood pressures dropped an average of 12 to 14 percent.

"Phthalide was found to relax the muscles of the arteries that regulate blood pressure, allowing the vessels to dilate," says Dr. Elliott. In addition, the chemical reduced the amount of "stress hormones," called catecholamines, in the blood. This may be helpful because stress hormones typically raise blood pressure by causing blood vessels to constrict.

If you have high blood pressure and would like to give celery a try, try this strategy recommended by Asian folk practitioners. Eat four to five stalks every day for a week, then stop for three weeks. Then start over and eat celery for another week.

But don't overdo it and start eating celery by the pound, Dr. Elliott warns. Celery does contain sodium—one stalk contains 35 milligrams—and for some people this can cause blood pressure to go up rather than down. "Eating a ton of celery can be dangerous if you have salt-sensitive hypertension," he warns.

BLOCKING CANCER CELLS

Who'd have thought that crunching celery might help prevent cancer? Celery contains a number of compounds that researchers believe may help prevent cancer cells from spreading.

For starters, celery contains compounds called acetylenics. "Acetylenics have been shown to stop the growth of tumor cells," says Robert Rosen, Ph.D., associate director of the Center for Advanced Food Technology at Cook College, Rutgers University, in New Brunswick, New Jersey.

In addition, celery contains compounds called phenolic acids, which block the action of hormonelike substances called prostaglandins. Some prostaglandins are thought to encourage the growth of tumor cells, says Dr. Rosen.

Getting the Most

Leave on the leaves. While celery stalks are certainly a healthful snack, it's the leaves that contain the most potassium, vitamin C, and calcium.

Eat it the way you like it. While many foods lose nutrients during cooking, most of the compounds in celery hold up well during cooking. Eating a cup of celery, raw or cooked, provides about 9 milligrams of vitamin C, 15 percent of the Daily Value (DV); 426 milligrams of potassium, 12 percent of the DV; and 60 milligrams of calcium, 6 percent of the DV.

Sprinkle on the seeds. Celery seeds, which are found in the spice section of supermarkets, provide a nutritional bonus. One tablespoon of seeds, which can be added to soups, stews, or casseroles, contains 3 milligrams of iron, 17 percent of the DV.

WARM CELERY AND RED PEPPER SALAD

5   large stalks celery
1   teaspoon olive oil
¼   cup thinly sliced roasted sweet red peppers
1   tablespoon white-wine vinegar
2   teaspoons sugar
¼   teaspoon celery seeds

PER SERVING
calories **33**
total fat **1.3 g.**
saturated fat **0.2 g.**
cholesterol **0 mg.**
sodium **107 mg.**
dietary fiber **0.9 g.**

Pull the leaves off the celery stalks. Chop the leaves and set aside. Cut the stalks into ⅛" diagonal slices.

Warm the oil in a large no-stick skillet over medium heat. Add the celery and cook, tossing frequently, for 1 to 2 minutes, or until crisp-tender. Add the peppers and toss to combine.

Stir in the vinegar, sugar, and celery seeds. Cook for 10 seconds, or until the sugar dissolves. Remove from the heat and stir in the reserved leaves.

Makes 4 servings

CELIAC DISEASE
LIVING WITHOUT THE LOAF

It's hard to resist the aroma and taste of fresh-from-the-oven bread. But for people with celiac disease, giving into temptation means intestinal misery.

Celiac disease, also known as celiac sprue, is caused by a sensitivity to gluten, a protein found in wheat, barley, oats, and rye. In people with celiac disease, even small amounts of gluten can damage millions of villi, the fingerlike projections lining the small intestine that contain many digestive enzymes and that absorb nutrients and fluids. Once the villi are damaged, they're less able to absorb nutrients from food. That's why doctors say that people with celiac disease are "starving in the midst of plenty."

Taking control of celiac disease is a two-step process. The first step, of course, is to avoid the thing that's making you sick. "Eliminate gluten from your diet and you get better," says Frederick F. Paustian, M.D., a gastroenterologist at the University of Nebraska Medical Center and a member of the Celiac Sprue Association medical advisory board, both in Omaha.

The second step is to work with your doctor to correct any nutritional deficiencies you may already have. For example, because people with active celiac disease have difficulty absorbing fats, they may be deficient in fat-soluble vitamins such as vitamins A, D, E, and K. They may have low levels of iron and calcium as well, says Dr. Paustian.

Without treatment, celiac disease can be extremely serious. But once you know you have it, it's easy to treat. "People with celiac disease can choose to be well by making the right dietary choices," says Leon Rottmann, Ph.D., executive director of the Celiac Sprue Association.

There are many whole grains and flours, for example, that don't contain gluten. Gluten-free flours include corn flour, potato flour, rice flour, soy flour, tapioca, arrowroot, and milo. You can even find pea, bean, and lentil flours, none of which contain gluten, at health food stores. Baking with gluten-free flours is tricky because they don't "handle" like regular flours. It takes some trial and error to learn tricks for handling each type of flour. Here are some tips.

- Corn flour can be blended with other gluten-free flours and used to make cornbread.
- Potato flour is usually used as a thickening agent in casseroles and soups, while its relative, potato starch flour, makes a great sponge cake.

HIDDEN DANGERS

For people with celiac disease, staying away from bread and the gluten it contains is an obvious solution. But there are many sources of gluten that aren't so obvious.

For instance, there may be a wheat-derived thickening agent in ice cream that is a source of gluten, says Frederick F. Paustian, M.D., a gastroenterologist at the University of Nebraska Medical Center and a member of the Celiac Sprue Association medical advisory board, both in Omaha.

Gluten is found in many other processed foods as well, among them yogurt with fruit, ketchup, lunch meats, cheese spreads, salad dressings, and canned soups. Some food labels may list gluten as an ingredient. Others refer to it by other names. Here's what you need to watch out for.

- Distilled white vinegar
- Hydrolyzed vegetable protein
- Malt or malt flavoring
- Modified starch or modified food starch
- Monoglycerides and diglycerides
- Products that list "natural" or "artificial" flavorings
- Red or yellow food dyes
- Vegetable gum or vegetable protein

- Rice flour, with its rather bland flavor, is often mixed with other gluten-free flours, especially potato starch flour.
- Pea, bean, and lentil flours can be used as direct substitutes for wheat flour, as long as egg whites and cottage cheese are added as softeners. They're also good for thickening gravies, soups, and sauces.

People with celiac disease are often unable to drink milk or eat cheese because they lack the enzyme (lactase) that is needed to digest a sugar (lactose) found in dairy foods. Yogurt, however, is a good alternative. "Yogurt contains a type of bacteria that breaks down the lactose," explains Dr. Paustian. "So people with celiac disease can get the benefit of the milk protein as well as the calcium present in yogurt."

An interesting point is that when people with celiac disease have maintained gluten-free diets, they may find that they're able to digest dairy foods without having problems, due to the regrowth of villi in the small intestine.

People with celiac disease are often deficient in calcium and magnesium, says Dr. Paustian. So it's important to eat plenty of magnesium-rich foods, like potatoes, avocados, and beans, along with calcium-rich foods such as yogurt.

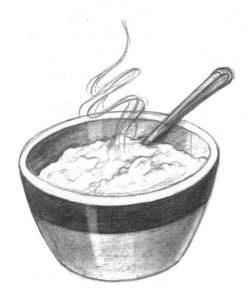

CEREAL
A HEALTHY WAY
TO START THE DAY

HEALING POWER

CAN HELP:
Prevent cancer
and heart disease

Keep digestion regular

Protect against birth
defects

The cereal aisle in the supermarket can seem more like a playground than a place to buy real food. Many of the colorful boxes are festooned with cartoon characters, puzzles, and promises of prizes inside. And the cereal inside those boxes is often no more substantial. Many popular cereals are essentially sugary snacks, containing as much sweetness per serving as an equal amount of your favorite dessert.

But if you read the labels and push on past the worst offenders, you'll find that breakfast cereals, both hot and cold, can be very healthful foods. Many cereals are extraordinarily high in dietary fiber, and almost all are fortified with nutrients such as folic acid. "Cereals are the ideal breakfast," says Pat Harper, R.D., a nutrition consultant in the Pittsburgh area. "They're convenient, quick, and wonderfully nutritious."

A SPOONFUL OF NUTRITION

One of the best things about having a bowl of cereal in the morning is that every spoonful is like a mini-multivitamin. Even the marshmallow-filled, cocoa-covered concoctions for children, although they're too sugary to be truly healthful, are often fortified with a host of essential vitamins and minerals that you might not get enough of any other way. "We'd be in big trouble without fortified and enriched foods like breakfast cereals," says Paul Lachance, Ph.D., professor of nutrition and chairman of the department of food science at Rutgers University in New Brunswick, New Jersey. "That's where we get up to 25 percent of many important nutrients. Their contribution to our health is very real."

Breakfast cereals are so healthful, in fact, that doctors often recommend them for older people, who may not be eating as well as they used to and are missing out on essential vitamins and minerals, says William Regelson, M.D., professor of medicine at Virginia Commonwealth University, Medical College of Virginia School of Medicine in Richmond.

Cereals are particularly important when it comes to getting enough B vitamins, like thiamin, niacin, riboflavin, vitamin B_6, and folate . The B vitamins, which are essential for turning food into energy and keeping the blood and nervous system healthy, are often difficult to get from foods alone. This is particularly true of folate, which may help prevent birth defects. Cereals that are fortified with folic acid (the supplement form of folate), which typically contain 25 percent of the Daily Value (DV), make it easier to get enough of this essential nutrient, Harper says.

To get the most B vitamins, however, it's important to spoon up all the milk when the cereal is gone. When cereals are fortified, the vitamins are literally sprayed on the cereal, and some will end up in the milk in the bottom of the bowl.

FLAKES OF FIBER

Doctors agree that dietary fiber is the key to a healthful diet, not only because it keeps digestion regular but also because it's been shown to lower cholesterol. In excess amounts, cholesterol can stick to artery walls, narrowing blood vessels and increasing the risk of heart disease.

Eating cereal is a good way to get enough of the rough stuff. A serving of Wheaties or Cheerios, for example, has 3 grams of fiber. Oat bran is even better. One serving provides 6 grams of fiber, 24 percent of the DV. Other first-rate fiber contenders include Fiber One, with 13 grams per serving, and Uncle Sam cereal, with 10 grams per serving.

In one study, people who got just 3 grams of soluble fiber from oat bran were able to reduce their cholesterol levels five to six points.

The same cereal that's good for your heart can also lower your risk of colon cancer. This is because the fiber in cereal causes stool to move through the intestine more quickly. The faster stool moves, the less time there is for harmful substances to irritate the colon wall, says Beth Kunkel, R.D., Ph.D., professor of food and nutrition at Clemson University in South Carolina.

"The 25 to 30 grams of fiber that is recommended is always a little tough

IN THE KITCHEN

The problem with starting the day with hot cereals like oatmeal, Cream of Wheat, and Cream of Rice is that in their plain, unadulterated state, they can leave your taste buds fast asleep. To get the benefits of hot cereals along with some zing, here are some tips you may want to try.

- Substituting orange or apple juice for the cooking water adds a hint of fruity sweetness to hot cereals, along with a nutritional boost.

- You can also use skim milk instead of water when cooking hot cereals. Milk adds a touch of creaminess, along with a healthful shot of calcium. Cooking a half-cup of oatmeal in 1 cup of skim milk will deliver 320 milligrams of this important mineral.

- Adding fruit to hot cereals is an easy way to boost the flavor. With hard fruits like apples or pears, simply grate the fruit directly into the cooked cereal. Bananas, berries, and other soft fruits can also be dropped in after cooking. When using dried fruits like raisins, however, add them at the beginning of the cooking time so that they become plump and juicy.

to get in the diet," Harper adds. "By choosing high-fiber cereals more often, you'll have a better chance of getting the fiber you need."

THE BEST PICKS

Even though many breakfast cereals are high in fiber, others are only middling, and some contain negligible amounts. Here are a few tips to help you find the most fiber in each serving.

Follow the "rule of five." With so many high-quality cereals to choose from, there's simply no reason to settle for second best, Harper says. Cereals that have at least 5 grams of fiber per serving are good choices, so she recommends setting a 5-gram minimum.

Shop for variety. Different cereals contain different types of dietary fiber. To get the best fiber kick, it is a good idea to mix cereals, Harper says. Wheat and rice cereals, for example, are high in insoluble fiber, which is the best kind for preventing constipation and reducing the risk of colon cancer. Oatmeal, on the other hand, contains mainly soluble fiber, which is the cholesterol-lowering kind. Still other cereals, such as those that mix grains and fruit, contain both types of fiber, she adds.

Buy the bran. Hot cereals such as corn, wheat, or oat bran are excellent sources of fiber, Harper says. In fact, any cereal that contains the outer portions of grains will contain more fiber than its "lighter" counterparts. So when buying cereals, look for those that say "bran" or "whole grain" on the label.

Keep your guard up. Don't reach for a box just because it says "oats" or "wheat," advises Michael H. Davidson, M.D., president of the Chicago Center for Clinical Research. Manufacturers can put almost anything on (or in) a box of cereal. A cereal labeled "wheat," for instance, could have only a trace of the grain and almost no fiber, Dr. Davidson says. So before putting any cereal in your cart, read the label.

Mix and match. Even if you don't love the taste of many high-fiber cereals, you can make them a little more pleasing by mixing them half-and-half with cereals you do like. "You'll get the benefit of the fiber with the taste of your favorite cereal," Harper says.

Eat them anytime. Even though cereals are usually eaten at breakfast, there's no reason to limit yourself, Harper says. Because they're high in fiber, they'll help keep you satisfied, whether you're eating them for a quick lunch, a late dinner, or as an afternoon snack. Plus, most high-fiber cereals are low in fat, which is another bonus. In fact, many people keep a box of cereal at work and dip in throughout the day.

HEARTY CEREAL WITH APRICOTS

1 **cup skim milk**

½ **cup uncooked Ralston or Wheatena whole-wheat cereal**

¼ **teaspoon ground cinnamon**

⅛ **teaspoon salt**

1 **teaspoon packed light brown sugar (optional)**

¼ **cup chopped dried apricots**

PER SERVING

calories	**307**
total fat	**1.4 g.**
saturated fat	**0.4 g.**
cholesterol	**4 mg.**
sodium	**135 mg.**
dietary fiber	**9.3 g.**

In a 2-cup glass measuring cup, combine the milk, cereal, cinnamon, salt, brown sugar (if using), and about half the apricots. Stir to mix. Microwave on high power for 45 seconds to 1 minute, or just until the mixture starts to boil; stop and stir after 30 seconds. Let stand for 1 minute; stir.

Transfer to a cereal bowl and sprinkle with the remaining apricots.

Makes 1 serving

Cook's Note: You can also cook this cereal in a small saucepan on the stove. Bring the ingredients to a simmer over medium heat, then remove from the heat, cover, and let stand for 2 minutes. You can easily increase the recipe to make more servings.

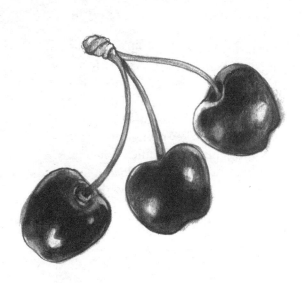

CHERRIES
PICK A LITTLE PREVENTION

HEALING POWER
CAN HELP:
Relieve gout

Prevent a variety
of cancers

Reduce the risk
of heart disease
and stroke

With their hard little pits and rich, shirt-staining colors, cherries take a bit more work to eat than many fruits. But research suggests that cherries, which contain a compound called perillyl alcohol, are worth the bother—and then some.

"Perillyl alcohol is about the best thing we've ever seen for curing mammary cancer in laboratory animals," says Michael Gould, Ph.D., professor of human oncology at the University of Wisconsin Medical School in Madison. In fact, it shows so much promise that it's being tried in cancer patients at the University of Wisconsin.

Perillyl alcohol belongs to a group of compounds called monoterpenes. Limonene, found in the peel of citrus fruits, is another member of this family. These compounds have been shown in studies to block the formation of a variety of cancers, including those of the breasts, lungs, stomach, liver, and skin. Expectations for perillyl alcohol are high, in part, because it is 5 to 10 times more potent than limonene, which itself has been proven to be very effective.

It's not yet known how much perillyl alcohol there is in cherries, adds Pamela Crowell, Ph.D., assistant professor of biology at Indiana University School of Medicine in Indianapolis. Even in small amounts, however, the compound probably has some beneficial effects. So cherries, when eaten as part of a well-rounded diet, can play a small but important role in helping the body ward off cancer.

In the Kitchen

Fresh cherries are at their ever-loving, mouth-watering best from May through July. To get the sweetest taste from the harvest, here are some tips you may want to try.

Check the stems. When buying cherries, make sure that the stems are green. Dark-colored stems are a tip-off that cherries have been sitting in the bin too long.

Buy in small quantities. Cherries are highly perishable. Even when properly stored in the refrigerator, they'll only keep for a few days. So plan on buying only what you're going to eat right away.

Store them dry. Washing cherries ahead of time can cause them to spoil in the refrigerator. So it's best to store them dry, then wash them as needed.

It's important, however, to wash them thoroughly. Cherries are often coated with a mixture of insecticides, antifungal oils, and moisture seals that producers use to keep them fresh.

Use up the extras. When you're tired of munching cherries, you may want to try a little juice. Simply wash, stem, pit, and crush the cherries. Heat them in a saucepan, then press the mixture through a strainer. Refrigerate several hours, then pour off the clear juice and add sugar to taste.

VITAMIN C AND MORE

There's more to cherries than exotic new compounds. They also contain a variety of healing compounds. For example, a half-cup of sour cherries has 5 milligrams of vitamin C, about 8 percent of the Daily Value (DV). They also provide vitamins A and E. Sweet cherries also contain these nutrients, but not as much of vitamins A and E as their mouth-puckering kin.

The vitamin E in cherries is of particular interest, since one study of post-menopausal women found that those who consumed the most vitamin E had the least risk of heart disease. And there was an interesting twist. The women who got their vitamin E naturally—solely from food—had less risk than women who were also taking vitamin E supplements.

The problem with vitamin E is that it's difficult to get the DV of 30 international units from food alone. In fact, the only foods with a lot of vitamin E are high-fat cooking oils and nuts, which you don't want a lot of. Cherries are one of the better food sources for vitamin E.

Finally, cherries contain a compound called quercetin. Like vitamin C and other antioxidants, quercetin helps block the damage caused by free radicals, unstable oxygen molecules in the body. Studies show that quercetin and similar-acting compounds may significantly reduce the risk of stroke and also cancer.

A Pitted Pleasure

The maraschino cherry is perhaps the only fruit that spends most of its life in a jar. Used to add a jot of color to fruit cocktails and a swirl of sweetness to Shirley Temples, maraschino cherries don't have much in common with their on-the-tree kin.

Made by steeping pitted cherries in a flavored sugar syrup, maraschino cherries have never gotten much respect, not only because of their sticky-sweet taste but also because their fire engine–red color originally came from harmful dyes.

Even though safer dyes are now being used, maraschino cherries, which were originally flavored with maraschino liqueur, aren't exactly a healthful food. They're essentially devoid of nutrients and fiber, and they're high in calories, with 60 calories in a 1-ounce serving—about 10 calories per cherry.

Of course, it's unlikely that you'd ever eat more than one or two maraschino cherries at a time, so they really won't do you any harm. Go ahead and enjoy them. Just be sure to lick the red from your lips when you're done.

Relief for Gout

Folklore is full of stories about people who relieved the agonizing pain of gout by eating cherries or drinking cherry juice daily. While the Arthritis Foundation says that there's no evidence to suggest that cherries really can ease the ache of gout, many gout sufferers swear by them.

A survey by *Prevention* magazine found that 67 percent of readers who tried cherries for gout had good results. And Steve Schumacher, a kinesiologist in Louisville, Kentucky, enthusiastically recommends them. He advises people with gout to quit eating red meats and organ meats and also to drink two to three glasses of cherry juice a day. He recommends using pure black-cherry juice diluted with an equal amount of water.

"Those who have followed this diet faithfully have all gotten results, some within 48 to 72 hours, and some within a week, depending on the severity," Schumacher says.

Getting the Most

Eat them raw. Because cooking destroys some of the vitamin C and other nutrients in cherries, it's best to eat them raw to reap their full nutritional bounty.

Prepare them for baking. While it's easy to eat sweet cherries raw, that's really not an option for the sour kinds. Still, they're high enough in a variety of nutrients that they'll keep some of their value even after baking.

CHERRY TOPPING

1 tablespoon cornstarch
¾ cup apple juice
2 tablespoons honey
½ teaspoon vanilla
3½ cups Bing cherries, stemmed and pitted
¼ teaspoon ground cinnamon
⅛ teaspoon ground cardamom (optional)

PER ½ CUP

calories	77
total fat	0.7 g.
saturated fat	0.2 g.
cholesterol	0 mg.
sodium	1 mg.
dietary fiber	1.1 g.

Place the cornstarch in a medium saucepan. Whisk in the apple juice to dissolve the cornstarch. Whisk in the honey and vanilla.

Add the cherries, cinnamon, and cardamom (if using). Cook over medium-low heat, stirring frequently, for 4 to 5 minutes, or until the sauce thickens and turns transparent. Remove from the heat. Serve warm.

Makes about 4 cups

Cook's Notes: Serve over pancakes, waffles, or nonfat frozen yogurt.

The sauce can be refrigerated in a covered container for up to 3 days. Reheat gently in the microwave or in a saucepan before serving.

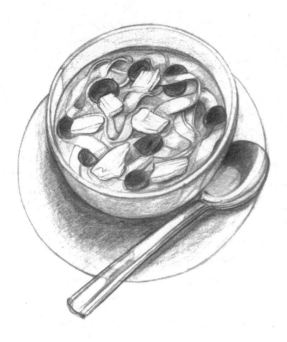

Chicken Soup

Food for Body and Soul

Healing Power

Can help:
Relieve nasal congestion

Soothe irritated airways

Put a chicken in a pot with water, onions, carrots, peppercorns, and a little salt. Cook until it falls apart. Strain. Discard fat. Feed the overdone chicken and vegetables to a hungry pet. Add a whole chili pepper to the broth, half a large garlic clove, and thin slices of lemon. Serve steaming hot. This is the cure for the common cold."

Grandma's traditional favorite? Not quite. This recipe was created by Pauline M. Jackson, M.D., a psychiatrist at Gunderson Lutheran Medical Center in La Crosse, Wisconsin, and a firm believer in the soothing powers of chicken soup. "It's hot, it tastes good, and it reminds you of Mom," she says.

You don't need a panel of experts to tell you that chicken soup is soothing when you're sick. But evidence suggests that it's more than a feel-good food. When you're honking and sniffling with a cold or other upper respiratory infection, says Dr. Jackson, virtually no remedy is more effective than chicken soup.

Breathing Easy

The classic chicken soup study was conducted in 1978 by three lung specialists at Mount Sinai Medical Center in Miami Beach, Florida. Intrigued by the healing mystique surrounding the savory brew, they had 15 people with colds sip either hot chicken soup, hot water, or cold water. Then they measured how quickly and easily mucus and air flowed through the patients' noses. The result was that chicken soup eased nasal congestion better than both hot water and cold water.

Chicken soup may relieve cold symptoms, speculated the researchers, because the heat "increases nasal mucous velocity." In other words, it makes your nose run, possibly reducing the amount of time that cold germs spend in your nose and helping you recover more quickly.

So why didn't the hot water work just as well at relieving colds as the chicken soup did? The soup's healing secret may lie in its savory aroma and taste, which "appear to possess an additional substance for increasing nasal mucous velocity," the researchers reported. What this substance might be, however, remains a mystery.

More recently, Stephen Rennard, M.D., professor in the department of internal medicine at the University of Nebraska Medical Center in Omaha, tested chicken soup that was prepared by his wife from her grandmother's recipe. He found that the soup reduced the action of neutrophils—white blood cells that are attracted to areas of inflammation and that may cause common cold symptoms like irritated airways and mucus production.

Researchers also suspect that part of the healing power of chicken soup lies in the bird itself. Chicken contains a natural amino acid called cysteine, which is chemically similar to a drug called acetylcysteine, says Irwin Ziment, M.D., professor of medicine at the University of California, Los Angeles. Doctors use acetylcysteine to treat people with bronchitis and other respiratory infections. "Acetylcysteine was originally derived from chicken feathers and chicken skin," notes Dr. Ziment.

IN THE KITCHEN

When a cold hits, so might a yearning for homemade chicken soup. But who wants to get out of a cozy sickbed to make it from scratch? You won't have to if you make and freeze a batch of chicken stock before a flu bug bites.

Making stock isn't difficult. Put some skinless chicken parts in a large pot, cover with cold water, add a carrot, onion, a garlic clove, and a bay leaf, and simmer for a few hours. Strain out the solids and set the stock aside to cool.

To reduce the fat in stock, first ladle it into shallow containers and let cool for up to 2 hours. Then refrigerate overnight. The fat will solidify into a thin sheet that can be peeled right off.

Frozen stock will keep for up to six months. For convenience, freeze it in ice-cube trays rather than large containers; the small, frozen cubes will defrost more quickly than large blocks.

Getting the Most

Sip it often. The therapeutic effects of chicken soup last about 30 minutes, according to the Miami Beach study. So it's a good idea to make a large batch and keep it handy for reheating so that you can sip a cup when symptoms flare up.

Opt for convenience. If you can coax a sympathetic spouse into whipping up a pot of homemade, aromatic soup, enjoy the pampering. But home-cooked broth really isn't mandatory, says Dr. Ziment. Canned chicken soup can also be helpful in breaking up congestion.

Heat it up. Adding hot spices to chicken soup—a clove of garlic, say, or a diced chili pepper or some fresh grated ginger—will speed up chicken soup's de-clogging power, says Dr. Ziment.

SPICY CHICKEN NOODLE SOUP

1   **package (9 ounces) fresh angel hair pasta**

9   **cups defatted homemade chicken broth**

6   **cloves garlic, coarsely chopped**

1   **piece fresh ginger (1½″ long), unpeeled, cut into 2 or 3 chunks**

3   **dried small hot red peppers**

8   **ounces skinless, boneless chicken breast, cut into bite-size pieces**

4   **scallions, finely chopped**

PER SERVING

calories	**198**
total fat	**3.7 g.**
saturated fat	**1.3 g.**
cholesterol	**28 mg.**
sodium	**274 mg.**
dietary fiber	**1.5 g.**

Place the pasta in a large heat-proof bowl. Pour enough boiling water over the pasta to cover it. Stir gently with a fork to break up the noodles. Set aside.

In a large saucepan, combine the broth, garlic, ginger, and peppers. Bring to a boil over high heat. Reduce the heat to low and simmer for 10 minutes. Add the chicken and cook for 5 minutes, or until the chicken is no longer pink in the center. Test by cutting one piece in half.

Drain the noodles and add to the saucepan. Cook, stirring with a fork, for 1 to 2 minutes, or until the noodles are tender and heated through.

Remove the ginger and peppers from the soup; discard. Ladle the soup into bowls, and sprinkle with the scallions.

Makes 6 servings

Cook's Note: If you don't have any homemade chicken broth, substitute 6 cups defatted reduced-sodium canned broth and 3 cups water.

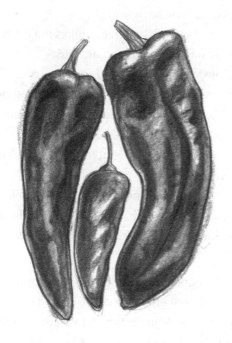

CHILI PEPPERS
RED-HOT HEALERS

HEALING POWER
CAN HELP:
Clear sinuses
and relieve congestion

Prevent ulcers

Reduce the risk
of heart disease
and stroke

According to an old saying, "Whatever doesn't kill you makes you stronger." This might be the perfect motto for the chili pepper. Not only can many people withstand the heat, they actually enjoy it. Chili pepper fans savor the heat at every opportunity, not just in traditional favorites like tacos and burritos but also in foods such as omelets, stews, and even salads.

More is involved than just a little culinary spice. These thermogenic morsels are prized around the globe for their healing power as well as their firepower. Hot chilies have long been used as natural remedies for coughs, colds, sinusitis, and bronchitis, says Irwin Ziment, M.D., professor of medicine at the University of California, Los Angeles. There's some evidence that they can help lower low-density lipoprotein (LDL) cholesterol, the type associated with stroke, high blood pressure, and heart disease. There's also some evidence that chilies can help prevent—of all things—stomach ulcers.

HEAT UP A COLD
Chili-lovers have long asserted that hot peppers, from serranos to jalapeños, are the ultimate decongestant, clearing a stuffy nose in the time it takes to gasp "Yow!" In fact, the fiery bite of hot chilies (or chili-based condiments like

Rub Away Pain

You love the fiery bite of chilies in your salsa. But on your skin?

You bet. When applied as a cream, capsaicin, the stuff that gives chilies their heat, has been shown to ease the discomfort of psoriasis, nerve pain, and arthritis.

Capsaicin creams are thought to work by depleting nerve cells and receptors of substance P, a chemical that transmits pain and itch sensations to the brain. When capsaicin cream is applied to the skin, the nerves release a flood of substance P. Over time, the nerves are unable to replenish their supply. The less "fuel" they have, the less pain you feel.

Incidentally, you can't use capsaicin cream for simple muscle aches. The pain has to stem from the nerves, not the muscles themselves.

Capsaicin cream is available over the counter. But make no mistake. This stuff is strong. So consult your doctor before using it, says Rup Tandan, M.D., a neurologist at the University of Vermont in Burlington. Once you have your doctor's okay, follow Dr. Tandan's tips.

- Try a milder concentration first. Zostrix has a concentration of 0.025 percent. Zostrix HP has three times the power, with a concentration of 0.075 percent.
- Apply the cream with a rubber glove or a rubber finger guard. "If you don't and you accidentally put your finger in your eye, it can be bad," says Dr. Tandan.
- Use a very small amount of cream. "If you can see it on your skin, you've used too much," says Dr. Tandan.
- Don't apply the cream within two hours of a hot bath or shower. "Heat increases the cream's effect and can cause even more pain," says Dr. Tandan.
- Don't give up. "Your skin may burn for a few days as it gets used to the cream," says Dr. Tandan. The pain will diminish quickly and, in most cases, the cream will begin working in about two weeks.

Tabasco sauce) can work as well as over-the-counter cold remedies, says Dr. Ziment. "Some of the foods used to fight respiratory diseases for centuries, including hot peppers, are very similar to the drugs we now use."

The stuff that makes hot peppers so nose-clearing good is capsaicin, a plant chemical that gives hot peppers their sting. Chemically, capsaicin is similar to a drug called guaifenesin, which is used in many over-the-counter and prescription cold remedies such as Robitussin, says Dr. Ziment.

Of course, eating a chili pepper has more of an immediate impact than taking a spoonful of medicine. When hot pepper meets tongue, the brain is slammed with an onslaught of nerve messages. The brain responds to this "Ow!" message by stimulating secretion-producing glands that line the airways. The result is a flood of fluids that makes your eyes water, your nose run, and the mucus in your lungs loosen, says Dr. Ziment. In other words, chili peppers are a natural decongestant and expectorant.

It doesn't take a lot of pepper to get the healing benefits. Adding 10 drops of hot-pepper sauce to a bowl of chicken soup can be very effective, says Paul Bosland, Ph.D., professor in the department of horticulture at New Mexico State University in Las Cruces and founder of the Chile Pepper Institute at the university. "Most of us here in New Mexico do this when we're sick," he says. "We all feel better after we've had a little bit of chili pepper."

Dr. Ziment recommends treating a cold with a warm-water gargle to which you've added 10 drops of Tabasco sauce. "This remedy can be quite effective, particularly if you want to clear your sinuses," he says.

HELP FOR HEART AND STOMACH

Besides unblocking clogged airways, chilies may also cut blood cholesterol, says Earl Mindell, R.Ph., Ph.D., pharmacist and professor of nutrition at Pacific Western University in Los Angeles and author of *Earl Mindell's Food as Medicine*. "When laboratory animals were fed a diet high in capsaicin and low in saturated fat, it helped reduce their 'bad' LDL cholesterol," says Dr. Mindell.

Eating chili peppers also appears to have a blood-thinning effect. Researchers at Max Planck Institute in Germany found that chilies can hinder the formation of blood clots by increasing the amount of time it takes for blood to coagulate. This could play a role in helping prevent blood clots that lead to heart attack and stroke, says Dr. Mindell.

For years, doctors advised people prone to ulcers to abstain from spicy foods. Research now suggests the opposite: that chili peppers may help prevent ulcers from occurring.

Capsaicin appears to shield the stomach lining from ulcer-causing acids and alcohol by stimulating the flow of protective digestive juices. Researchers at National University Hospital in Singapore found that people who consumed the most chili powder had the fewest ulcers, leading them to speculate that chili, or capsaicin, was the protective factor.

RED-HOT VITAMINS

Getting more hot chilies into your diet may strengthen your personal anti-aging arsenal. That's because they're a rich source of the antioxidants vitamin C and beta-carotene (which is converted into vitamin A in the body).

These antioxidants help protect the body by "neutralizing" free radicals, harmful oxygen molecules that naturally accumulate in the body and cause cell damage. Upping your intake of antioxidant vitamins, researchers believe, may

In the Kitchen

Cooking with hot peppers is like riding a Harley. You have to do it very carefully.

"Approach hot peppers with respect," says Bill Hufnagle, author of *Biker Billy Cooks with Fire*. "People tell me the most unusual stories about their experiences with hot peppers—where they touched, whom they touched, and what happened," says Hufnagle.

To enjoy the heat of peppers without getting burned, follow Hufnagle's tips.

Protect your hands. When you're cooking with very hot peppers—"anything hotter than a jalapeño," Hufnagle says—put on a pair of disposable plastic gloves. (If you have sensitive hands, you may want to wear gloves even when working with milder peppers.) When you're done, thoroughly rinse the tips of the gloves with soapy water before taking them off to avoid transferring the pepper oil to your fingers. Then immediately wash your hands, says Hufnagle.

Use plenty of soap. Chili oil sticks to the skin, and water alone won't get it off. You need to use plenty of soap as well. "You might want to wash your hands more than once, depending on the kind of pepper you were working with and how much of it you handled," says Hufnagle.

Protect against pepper dust. When grinding or crushing dried hot peppers, wear a dust mask and goggles. "The dust can get in your throat and eyes," says Hufnagle.

Crush them by hand. It may be convenient to grind dried hot peppers in a blender or coffee grinder—but you won't appreciate the aftershocks. "How thoroughly can you wash a coffee grinder or blender, anyway?" says Hufnagle. "If you use them to grind peppers, you're going to have some nice hot coffee—or milk shakes." At the very least, you may want to consider getting a separate grinder to use on dried hot peppers only.

help prevent damage that can lead to cancer, heart disease, and stroke as well as such things as arthritis and a weakened immune system.

One red chili packs 3 milligrams of beta-carotene, between 30 and 50 percent of the amount recommended by most experts. Studies show that people who consume more beta-carotene-rich foods get less cancer and heart disease.

Getting the Most

Enjoy them raw. Although raw chilies can be uncomfortably hot for some people, that's the best way to get the most vitamin C; cooking destroys the stores of this vitamin, says Dr. Bosland. On the other hand, capsaicin isn't affected by heating, so if that's what you're after—to help relieve congestion, for example—cook the peppers to your taste.

Munch the membrane. Inside the chili is a thin membrane that connects the seeds to the flesh. Most of the capsaicin in chili peppers is located in the membrane, experts say.

Preserve the powder. Storing chili powder at room temperature will eventually deplete its beta-carotene. "Keep chili powder in a dark, cool place, like in the freezer," says Dr. Bosland.

Eat for comfort. The hottest chili pepper isn't necessarily the most healing, so don't make yourself suffer. From wild to mild, here are a few chilies you may want to try.

- Habanero pepper and Scotch bonnet are among the most mouth-blistering peppers.
- Jalapeño and Fresno peppers weigh in at 50 percent firepower, compared to the habanero.
- Hungarian cherry and Anaheim peppers emit more of a glow than a flame and are a good choice for tamer palates.

FIERY CHILI PEPPER SALSA

2 medium tomatoes, coarsely chopped

2 small jalapeño peppers, cut in half lengthwise and very thinly sliced (wear plastic gloves when handling)

¼ cup minced red onions

2 tablespoons minced fresh cilantro

2 tablespoons freshly squeezed lime juice

⅛ teaspoon salt

In a small bowl, combine the tomatoes, peppers, onions, cilantro, lime juice, and salt. Mix well. Let the salsa stand for at least 30 minutes to allow the flavors to blend.

Makes 1⅓ cups

Cook's Notes: The salsa can be covered and stored in the refrigerator for several days.

Serve with nonfat corn chips or as a condiment for baked potatoes or grilled poultry or meat.

PER ⅓ CUP

calories	**29**
total fat	**0.2 g.**
saturated fat	**0 g.**
cholesterol	**0 mg.**
sodium	**74 mg.**
dietary fiber	**0.8 g.**

CHOLESTEROL CONTROL
KEEP YOUR ARTERIES CLEAN

When you consider that haggis, a favorite food in Scotland, is made of the innards of various animals mixed with animal fat and that many of the people there never eat vegetables, it's easy to understand why the Scots have one of the highest mortality rates from cardiovascular disease in the world. Of course, Americans are more likely to eat hamburgers than haggis, but when it comes to cardiovascular health, we're only a few chest-clutching steps behind the Scots.

The reason, to a large extent, is high cholesterol. Having high cholesterol levels is one of the primary risk factors for heart attack, stroke, and other vascular diseases. Over half of American adults have cholesterol levels over 200. Twenty percent of us have cholesterol levels of 240 or above.

If there's any good news in these statistics, it's this: While elevated cholesterol puts you at higher risk for heart disease, it's a risk that you can control every day. Eating a low-fat, low-cholesterol diet is an efficient way to reduce the amount of cholesterol in your blood. Moreover, making even small reductions in cholesterol can add up to big health benefits. For each 1 percent that you lower your total cholesterol, you lower your risk of having a heart attack by 2 percent.

UNDERSTANDING CHOLESTEROL

By itself, cholesterol isn't the toxic sludge that people think it is. Indeed, the body uses cholesterol, which is produced in the liver, to make cell membranes, sex hormones, bile acids, and vitamin D. You couldn't live without it.

In large amounts, however, this essential substance, which is found in animal foods such as meats, milk, eggs, and butter, quickly becomes dangerous. This is particularly true of a form of cholesterol called low-density lipoprotein (LDL), the "bad" cholesterol.

As LDL cholesterol circulates in the bloodstream, it undergoes a process called oxidation. Essentially, this means that it spoils and turns rancid. Your immune system quickly spots the decaying LDL and reacts to it as it would to any other invader. Immune cells gobble up the cholesterol molecules. Once engorged, they stick to the walls of arteries, hardening into a dense, fatty layer called plaque. When enough plaque accumulates, there's less room for blood to flow. Eventually, blood flow may slow or even stop. When this occurs in arteries supplying the heart, the result is a heart attack. When it occurs in arteries supplying the brain, the result is a stroke.

Your body has a mechanism for dealing with this threat. A second form of cholesterol, called high-density lipoprotein (HDL), transports the dangerous cholesterol out of the blood and to the liver for disposal. Normally, it does a good job. But when cholesterol levels get too high, the HDL cholesterol can't keep up, and LDL gradually rises to dangerous levels.

Ideally, you want to have high levels of HDL and low levels of the dangerous LDL. The National Cholesterol Education Program recommends keeping total cholesterol below 200 milligrams per deciliter of blood. More specifically, LDL should be below 130, and HDL should be above 65.

One way to help keep your blood cholesterol within healthy limits is to eat no more than 300 milligrams of dietary cholesterol a day (a little more than the amount in 1½ egg yolks). But as mentioned, the body makes cholesterol on its own. That's why limiting the amount of cholesterol in your diet is only part of the solution.

How Diet Helps

When John A. McDougall, M.D., medical director of the McDougall Program at St. Helena Hospital in Napa Valley, California, and author of *The McDougall Program for a Healthy Heart*, was a medical resident in the late 1970s, he worked with a Chinese physician who told him that in Hong Kong, "heart attacks were so rare that whenever one occurred, doctors all over the city rushed to the autopsy lab to see this medical curiosity."

Can you imagine American physicians being surprised by a heart attack? Quite the contrary. Every year at least 1.5 million Americans will have heart attacks. A third of them will die, making heart attack America's single largest killer.

What explains the tremendous difference between the two countries? To a large extent it's due to cholesterol. More specifically, it's due to the types of diets that cause cholesterol to go up or down. Among Chinese who eat a traditional diet, for example, the average cholesterol level is a healthy 127. Among Americans, who generally eat a lot of red meats and fatty processed foods, the average is 100 points higher.

According to Dr. McDougall, the traditional Asian diet, which is high in vegetables, fruits, and grains and low in red meats and dairy foods, is nearly perfect for lowering cholesterol.

It can work in this country, too. The Lifestyle Heart Trial found that when people followed a low-fat vegetarian diet (much like the traditional Asian diet), they had a drop in total cholesterol of 24 percent. Better yet, levels of dangerous LDL cholesterol fell an average of 37 percent—in one year.

It Begins with Fat

Even though it's important to reduce the amount of cholesterol in your diet, the real culprit lies elsewhere. "The component in food that has the biggest effect on blood cholesterol levels is saturated fat," says Mark Kantor, Ph.D., associate professor of nutrition and food science at the University of Maryland in College Park. Saturated fats, which are found mostly in animal foods such as red meats, whole and 2 percent milk, egg yolks, butter, and cheese, can increase the amount of LDL cholesterol in the bloodstream as well as the total amount of cholesterol.

Every day, the average American eats the fat equivalent of a full stick of butter. That's three times as much as the Japanese. Clearly, this is one instance where it's better to be below average.

If you haven't already begun reducing the amount of saturated fat in your diet, consider the evidence. In a study conducted by researchers at the U.S. Department of Agriculture's Lipid Nutrition Laboratory in Beltsville, Maryland, and George Washington University in Washington, D.C., men with normal or borderline-high cholesterol levels alternated between a high-fat diet (41 percent of calories from fat), a low-fat diet (19 percent of calories from fat), and their usual diets. When the men switched from the high-fat to the low-fat plan, almost 80 percent saw their cholesterol fall 20 points after six weeks.

Although the Daily Value (DV) for fat is 30 percent of total calories, Dr. Kantor and other health experts say that going lower, to 25 percent of total calories, with no more than 7 percent from saturated fats, is even better.

Along with cheese, milk, and convenience foods, red meats are the most common source of fat in the American diet. You don't have to make drastic changes, however, since even small reductions in saturated fat can result in a significant reduction in cholesterol levels, says Dr. Kantor. Replacing a hamburger with an equal amount of fish twice a week could save you from eating about 4 pounds of fat a year. Eating two fewer slices of American cheese a week would save you a pound of fat a year.

Although the saturated fats in animal foods tend to cause the most problems, the fats found in cooking oils can also make your cholesterol levels creep upward. The American Heart Association recommends limiting the amount of oil you consume in a day to between 5 and 8 teaspoons.

One of the easiest ways to cut back on cooking oils is simply to avoid eating fried foods. Instead, take advantage of steaming and microwaving. Since these techniques cook with moist heat, they require little or no added fat to keep food moist and tender.

Another way to reduce the amount of fat in your diet is to approach dairy foods with caution. Milk has a reputation as a wholesome food, but when it's the full-fat kind, it can dump a lot of fat into your system. It's fine to enjoy milk,

THE MONOUNSATURATED EDGE

Even though it's a good idea to reduce the amount of fat in your diet, there's one type of fat that you can feel good about eating. Research suggests that having moderate amounts of monounsaturated fat, the kind found in avocados and olive oil, can lower levels of harmful low-density lipoprotein (LDL) cholesterol, while leaving the beneficial high-density lipoprotein (HDL) untouched.

Researchers have known for a long time that people in Greece, Spain, and other Mediterranean countries where olive oil is used every day have some of the lowest rates of heart disease in the world. Indeed, even when their cholesterol levels are fairly high, they're about half as likely to die of heart disease as an American with the same cholesterol reading. Research suggests that olive oil may somehow improve the liver's ability to remove LDL cholesterol from the bloodstream.

Even so, olive oil can't take credit for all the benefits. People in the Mediterranean also eat a lot of fresh fruits and vegetables, plus they walk more than Americans and are less likely to be overweight.

If you do decide to add more olive oil to your diet, use it in moderation, adds Mark Kantor, Ph.D., associate professor of nutrition and food science at the University of Maryland in College Park. It may be better than other oils, but it's still 100 percent fat. "Cut back on all fats," Dr. Kantor says, "and consume olive oil in moderation. Don't increase the total amount of oil in your diet."

but keep it low-fat. Use skim or 1 percent milk as well as low-fat yogurt.

Perhaps the easiest way to eat less fat is simply to eat more fruits and vegetables. Not only are these foods high in vitamins and minerals, they'll help fill you up so that you eat less of other foods that contain more fat. Having an extra serving of broccoli at supper, for example, means that you'll probably eat a little less meat, and that will pay off in lower cholesterol.

HELP FROM FIBER

You know that eating whole grains, beans, and fresh fruits will help keep your digestive system in top shape, but you may want to eat these foods to reduce cholesterol, too. They're filled with soluble fiber, a substance that forms a gummy gel in the digestive tract, which helps lower cholesterol.

A study of people in China, conducted by researchers from Johns Hopkins University in Baltimore, found that cholesterol levels in men who ate about 3 ounces of oats a day were 11 percent lower than those of men who rarely ate oats. In addition, the blood pressures of the men who ate oats were 8 percent lower.

"This study suggests that eating a high-fiber diet can have a beneficial effect on blood cholesterol and blood pressure," says Jiang He, M.D., Ph.D., an epidemiologist in the School of Hygiene and Public Health at Johns Hopkins. "It further suggests that adopting a high-fiber diet could reduce the death rate from cardiovascular disease in the United States."

In another study, researchers at the University of Kentucky in Lexington looked at two groups of people following a low-fat diet. People in one group ate 15 grams of fiber a day, while those in the second group had an extra 35 grams. After a year, the cholesterol levels of those on the higher-fiber diet had dropped 13 percent.

The DV for fiber is 25 grams. In practical terms, this means eating 2 to 4 servings of fruit, 3 to 5 servings of vegetables, and 6 to 11 servings of breads, cereals, and grains a day, says Joanne Curran-Celentano, R.D., Ph.D., associate professor of nutritional sciences at the University of New Hampshire in Durham. "Eating oatmeal or oat bran cereal several times a week will add even more soluble fiber to your diet," she adds. Other good sources of soluble fiber include pinto beans, red kidney beans, brussels sprouts, and sweet potatoes.

THE ASIAN SUPERFOOD

We feed soybeans to chickens. But in Asian countries, people eat soybeans as well as soy foods such as tofu nearly every day. These foods contain compounds that help lower cholesterol, and this may explain, at least in part, why cholesterol levels in Japan are so much lower than they are here in the United States.

Studies have shown that replacing protein from animal sources with about 1½ ounces of soy protein a day can lower total cholesterol by 9 percent. It lowers dangerous LDL cholesterol even more, by 13 percent.

Tofu and other soy foods contain compounds called phytoestrogens, says James W. Anderson, professor of medicine and clinical nutrition at the Veterans Administration Medical Center at the University of Kentucky College of Medicine in Lexington. Researchers believe that these compounds help transport LDL cholesterol from the bloodstream to the liver, where it's broken down and excreted. They also may prevent the LDL from oxidizing, making it less likely to clog the coronary arteries.

To get the cholesterol-lowering benefits of soy, you need to eat two or three servings of soy foods a day, says Dr. Anderson.

CLOVES OF PROTECTION

Garlic-lovers say that you can't eat too much of the "stinking rose," and it seems that they're right. Research suggests that this pungent bulb can significantly lower cholesterol.

Garlic contains a compound called allicin that changes the way in which the body uses cholesterol, says Stephen Warshafsky, M.D., assistant professor of medicine at New York Medical College in Valhalla. When Dr. Warshafsky analyzed data from five of the most reliable scientific studies on garlic and cholesterol, he found that eating one-half to one clove of garlic a day lowered blood cholesterol an average of 9 percent.

When using garlic, it's a good idea to mince or crush it, since this releases more of the allicin. Even if you eat a lot of garlic, however, don't count on it to be a magic bullet against cholesterol. "Eating garlic on top of a diet high in saturated fat and cholesterol is unlikely to do you any good," says Dr. Kantor.

HELP FROM THE DEEP

In addition to knowing your cholesterol levels, there's another number to watch: your level of blood fats called triglycerides. People with high levels of triglycerides are more likely to have low levels of protective HDL. Conversely, lowering your level of triglycerides can help decrease your risk of heart disease.

Salmon, tuna, and other fish contain fats called omega-3 fatty acids, which have been shown to lower triglycerides. In a study at the University of Western Australia in Perth, two groups of men followed a low-fat diet. Those in one group ate a variety of protein foods, while those in the second group ate 3 to 5 ounces of fish a day. After three months, men in both groups had drops in cholesterol. But the men who ate fish also experienced a 23 percent reduction in triglycerides.

Omega-3's may do more than lower triglycerides. Research suggests that they may raise levels of beneficial HDL cholesterol as well. Men in the Australian study who ate fish had a 15 percent increase in HDL. It appears that as fish is added to a low-fat diet, triglycerides go down and HDL levels go up.

Finally, fish is also low in calories and saturated fat, making it a perfect addition to a cholesterol-reducing diet. To get the maximum benefits from omega-3's, plan on eating 3 to 4 ounces of fish two times a week, recommends Dr. Curran-Celentano.

Incidentally, if you're a fan of canned tuna, you're in luck since it also contains omega-3's. However, be sure to buy tuna packed in water. Three ounces contains 111 calories and less than 1 gram of fat, while the same amount of tuna canned in oil contains 168 calories and nearly 7 grams of fat.

COLDS AND FLU
FOODS THAT FIGHT INFECTION

The only way to avoid colds and flu entirely would be to become a hermit, living far from the sneezes of co-workers, the runny noses of children, and the coughs of strangers on city streets.

Since secluding yourself on a desert island won't pay the bills, however, one of the best strategies is to eat all the immunity-boosting foods you can find. As it turns out, there are plenty to choose from. Research has found that some of the foods we eat every day contain powerful compounds that can help stop viruses from taking hold. Even when you're already sick, choosing the right foods will ease the discomfort and possibly help you get better more quickly.

EAT FOR IMMUNITY

Colds and flu get their starts when just a few viruses slip into your system. Once they're inside, they immediately set to work making more viruses. If your immune system doesn't stop them early on, they multiply to enormous numbers, and that's when you start feeling sick.

One way to stop this microbial invasion is to eat more fruits and vegetables. These foods contain a variety of substances that strengthen the immune system, making it better able to destroy viruses before they make you sick. Research has shown, for example, that many fruits and vegetables contain a compound called glutathione, which stimulates the immune system to release large numbers of macrophages, specialized cells that seize viruses and mark them for destruction. Avocados, watermelons, asparagus, winter squash, and grapefruit are all rich in glutathione. Okra, oranges, tomatoes, potatoes, cauliflower, broccoli, cantaloupe, strawberries, and peaches are also good sources.

Another powerful compound in many fruits and vegetables is vitamin C. Doctors have been debating for years whether vitamin C can help prevent colds—and they're still debating. When you're already sick, however, getting extra vitamin C in your diet has been proven to relieve cold symptoms and help you get better more quickly.

Vitamin C lowers levels of histamine, a defensive chemical released by the immune system that is responsible for causing stuffiness and other cold and flu symptoms. At the same time, vitamin C appears to strengthen white blood cells, which are essential for fighting infection.

After reviewing 21 scientific studies published since 1971, researchers at the University of Helsinki in Finland concluded that getting 1,000 milligrams of vitamin C a day can reduce cold symptoms and shorten the duration of the illness by 23 percent.

Of course, you'd have to eat a lot of oranges, broccoli, and other foods rich in vitamin C to get that much of this important nutrient. A better strategy is to drink a lot of juices, says Won Song, R.D., Ph.D., associate professor of human nutrition at Michigan State University in East Lansing. Orange juice, which has 61 milligrams of vitamin C in a 6-ounce serving, is probably your best choice, although cranberry and grapefruit juices also contain a lot of vitamin C.

BULBS OF HEALTH

Garlic has been used throughout history for treating virtually every type of infection. Now there's increasing evidence that it can help protect against colds and flu as well.

Garlic contains dozens of chemically active compounds. Two of them, allicin and allin, have been shown to kill germs directly. Plus, garlic appears to stimulate the immune system to release natural killer cells, which destroy even more germs.

To get the benefits of garlic, however, you have to eat a lot of it—as much as an entire bulb a day to combat colds and flu, says Elson Haas, M.D., director of the Preventive Medical Center of Marin in San Rafael, California, and author of *Staying Healthy with Nutrition*.

Unless you have developed a taste for it, you probably can't eat that much raw garlic. Microwaving or baking garlic until it's tender, however, will take away some of the burn and sweeten the taste, says Irwin Ziment, M.D., professor of medicine at the University of California, Los Angeles. "The softened garlic still seems to be quite potent," Dr. Ziment adds.

HOT AND HELPFUL

Research has shown that two traditional treatments for colds and flu—a cup of hot tea followed by a steaming bowl of chicken soup—are among the most-potent home remedies there are. Both of these foods, along with chili peppers and other spicy foods, contain compounds that can relieve congestion and keep the immune system strong.

Tea, for example, contains a compound called theophylline, which helps break up congestion, says Steven R. Mostow, M.D., chairman of the American Thoracic Society Committee on the Prevention of Pneumonia and Influenza in Denver. Tea also contains quercetin, a compound that may help prevent viruses from multiplying.

Chicken soup is another folk remedy that has been proven to be effective. In fact, having a bowl of chicken soup is one of the best ways to relieve stuffiness and other cold and flu symptoms. In laboratory studies, for example, researchers at the University of Nebraska Medical Center in Omaha found that chicken soup was able to prevent white blood cells from causing inflammation and congestion in the airways.

It's important, however, to use homemade chicken soup, Dr. Mostow adds. Doctors aren't sure why, but canned chicken soup doesn't work as well as homemade, and broth made from bouillon doesn't work at all.

When a cold has your nose so stuffy that you feel like you're breathing through a thick blanket, you may want to take a bite of hot pepper. Jalapeños, ground red pepper, and their fiery kin contain a compound called capsaicin. This compound, which is similar to a drug in cold and flu medications, will help you breathe easy again, says Dr. Ziment.

You don't need fresh peppers to get the benefits, adds Dr. Haas. Mixing ¼ teaspoon of ground red pepper in a glass of water and drinking it can be very effective. "It's heating, but not irritating," Dr. Haas says.

CONSTIPATION
THE FIBER EXPRESS

There's not much that people don't talk about these days. Spend a few minutes around the water cooler, and you'll hear about sex, divorce, and the details of a colleague's prostate surgery.

The one thing people don't talk about, even with their doctors, is constipation. If they did, constipation probably would no longer be the most common digestive complaint, because they'd find out that it's easy to treat. For most people, getting more fiber and fluids in their diet can put an end to constipation for good.

JUST PASSING THROUGH

Unlike vitamins and minerals, fiber isn't absorbed by the digestive tract. Instead, it spends a long time in the intestine, absorbing large amounts of fluid. And that's precisely its constipation-fighting secret.

When fiber absorbs water, stools gradually swell, getting bigger and wetter. Unlike small stools, which can accumulate for days before moving on, large stools are moved out of the intestine much more quickly, says Marie Borum, M.D., assistant professor of medicine at George Washington University Medical Center in Washington, D.C. And because large stools are much softer than small ones, there's less straining when they do move, she adds.

All fruits, vegetables, legumes, and whole-grain foods contain healthful amounts of fiber. Doctors once believed that insoluble fiber, the kind found mainly in whole wheat, was the only choice for beating constipation. As it turns out, however, both insoluble and soluble fiber, the kind found primarily in legumes, oats, and many fruits, can help keep the intestine working smoothly. "Both types of fiber add bulk, soften the stool, and speed transit time," says Dr. Borum.

The reason that constipation is so common is that most Americans simply don't get enough fiber. On average, we only get about 11 grams a day, a lot less than the Daily Value (DV) of 25 grams, says Pat Harper, R.D. a nutrition consultant in the Pittsburgh area. Since virtually all plant foods contain healthy quantities of fiber, you don't have to work very hard to get the necessary amounts. A 1-cup serving of Wheaties has 3 grams of fiber, 12 percent of the

Good Morning, Joe

Coffee drinkers have always known that a morning cup of their favorite jolt does more than pop their eyes open. It appears to wake up the digestive tract as well.

It's not your imagination. The caffeine in coffee stimulates the large intestine, causing it to contract, says Pat Harper, R.D., a nutrition consultant in the Pittsburgh area. "A cup or two of coffee in the morning can help you stay regular," she says. In fact, some doctors recommend that anyone who is constipated try drinking a cup of coffee rather than taking an over-the-counter laxative.

The problem with coffee, of course, is that when you drink a lot of it, it removes more fluids from your body than it puts in. It's fine to use coffee as a morning wake-up call, Harper says. It's a good idea, however, to limit yourself to fewer than five cups a day.

DV, and Kellogg's Raisin Bran has 8 grams in the same size serving, 32 percent of the DV. A half-cup of cooked kidney beans has 3 grams of fiber, 12 percent of the DV, and an apple also has about 3 grams.

There is one problem with adding more fiber to your diet. When your body isn't used to it, it can cause cramping and gas, Dr. Borum warns. To get the benefits without the grief, she recommends that you gradually add fiber to your diet over a period of several months. "A lifetime of not getting enough fiber can't be fixed in a week," she says. But if you gradually increase the amount of fiber you get each day, you probably won't have any discomfort at all, she adds.

Water Works

We often think of water as being sort of an add-on to a healthful diet, not an essential ingredient in its own right. But not getting enough water is a very common cause of constipation, Dr. Borum says. After all, stools can absorb large amounts of water. When they don't get enough, they get hard, sluggish, and more difficult to pass. This is particularly true when you're eating more fiber, which must be accompanied by fluids in order to keep things moving smoothly.

You can't depend on thirst to tell you when it's time to drink, Dr. Borum adds. The thirst mechanism isn't all that sensitive to begin with, and often it stays silent even when your body needs more fluids. What's more, the urge to drink naturally gets weaker with age, which is one reason that constipation is more common in older folks.

To avoid walking on the dry side, Dr. Borum recommends drinking at least six to eight full glasses of water a day. Or, if you don't want to drink that much water, make up the difference by having soups or juices.

Beverages containing alcohol or caffeine, however, don't count toward your daily fluid total because they're diuretics, meaning that they actually remove more fluids from your body than they put in, says Dr. Borum.

PRUNING THE PROBLEM

Prunes are probably the oldest home remedy for constipation—and, researchers have discovered, one of the most effective.

Prunes contain three ingredients that help keep digestion on track. For starters, they're very high in fiber, with 3 grams of the rough stuff, about 12 percent of the DV, in just three prunes. They also contain a compound called dihydroxphenyl isatin, which stimulates the intestinal contractions that are necessary for regular bowel movements. Finally, prunes contain a natural sugar called sorbitol, which soaks up enormous amounts of water in the digestive tract and helps keep the system active.

Even if you don't care for prunes, you can get some of the same benefits by eating raisins. In one study, for example, people were given 4½ ounces of raisins a day. At the end of the study, the average time it took for stools to move through the digestive tract was cut in half, from two days to one.

Like prunes, raisins are very high in fiber, with a snack-size box providing about 2 grams, 8 percent of the DV. In addition, they contain a compound called tartaric acid, which acts as a natural laxative, Dr. Borum explains.

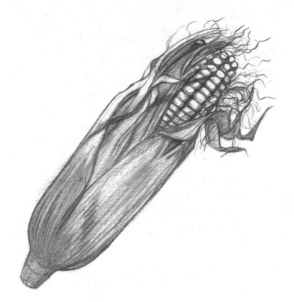

CORN
KERNELS AGAINST CHOLESTEROL

HEALING POWER

CAN HELP:
Lower cholesterol

Boost energy levels

In Mitchell, South Dakota, right in the middle of the corn belt, residents pay homage to the harvest. Their shrine is the Corn Palace, a mansion built in 1892 that's decorated—murals, minarets, towers, and all—with 3,000 bushels of corn.

It isn't necessary to take corn that seriously, but it does deserve a place of honor at your dinner table. Because corn is high in fiber, it can help lower cholesterol. And because it's very high in carbohydrates, it provides quick energy while delivering virtually no fat.

"Corn is really an excellent basic food source," says Mark McLellan, Ph.D., professor of food science at Cornell University and director of Cornell's Institute of Food Science in Geneva, New York. "When combined with other vegetables in the diet, it is a good source of protein, carbohydrates, and vitamins."

KERNELS AGAINST CHOLESTEROL

Corn contains a type of dietary fiber called soluble fiber. When you eat corn, this fiber binds with bile, a cholesterol-laden digestive fluid produced by the liver. Since soluble fiber isn't readily absorbed by the body, it passes out in the stool, taking the cholesterol with it.

You've heard a lot about how oat and wheat bran can lower cholesterol.

Corn bran is in the same league. In a study at Illinois State University in Normal, researchers put 29 men with high cholesterol on low-fat diets. After two weeks on the diet, some of the men were each given 20 grams (almost ½ tablespoon) of corn bran a day, while others received a similar amount of wheat bran. During the six-week study, those on the corn bran plan had a drop in cholesterol of more than 5 percent and about a 13 percent drop in triglycerides, blood fats that in large amounts can contribute to heart disease. Those who were given wheat bran showed no change beyond the initial drop caused by being on a low-fat diet.

A Bushel of Nutrients

The beauty of corn is that it provides a lot of energy while delivering a small number of calories—about 83 per ear.

Corn is an excellent source of thiamin, a B vitamin that's essential for converting food to energy. An ear of corn provides 0.2 milligram of thiamin, 13 percent of the Daily Value. That's more than you'll get in three slices of bacon or 3 ounces of roast beef.

And since fresh sweet corn consists primarily of simple and complex carbohydrates, it's a superb energy source, says Donald V. Schlimme, Ph.D., professor of nutrition and food science at the University of Maryland in College Park. "It fulfills our energy needs without providing us with a substantial amount of fat," Dr. Schlimme says. What little fats there are in corn are the polyunsaturated and monounsaturated kinds, which are far healthier than the saturated fats found in meats and dairy foods.

Getting the Most

Shop by color. Not all corn is created equal. Whereas yellow corn has more than 2 grams of fiber per serving, white corn more than doubles that, with a bit more than 4 grams per ear.

In the Kitchen

Corn on the cob is so easy to prepare, it's essentially Nature's fast food. Just strip off the husk and corn silk, drop the ears in a steamer, and wait until it's done a few minutes later. To maximize the taste, here are a few tips you may want to try.

Cook it right away. When corn sits around, its natural sugar turns into starch, giving up the natural sweet taste. So it's best to cook corn as soon after it was picked as possible.

Hold the salt. When cooking corn in boiling water, don't add salt. This will draw moisture from the kernels, making them tough and hard to chew.

Strip the kernels. When you have a craving for fresh corn but don't want to wrestle with the cob, just strip the kernels off. Hold the cob upright in a bowl. Using a sharp knife, slice downward, cutting away a few rows at a time. When all the kernels are removed, scrape the dull side of the blade down the sides of the cob to extract the sweet, milky juice.

Make sure it's mature. When you buy corn at the supermarket, look for ears that have full, plump kernels. "Purchase it at the optimum stage of maturity," Dr. Schlimme advises. "Under those conditions, the level of nutrients is higher."

To see if corn is ripe, puncture one of the kernels with your fingernail. If the liquid that comes out isn't milky-colored, the corn is either immature or overripe, and you should pass it by.

Steam it. Corn on the cob is traditionally boiled, but that's perhaps the worst way to prepare it since boiling curtails corn's nutritional power. "You lose fewer nutrients when you steam corn," Dr. Schlimme says. "Putting it in boiling water, which is the way most people prepare sweet corn, leaches out more water-soluble nutrients than steaming does."

Get the whole kernel. No matter how diligent you are when eating corn on the cob, you invariably leave a lot behind. To get the most out of each kernel, you're better off buying frozen or canned corn. Or you can cut the kernels from the cob with a knife. Unlike eating it right off the cob, "you get more of the corn's benefit by having a mechanical cut that takes the entire kernel off," Dr. McLellan says.

Buy it vacuum-packed. While canned corn can be almost as nutritious as fresh, it loses some of its value when it's packed in brine, a salty liquid that leaches nutrients from food during processing, says Dr. Schlimme. To get the most vitamins, look for vacuum-packed corn, which doesn't contain brine. Corn that's vacuum-packed (it will say so on the label) usually comes in short, squat cans, he says.

CORN SALAD WITH HONEY DRESSING

1   bag (16 ounces) frozen corn
1   small sweet red pepper,
    finely diced
1   tablespoon chopped fresh
    chives
3   tablespoons cider vinegar
1   tablespoon honey
½   teaspoon celery seeds
⅛   teaspoon salt

PER SERVING
calories **112**
total fat **0.2 g.**
saturated fat **0 g.**
cholesterol **0 mg.**
sodium **74 mg.**
dietary fiber **3 g.**

Place the corn in a colander and rinse with hot water to thaw. Place in a large bowl and add the peppers and chives. Toss to combine.

In a small saucepan, combine the vinegar, honey, celery seeds, and salt. Cook over medium heat for 1 to 2 minutes, or until the honey thins out. Pour over the corn and toss to coat. Serve immediately or chill.

Makes 4 servings

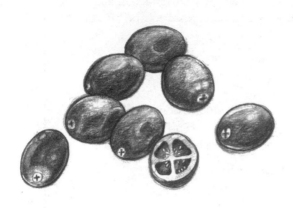

CRANBERRIES
A SAUCE FOR ALL SEASONS

HEALING POWER

CAN HELP:
Prevent and treat
urinary tract infections

Protect cells
from cancerous changes

Reduce the risk
of heart disease
and stroke

Pity the lowly cranberry. Like swallows returning to San Juan Capistrano, this Thanksgiving staple finds its way back into our diet every year—then gets lost after the holiday season is over.

And that's a pity. Cranberries contain a number of compounds that show early promise against cancer and heart disease. What's more, cranberry juice has finally earned the scientific stamp of approval for its traditional role in relieving bladder infections.

A ROLE AGAINST CANCER

Along with raspberries, strawberries, and blackberries, cranberries are a good source of ellagic acid, an antioxidant compound that has raised high hopes in cancer researchers.

In laboratory tests, ellagic acid has been shown to help prevent mutations in DNA, the genetic stuff that instructs our cells how to function. In addition, ellagic acid has been shown to disarm cancer-causing agents and also to help prevent tumors from growing.

Indeed, one tantalizing aspect of this compound is its apparent ability to battle carcinogens on both ends—before and after they take hold. "Ellagic acid has what we call anti-initiating activity. It inhibits the genetic damage that starts

166

the cancer process," says Gary D. Stoner, Ph.D., director of the cancer chemo-prevention program at the Ohio State University Comprehensive Cancer Center in Columbus. Even after a carcinogen has been introduced into cells, he says, ellagic acid helps prevent the cells from becoming cancerous.

Pure ellagic acid—the form in which it's used in laboratory studies—doesn't get into the bloodstream very well. However, Dr. Stoner's research suggests that this compound is better absorbed in its natural state in food—good news for those who enjoy their cranberries year-round.

POWER FROM FLAVONOIDS

Another way in which cranberries will help keep you healthy is by putting more flavonoids into your diet. Flavonoids are plant pigments that put the reds and yellows into fruits and vegetables and that have powerful antioxidant abilities—that is, they help block damage from free radicals, harmful oxygen molecules that can lead to cancer, heart disease, and other serious conditions.

Cranberries contain two powerful flavonoids—quercetin and myricetin. The darker cranberry varieties, like Stevens, Early Black, and Ben Lear, contain a third compound called kaempferol. Each of these compounds has been shown in studies to help prevent genetic changes that can lead to cancer.

Here's a bonus. Flavonoids, in general, and quercetin, in particular, are thought to play a role in preventing artery disease, perhaps because their antioxidant ability helps prevent damage to the linings of blood vessels.

Large studies in Finland, the Netherlands, and the United Kingdom have shown that people with very low intakes of flavonoids have high risks of coronary disease. In one study of middle-age men in the Dutch town of Zutphen, those who ate a lot of fruits and vegetables—and consequently had a high intake of flavonoids—had a 73 percent lower risk of stroke than men who consumed few fruits and vegetables.

HELP FOR URINARY COMPLAINTS

For ages now, grandmothers and mothers—and a few wise doctors—have recommended cranberry juice to clear up urinary tract infections. Now, scientists are coming on board. A 1994 Harvard Medical School study of elderly women found that those who drank about 10 ounces of cranberry juice cocktail daily for six months had significantly lower amounts of bacteria in their urine and were almost 60 percent less likely to develop infections than women who drank a noncranberry impostor.

Among women who already had infections, those drinking cranberry juice were nearly 75 percent more likely to have their infections clear up.

One long-held belief was that if you could make urine more acidic, bacteria would have a tougher time growing. This was thought to be why cranberry juice helped prevent urinary tract infections. Following the same line of reasoning, doctors sometimes recommended high doses of vitamin C, up to 1,000 milligrams a day, for people with bladder or other urinary infections.

According to Mark Monane, M.D., assistant professor of medicine at Harvard Medical School, who was involved with the study, it wasn't the acidity of cranberries that helped keep bacteria in check. Rather, it appeared to be two compounds in the juice—fructose and a second compound yet to be identified—that helped prevent bacteria from adhering to the lining of the bladder and urethra.

Incidentally, Israeli researchers found that juice from blueberries—a close cousin of cranberries—had the same results.

In his book, *Doctor, What Should I Eat?*, Isadore Rosenfeld, M.D., clinical professor of medicine at New York Hospital–Cornell Medical Center in New York City, suggests women who have urinary tract infections drink two glasses (8 ounces each) of cranberry juice a day in addition to taking any antibiotics prescribed by their doctors. For women who are prone to infections and want to prevent them, drinking one glass every day will help ward off trouble.

Getting the Most

Eat them with relish. Since raw cranberries contain considerably more healing compounds than cooked, you may want to try a cranberry relish. Put a pound of cranberries, two apples, and a large orange in a food processor and process until coarse. Mix in honey or sugar to taste, refrigerate for several hours, and serve.

Have a drink. Because raw cranberries have a tart taste and tough texture, you're unlikely to eat them raw. But you can still get the nutritional payload by drinking the juice.

Commercial cranberry juice cocktail drinks are loaded with vitamin C, with one glass containing a full day's supply. Unfortunately, most also have a full day's supply of sugar and are never more than 30 percent juice.

An alternative to supermarket juice is the juice found in health food stores. You can buy either pure cranberry juice or concentrated cranberry extract, which is used to make cold drinks or hot teas.

CRANBERRY RELISH

1	**bag (12 ounces) cranberries**
1	**medium apple**
1	**thin-skinned navel orange**
½	**cup sugar**
⅛	**teaspoon ground ginger**

PER ¼ CUP

calories	**70**
total fat	**0.1 g.**
saturated fat	**0 g.**
cholesterol	**0 mg.**
sodium	**0 mg.**
dietary fiber	**1.7 g.**

Place the cranberries in a colander. Rinse well with cold water. Discard any soft cranberries.

Place in a food processor. Core the apple and cut into chunks. Add to the food processor. Cut the orange, including the rind, into chunks. Add to the food processor. Process, scraping down the bowl once or twice, until finely chopped.

Transfer to a medium bowl. Add the sugar and ginger and stir to mix. Let stand for at least 15 minutes. Stir before serving.

Makes 2½ cups

Cook's Notes: For a sweeter relish, peel the orange.

The relish can be refrigerated in a covered container for up to 2 days.

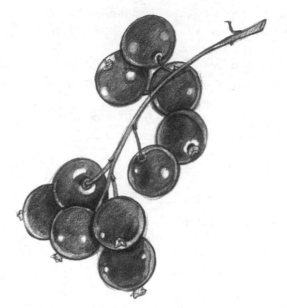

CURRANTS
A GREAT SOURCE OF C

HEALING POWER
CAN HELP:
Protect against cancer

Reduce cholesterol

Lower the risk
for heart disease

Prevent constipation

The British adore currant jams and jellies. The French favor black currant liqueur. And until the turn of the century, Americans delighted in fresh currants as well as currant jellies and sauces.

Today, unless you're lucky enough to have a currant shrub in your backyard, fresh currants are as scarce in the United States as icicles in July. (Don't be fooled by the black "currants" sold in supermarkets—they're really zante grapes.)

What ended our craving for currants? In the early 1900s, the U.S. Department of Agriculture banned the cultivation of currants because the shrubs harbored a fungus that was destroying white pines. Even though the ban was lifted in the 1960s, currants never really made a comeback.

This is unfortunate because currants are a superb source of vitamin C and fiber. What's more, they contain a compound with powerful cancer-fighting potential.

AN ARSENAL OF HEALTH

Even though currants are extraordinarily high in vitamins—a half-cup of black currants, for example, has 101 milligrams of vitamin C, 168 percent of the Daily Value (DV)—that's not what gets researchers excited. The big news is that the berries contain a compound called ellagic acid, which shows promise for stopping cancer before it starts.

Ellagic acid is a member of a disease-fighting family of compounds known as polyphenols. (Raspberries, strawberries, and grapes also contain polyphenols.) In laboratory studies, ellagic acid has been shown to be a powerful antioxidant, meaning that it helps neutralize free radicals, harmful oxygen molecules that are missing electrons, says Gary D. Stoner, Ph.D., director of the cancer chemoprevention program at the Ohio State University Comprehensive Cancer Center in Columbus. Free radicals try to replace their missing electrons by taking electrons from healthy cells, causing cellular changes that can lead to cancer.

Ellagic acid has also been shown to block the effects of cancer-causing chemicals in the body at the same time that it stimulates the activity of enzymes that fight cancer growth. This two-pronged approach makes this compound a powerful ally for blocking cancer.

Doctors aren't sure how many currants you'd have to eat to reap the full benefits. Dr. Stoner speculates that four to six servings of fruits (including currants) and vegetables a day is enough to substantially lower your risk of developing cancer.

IN THE KITCHEN

Currants are mouth-puckeringly tart, which is why they're rarely eaten out of hand. Here are several sweeter uses for these bitey berries.

- Like cranberries, currants make a perfect sauce for livening up meat dishes. They're slightly sweeter than cranberries, however, so you'll want to add less sugar when making the sauce.
- Putting currants in fruit salads will add a tangy taste. For an even prettier plate, add a combination of red, white, and black currants.
- To make a tangy dessert, put currants in a bowl and top with sugar and just a bit of light cream.

DIGESTIVE AIDS

Like most berries, currants are high in fiber; the black, red, and white varieties all provide about 2 grams of the rough stuff, 8 percent of the DV. Fiber does more than control digestive problems like constipation and hemorrhoids. It also helps head off more serious health problems like high cholesterol and heart disease.

In fact, a study of 21,930 Finnish men found that those who got just 10 extra grams of fiber a day were able to reduce their risk of dying from heart disease by 17 percent. Eating one or two servings of currants a day, along with extra fruits and vegetables, will provide all the fiber you need to help keep your circulation in the swim.

Getting the Most

Check the roadsides. The one problem with fresh currants is that they're so hard to find. Since most supermarkets don't stock them, your best bet is to check out roadside stands or farmer's markets since growers will sometimes sell small amounts of these homegrown favorites.

Store them carefully. When you're lucky enough to get your hands on fresh currants, you'll want to make them last. The berries will stay fresh for two or three days when stored in an airtight container in the refrigerator. Or you can freeze them for use throughout the year.

CURRANT CHUTNEY

2   **cups fresh red currants**

2   **cups chopped green tomatoes**

2   **cups chopped tart apples**

1   **cup chopped onions**

½   **cup honey**

½   **cup cider vinegar**

2   **teaspoons minced garlic**

2   **teaspoons brown mustard seeds**

1   **serrano pepper, minced (wear plastic gloves when handling)**

1   **teaspoon grated fresh ginger**

1   **lime**

PER ¼ CUP

calories	**63**
total fat	**0.3 g.**
saturated fat	**0 g.**
cholesterol	**0 mg.**
sodium	**4 mg.**
dietary fiber	**1.6 g.**

In a large saucepan, combine the currants, tomatoes, apples, onions, honey, vinegar, ½ cup water, garlic, mustard seeds, peppers, and ginger. Bring to a boil over medium-high heat.

Slice the lime into 4 lengthwise wedges. Cut each wedge into thin crosswise slices. Add to the saucepan. Reduce the heat to medium low. Simmer the mixture for 15 to 20 minutes, or until the apples are tender and the mixture thickens slightly.

Cool. Refrigerate in a covered container for several days for the flavor to develop.

Makes 4 cups

Cook's Notes: The chutney can be refrigerated for several weeks or frozen for several months in a covered container.

Serve with grilled or broiled turkey breast, chicken drumsticks, or pork tenderloin.

DEFICIENCY DISEASES
FOOD OR CONSEQUENCES

Spirit, tell me if Tiny Tim will live," pleads a woeful Ebenezer Scrooge as he gazes at visions of Christmases to come. "I see a vacant seat," replies the Ghost, "in the poor chimney-corner, and a crutch without an owner, carefully preserved. If these shadows remain unaltered by the Future, the child will die."

As we know, the beloved Tiny Tim in Dickens' *A Christmas Carol* doesn't die but lives to romp through the streets of London. But sadly, many real-life children in the nineteenth century weren't so fortunate, especially those who, like Tiny Tim, may have had rickets, a bone-softening disease that occurs when the body doesn't get enough vitamin D. It was one of the most common crippling diseases of the time.

Perhaps the saddest thing about rickets, as with other deficiency diseases, is that they're entirely preventable. These diseases occur when people don't get even the bare-bones minimum of nutrients that the body needs to thrive.

Severe deficiency diseases are rare in this country, partly because of advances in food technology and distribution that have made it possible for most foods to be available all year long. In addition, manufacturers fortify many foods with vitamins and minerals. "Our food technology has really helped make these diseases a thing of the past," says Jack M. Cooperman, Ph.D., clinical professor of community and preventive medicine at New York Medical College in Valhalla.

But even though serious deficiency diseases are rare in this country, they still occur. People who are ill with digestive disorders or other conditions may not get all the nutrients they need. People who abuse alcohol are particularly prone to deficiency diseases, as are those who live in poverty. In many parts of the developing world, in fact, deficiency diseases regularly occur.

RICKETS: NORTHERN EXPOSURE

It's not surprising that Tiny Tim, who lived in London at a time when air pollution got so thick that the sun was barely visible, may have suffered from rickets. The only practical way to get enough vitamin D, with the exception of drinking fortified milk, is by spending time in the sun. In fact, doctors sometimes call vitamin D the sunshine vitamin.

Whenever sunshine touches the skin, the body uses the ultraviolet rays to manufacture vitamin D, which is essential for transporting calcium and phosphorus into the bones. If you don't get enough vitamin D, your bones get soft and weak, sometimes bowing under the body's own weight.

Ever since food manufacturers began fortifying milk with vitamin D, rickets has become much less common. But it's hardly gone. Not so long ago, in fact, seven children in Minneapolis were discovered to have rickets. "Getting enough vitamin D can be a big problem for people living in northern climates," says Dr. Cooperman.

You don't have to bake in the sun to get enough vitamin D, he adds. For most people, about 15 minutes of sunshine on the face and hands will provide the Daily Value (DV) of 400 international units of vitamin D. Don't try to do your sunning indoors, though, he adds, since window glass absorbs the necessary rays.

Even if you get plenty of sunshine, it's still a good idea to get a little extra vitamin D in your diet. Having one glass of fortified milk will provide about 100 international units, 25 percent of the DV.

BERIBERI: A LACK OF ENERGY

The word *beriberi*, which originated in the tiny country of Sri Lanka and means "I can't, I can't," became the name of an illness supposedly because a man with the disease was so weak that he couldn't rise to meet the physician who had come to help him.

Beriberi is caused by a deficiency of thiamin, a B vitamin that is essential for helping the body utilize energy. People who don't get enough thiamin become extremely weak and may experience symptoms such as swelling in the legs or a buildup of fluids in the heart.

Although rice and whole grains naturally contain a lot of thiamin, much of this nutrient is lost during processing. Since manufacturers put most of the thiamin back into foods after processing, however, beriberi has become very rare, at least in this country. (People who abuse alcohol, though, may still suffer from severe thiamin deficiencies.) Rice, flours, cereals, and breads are all fortified with thiamin. In addition, pork is naturally high in thiamin, with 3 ounces of tenderloin providing 0.8 milligram, 53 percent of the DV.

PELLAGRA: A FRIGHTENING MYSTERY

In 1914, the year World War I began, there was another threat facing Americans. For a brief time, a terrifying epidemic swept through the South, causing diarrhea, skin inflammation, and in many cases, death. More than 100,000 people were struck down, and worst of all, nobody knew what was the cause was.

It wasn't until 1937 that scientists understood that pellagra, as the disease was called, occurred when people didn't get enough niacin in their diets. The rural South was particularly hard-hit because people there relied on corn as their main grain, and corn contains a form of niacin that isn't available to the body.

Today, thanks to the fortification of flours and cereals, we've all but kissed pellagra goodbye since it's very easy to get the DV of 20 milligrams of niacin. Meats also contain niacin. A serving of skinless roast chicken breast, for example, contains 12 milligrams of niacin, 60 percent of the DV.

SCURVY: THE SAILOR'S BANE

Long before it was understood that certain foods are essential for preventing disease, sailors worldwide often suffered from scurvy, a vitamin C deficiency that causes slow wound healing, bleeding gums, pneumonia, and eventually death. Landlubbers also got scurvy, but because they were more likely to have fresh fruits and vegetables, they didn't get it anywhere near as often as their seafaring friends.

The amazing thing about scurvy is this: You can reverse it almost instantly by having several servings of foods that are rich in vitamin C. In fact, sailors who were all but depleted of vitamin C were often able to recover in a matter of days after including oranges or lemons in their diets.

Today, the people most at risk for scurvy are not sailors but the elderly, who may find it difficult to shop for (or to eat) the proper foods. In one study, French researchers found that 20 people living in a nursing home had extremely low levels of vitamin C—low enough to cause scurvy. The problem tends to be worse in people who take aspirin frequently for pain relief, because aspirin reduces the body's absorption of vitamin C by about 50 percent.

To make sure you get enough of this essential vitamin, just pour some orange juice. One 6-ounce glass contains 73 milligrams of vitamin C, 121 percent of the DV. Other excellent sources include citrus and tropical fruits, broccoli, and sweet peppers.

DENTAL HEALTH
A TOOTH-PROTECTION PLAN

Even though teeth are hard and bonelike, they're very much alive. Like your skin, muscles, or any other part of your body, they must be well-nourished to stay healthy. "In fact, selecting nutritious foods is probably as important as staying away from cavity-causing foods," says Dominick DePaola, D.D.S., Ph.D., president of Baylor College of Dentistry in Dallas.

While there's no substitute for regular brushing and flossing, choosing the right foods, particularly those that provide large amounts of calcium and vitamins A and C, will help keep your teeth and gums strong. At the same time, it's important not to bombard your teeth frequently with sugary, sticky snacks, which make it easy for cavity-causing bacteria to flourish, says Donna Oberg, R.D., a nutritionist with the Dental Health Program of the Seattle–King County Department of Public Health in Kent, Washington.

EATING FOR STRONG TEETH

Just as bones need calcium to stay strong, your teeth also depend on this essential mineral, especially during the early years. "Calcium-rich foods are extremely important," says William Kuttler, D.D.S., a dentist in private practice in Dubuque, Iowa. "Without calcium, teeth won't form," he explains. And in adults, calcium fortifies the bone that supports the teeth so they don't loosen over time.

Getting more dairy foods in your diet is about the best protection teeth can have. A glass of low-fat milk or a serving of yogurt, for example, each contains about 300 milligrams of calcium, about 30 percent of the Daily Value (DV). You can get somewhat smaller amounts from low-fat cheeses and some leafy green vegetables like turnip greens, bok choy, and curly endive.

You need more than just calcium for good dental health. You also need a variety of vitamins, including vitamins C and A. The body uses vitamin C to make collagen, a tough protein fiber that keeps the gums strong. Vitamin A is used to form dentin, a layer of bonelike material just beneath the surface of the teeth.

It's easy to get enough of both of these nutrients in your diet. A half-cup serving of cooked broccoli, for example, has 58 milligrams of vitamin C, almost

97 percent of the DV. A half-cup serving of cantaloupe has 34 milligrams, 57 percent of the DV, and a medium-size navel orange has 80 milligrams, 133 percent of the DV.

The best way to get vitamin A is by eating foods high in beta-carotene, which is converted to vitamin A in the body. Sweet potatoes are a great source, with a half-cup providing over 21,000 international units of vitamin A, more than four times the DV. Other good sources of beta-carotene include kale, carrots, and most of the yellow-orange winter squashes. (Despite its hue, acorn squash is a beta-carotene lightweight, with only 0.2 milligram in a half-cup.)

STICKY PROBLEMS

While some foods help keep the insides of the teeth healthy, others aren't so good for the outside. Sugary foods, for example, make it possible for large amounts of bacteria to flourish in the mouth. Over time, the bacteria and the acids they produce act almost like little dental drills, wearing away the surface of the teeth and allowing cavities to form, says Dr. Kuttler.

Even fruit juices, which many people drink as a healthful alternative to sodas, can be a problem. "Juice is a very concentrated source of sugar," Dr. Kuttler explains. In fact, researchers in Switzerland found that grapefruit and apple juices did slightly more damage to teeth than cola did.

While sweet foods can be a problem, sticky foods are even worse, Dr. Kuttler says. The reason for this is that because such foods stick to the teeth, they make it easy for bacteria to remain in the mouth for long periods of time.

You don't have to give up the occasional sweet. It's important, however, to take precautions. Just take a minute to brush your teeth after eating snacks or having a sweet drink. Even if you can't brush, simply rinsing out your mouth with water will help remove sugars before the bacteria have time to do damage.

It's not only what you eat but how you eat that plays a role in keeping teeth strong. Your mouth naturally produces saliva every time you chew, so the more you chew—during a meal, for example, or while chewing gum—the more saliva there is to wash away sugars from the teeth, says Dr. Kuttler. As a bonus, saliva also contains calcium and phosphorus, which help neutralize tooth-damaging acids that form in the mouth after eating.

While you're at the dinner table, you may want to consider having a little cheese. Researchers aren't sure why, but eating cheese appears to play a role in preventing tooth decay. It may be that cheese contains compounds that neutralize acids in the mouth before they do damage, Dr. Kuttler says.

DEPRESSION
EAT TO BEAT THE BLUES

It's hardly news that many of us, when we're feeling down, seek emotional comfort in foods, particularly such "comfort" foods as candy bars, snack cakes, or macaroni and cheese. But for some people, comfort foods are anything but comforting. The very foods they eat to make themselves feel better may actually make them feel worse—listless, moody, and fatigued.

Researchers have been studying the food-mood link for decades, but the connection is still uncertain. Studies have shown that for some individuals, diet can cause depression, according to Larry Christensen, Ph.D., chairman of the department of psychology at the University of South Alabama in Mobile and an expert on the effects of sugar and caffeine on mood. What you eat can lift your mood or, if you make the wrong choices, sink it. Moreover, what you don't eat can have as great an impact as what you do.

FOOD AND MOOD

Everything you do, from thinking and feeling to taking a walk, is influenced by nerve cells in the brain called neurons. You have billions of neurons—100 billion, in fact. In order to communicate, neurons depend on neurotransmitters, which are brain chemicals with intergalactic-sounding names like serotonin, dopamine, and norepinephrine.

These chemicals do more than just communicate; they can have a powerful effect on mood as well. When serotonin is in short supply, for example, depression—as well as insomnia and food cravings—may result. Conversely, high serotonin levels can impart feelings of calm and well-being, says Elizabeth Somer, R.D., author of *Food and Mood* and *Nutrition for Women*. Changing levels of dopamine and norepinephrine in the brain can have similar results.

Research has shown that a number of nutrients, among them the B vitamins, vitamin C, and the mineral selenium, convert amino acids from our diet into mood-lifting neurotransmitters. "It's quite clear that even borderline nutritional deficiencies can lead to depression," says Melvyn Werbach, M.D., assistant clinical professor of psychiatry at the University of California, Los Angeles, and author of *Healing through Nutrition* and *Nutritional Influences on Illness*.

Research has shown that vitamin B_6, found in leafy greens, fish, poultry, and whole grains, helps elevate serotonin to feel-good levels. Even though most people get plenty of B_6 in their diets, taking oral contraceptives or undergoing hormone replacement therapy may cause B_6 levels to decline.

Low levels of folate can also send serotonin levels into a free fall, says Dr. Werbach. Of all the nutritional deficiencies in this country, being low in folate is one of the most common. The consequences can be profound. Studies show that people who are clinically depressed often have low levels of folate in their bloodstreams.

In a study in England, researchers gave people with clinical depression 200 micrograms of folic acid—the amount in about ¾ cup of cooked spinach—or a placebo. After one year, those taking the folic acid saw their depression lift significantly—in some cases by as much as 40 percent, according to standard tests used to measure depression.

Beans and greens are especially high in folate (the naturally occurring form of folic acid) and vitamin B_6. A half-cup of canned chickpeas, for example, provides 0.6 milligram of vitamin B_6, 30 percent of the Daily Value (DV). A half-cup of cooked spinach provides 131 micrograms of folate, 33 percent of the DV.

Increasing your intake of the mineral selenium can also help bring you up when you're feeling down. In a study at University College in Swansea, Wales, where soils have low selenium levels and residents tend to be low in the mineral, people were given either 100 micrograms of selenium or a placebo every day for five weeks. Those taking the selenium showed a marked improvement in their moods. What's more, the greater their original selenium deficiency, the more their moods improved.

You can meet your selenium needs by eating more fish. Just eating a tuna sandwich will give you 138 micrograms, nearly twice the DV. Selenium is also found in whole-grain cereals and breads.

CARBOHYDRATES: NATURE'S CALMING TOUCH

Is life without your morning bagel not worth living? Does your passion for pasta know no bounds? Eat up—your moods will thank you for it.

In research pioneered by husband-and-wife researchers Richard Wurtman, Ph.D., and Judith Wurtman, Ph.D., both of the Massachusetts Institute of Technology in Cambridge, diets high in carbohydrate-rich foods have been shown to increase brain concentrations of the amino acid tryptophan. The tryptophan then is converted in the body to mood-boosting serotonin.

This may explain why, for many people, comfort foods that are high in carbohydrates can help ease feelings of depression, anxiety, and fatigue. For others, not eating carbohydrates may leave them grouchy and depressed.

"Some people, particularly women, may crave carbohydrates for their antidepressant effect," says Dr. Werbach. "This phenomenon does seem to exist, although not necessarily for everybody."

Of course, some people can eat pasta, potatoes, and bread by the bushel without noticing any particular difference. But for others, known to scientists as carbohydrate-cravers, the effects can be quite pronounced. It may be that carbohydrate cravings are the body's attempt to counteract low serotonin levels.

"Many people who eat spaghetti with marinara sauce and French bread for lunch get sleepy because that carbohydrate-heavy meal raises the serotonin level," Somer says. "But carbohydrate-cravers feel energized by that same meal."

STOPPING THE SWINGS

It's hardly news that some people experience mood swings at certain times—during the dark days of winter, for example, or for some women, just before their menstrual periods. And some people, it now appears, can improve their moods during these low times simply by eating more carbohydrates.

In a study conducted by researchers at Harvard University and the Massachusetts Institute of Technology, women suffering from premenstrual mood swings were asked to drink about 7½ ounces of a special formulated high-carbohydrate drink once a month, just before their periods. Within hours of having the drink, they experienced significant reductions in depression, anger, and confusion, the researchers found.

While the women in the study consumed a specially made drink, you can get a similar amount of high carbohydrates by eating a small portion of a carbohydrate-rich food such as a cup of low-fat yogurt, a baked potato, or a half-cup of raisins.

WHEN FOOD BRINGS YOU DOWN

You've probably experienced the droopy, let-down feeling that sometimes occurs after sipping a large cappuccino or bingeing on your favorite cookies. It's not your imagination. "Consuming too much sugar or caffeine definitely contributes to feelings of depression, for sensitive individuals," says Dr. Christensen.

Experts aren't sure why sugar gives some people the blues, but it may be related to the amount you consume, says Dr. Christensen. While indulging in an occasional candy bar or doughnut can trigger a "sugar buzz" that temporarily boosts your spirits, a steady diet of sugar seems to be linked with depression.

In one study led by Dr. Christensen and a colleague, 20 people with serious depression were asked to cut all sugar and caffeine from their diets. After three weeks, these folks were significantly less depressed.

While the effects of caffeine on mood haven't been studied extensively, there's evidence that cutting back on coffee (or other high-caffeine drinks) may lift your spirits, especially if you normally drink it by the potful.

Diabetes
The New Approach

It may sound strange, but there's never been a better time to have diabetes. Gone are the days when a doctor handed you a list of what you could and couldn't eat—the same list he gave to everyone else who came in the door. New evidence has significantly altered the one-size-fits-all dietary approach to this condition.

For example, even though it's best to eat sugar in moderation (and not just if you have diabetes), for most people with diabetes it's no longer forbidden. Some may be advised to cut back on fat and eat more carbohydrates; others will be told just the opposite. In fact, it's not unusual these days for two people with diabetes, even if they are the same age, same weight, and same overall condition, to have totally different diets for controlling it.

Yet one aspect of diabetes has stayed the same. Diet—what you eat, and in some cases, what you don't—is at the heart of any treatment plan. Along with maintaining a healthy weight and getting regular exercise, eating right helps keep blood sugar and fats at steady levels, which is the key to keeping problems under control.

Hunger amidst Plenty

Before seeing how you can use food to treat or prevent diabetes, here's a quick look at what this condition is. The fuel that keeps our bodies running is sugar. Doctors call it glucose. Soon after we eat, glucose pours into the bloodstream and is carried to individual cells throughout the body. Before it can enter these cells, however, it requires the presence of a hormone called insulin. And therein lies the problem.

People with diabetes either don't produce enough insulin or the insulin they do produce doesn't work efficiently. In either case, all that glucose in the bloodstream isn't able to get inside the cells. Rather, it hovers in the bloodstream, getting more and more concentrated as time goes by. Not only do individual cells go hungry, which can cause fatigue, dizziness, and many other symptoms, but all that concentrated sugar becomes toxic, eventually damaging the eyes, kidneys, nerves, immune system, heart, and blood vessels.

The most serious form of diabetes—and fortunately, the least common—

is Type I, or insulin-dependent, diabetes. It occurs when the body makes little or no insulin of its own. People with Type I diabetes must take insulin in order to replace their own missing supplies.

Far more common is Type II, or non-insulin-dependent, diabetes. People with this condition, which occurs mainly in those over 40, produce some insulin, but generally not enough. They may take oral medications, but generally don't require insulin injections, at least not in the early stages of the disease.

THE HEALING POWER OF FOOD

Experts have long recognized that what you eat can play a critical role both in preventing and controlling Type II diabetes. Perhaps the best way to understand the effects of diet on diabetes is to look at two similar groups of people who differ primarily in what they eat.

Consider the Pima Indians. Researchers discovered that Pimas who live in Mexico and eat a lot of corn, beans, and fruits are seldom overweight and rarely develop diabetes. By contrast, the Pima Indians in Arizona eat an Americanized diet that is high in sugar and fat. They commonly develop diabetes by age 50.

Just as a bad diet can help cause diabetes, a good one can help control or even prevent it. That's the strategy that Terry Shintani, M.D., director of preventive medicine at the Wainae Coast Comprehensive Health Center in Hawaii, used when he put some of his patients with diabetes on a native Hawaiian diet. This diet consists mainly of high-fiber, high-carbohydrate foods such as taro, poi, greens, and fruits and includes plenty of fish. It was extremely effective, Dr. Shintani says. In some cases, people no longer needed to take insulin.

FUEL UP WITH CARBS

Carbohydrates, which are found in most foods except meat, fish and poultry, are the body's main source of energy. There are two types. Complex carbohydrates, called starches, include foods like rice, beans, potatoes, and pasta. Simple carbohydrates, called sugars, include the natural sugars found in milk, fruits, and vegetables as well as white table sugar and honey. The body turns both complex and simple carbohydrates into glucose, which is either immediately converted into energy or stored until needed.

Most people with diabetes should eat a diet that's higher in carbohydrates, particularly the complex kind, than was formerly believed. While your doctor, dietitian, or nutritionist will determine your personal need for carbohydrates, most people should be getting approximately 50 percent of total calories from carbohydrates, says Stanley Mirsky, M.D., associate clinical professor of metabolic diseases at Mount Sinai School of Medicine in New York City and author of *Controlling Diabetes the Easy Way*.

Watching the Numbers

People with diabetes are generally advised to reduce their intake of dietary fats and get 50 to 60 percent of their calories from complex carbohydrates. For women, this means getting 240 to 300 grams of complex carbs a day; for men, it's 278 to 333 grams a day. Here are some of the best sources of carbohydrates.

Food	Portion	Fat (g.)	Carbohydrates (g.)
Grains and Grain Products			
Bagel	1 small	1.4	31.0
Barley, pearl, cooked	1/2 cup	0.4	22.3
Cheerios	1/2 cup	2	22
Cracklin' Oat Bran	1/2 cup	6	36
Macaroni, enriched	1 cup	0.9	39.7
Oatmeal, cooked	3/4 cup	1.8	18.9
Rice, brown	1/2 cup	0.8	23.0
Spaghetti, cooked	1 cup	0.9	39.7
Wheaties	1/2 cup	1	24
Whole-wheat bread	1 slice	0.7	13.8
Vegetables			
Broccoli, boiled	1/2 cup	0.3	4.0
Brussels sprouts, boiled	1/2 cup	0.4	6.8
Corn, frozen, cooked	1/2 cup	0.6	19.3
Cucumber	1/2	0.2	4.4
Kidney beans, boiled	1/2 cup	0.4	20.1
Tomato	1	0.4	5.7
Fruits			
Avocado	1/2	15.4	7.4
Cantaloupe, cubed	1 cup	0.5	13.4
Grapefruit, pink or red	1/2	0.1	9.5
Kiwifruit	1	0.3	11.3
Orange	1	0.2	15.4
Milk and Yogurt			
Buttermilk, cultured	1 cup	2.2	11.7
Milk, skim	1 cup	0.6	13.7
Yogurt, nonfat	8 oz.	0.4	17.4
Yogurt, plain low-fat	8 oz.	3.5	16

A helpful way to plan your meals is to use a system called carbohydrate counting. Once you know how many grams of carbohydrates you're allowed, it's up to you to decide how to "spend" them. For example, it's fine to enjoy an occasional candy bar or cheese Danish, as long as you count it toward your daily carbohydrate total, just as you would a plate of pasta or a cup of rice, says Joan V. C. Hill, R.D., director of Educational Service and Programs at Joslin Diabetes Center in Boston.

A Little More Fat

While most people with diabetes are advised to cut back on fat while increasing the amount of carbohydrates in their diets, for some it's just the reverse, Hill explains.

"We've been given the message that going low-fat is right for everybody. In fact, it may not be," she says. The reason is that carbohydrates raise blood sugar faster than protein or fat does. This in turn can increase levels of triglycerides, a type of fat that has been linked with a higher risk of heart disease in people with diabetes.

In contrast, consuming fewer carbohydrates and more monounsaturated fats will lower triglyceride levels, as well as the dangerous low-density lipoprotein cholesterol. Good sources of monounsaturated fats include olive oil, avocados, and many nuts.

Obviously, experts don't advise dousing your pasta with olive oil or eating avocados by the case. Eating too much of any type of fat, including the relatively healthful monounsaturated fats, is likely to cause weight gain, which is something that people with diabetes simply can't afford.

Healing Fiber

A high-fiber diet has been shown to relieve everything from constipation to heart disease. Research suggests that it can also play a powerful role in controlling blood sugar, says James W. Anderson, M.D., professor of medicine and clinical nutrition at the Veterans Administration Medical Center at the University of Kentucky College of Medicine in Lexington.

There are two types of fiber, soluble and insoluble. Insoluble fiber, which does not dissolve in water, speeds food through the intestine, thereby preventing constipation. It's the soluble form of fiber, however, that stabilizes blood sugar, says Dr. Anderson. Because it forms a gummy gel in the intestine, soluble fiber helps prevent glucose from being absorbed into the blood too quickly. This in turn helps keep blood sugar levels from rising or dipping too drastically.

In addition, soluble fiber seems to increase cells' sensitivity to insulin, so more sugar can move from the blood into the cells, says Belinda Smith, R.D., research dietitian at the Veterans Administration Medical Center.

In studies conducted by Dr. Anderson, people with Type II diabetes who ate a high-fiber (and high-carbohydrate) diet were able to improve their blood sugar control by an average of 95 percent. People with Type I diabetes on the same diet showed a 30 percent improvement.

It's not hard to increase your intake of soluble fiber. Simply eating more fruits and legumes will naturally give you a lot more of it. So will eating oat bran or oatmeal. You can also sprinkle a tablespoon of oat bran or wheat germ over salads, cereals, yogurt, or cottage cheese and eat fruits in their skins rather than peeling them.

Help from Vitamins

If you have diabetes, fruits and vegetables rich in vitamins C and E may be your ticket to healthier eyes, nerves, and blood vessels. These vitamins are known as antioxidants. They help protect your body's cells from free radicals, naturally occurring, cell-damaging molecules that may pose particular risks to people with diabetes.

What's more, vitamin C may provide even more direct benefits. In one study, Italian researchers gave 40 people with diabetes 1 gram of vitamin C every day. After four months, the patients' abilities to use insulin had significantly improved, perhaps because vitamin C helps insulin penetrate cells.

The Daily Value (DV) for vitamin C is 60 milligrams. Oranges and grapefruit are excellent sources of vitamin C, but they're not the only ones. One cup of chopped, cooked broccoli, for example, contains more than 116 milligrams, almost twice the DV. Half a cantaloupe has about 113 milligrams of vitamin C, and one sweet red pepper has 140 milligrams.

Vitamin E, which is good for the heart, may be particularly important for people with diabetes, who are two to three times more likely to develop heart disease than people who do not have the disease. And research suggests that, like vitamin C, it may help insulin work better. Finnish scientists studied 944 men and found that those with the lowest levels of vitamin E in their blood were four times more likely to have diabetes than those with the highest levels. Vitamin E may somehow help insulin carry sugar from the blood into cells in muscles and tissues, the researchers speculate.

Vitamin E also helps keep blood platelets, which are elements in blood that help it clot, from becoming too sticky. This is particularly important in people with diabetes, whose platelets tend to clump more readily and lead to heart disease.

Wheat germ is an excellent source of vitamin E, with ¼ cup containing 6 international units, 20 percent of the DV. Other good sources of this vitamin include sweet potatoes, avocados, shrimp, and chickpeas.

CHROME-PLATED PROTECTION

It's not just vitamins that can help control diabetes. The trace mineral chromium, found in broccoli, grapefruit, and fortified breakfast cereals, has been shown to improve the body's ability to regulate blood sugar, says Richard A. Anderson, Ph.D., a biochemist with the U.S. Department of Agriculture Human Nutrition Research Center in Beltsville, Maryland.

Tests show that people with diabetes have lower levels of chromium circulating in their blood than people without the disease. In one study, eight people who had difficulty regulating blood sugar were given 20 micrograms of chromium a day. After five weeks, their blood sugar levels fell by as much as 50 percent. People without blood sugar problems who were given chromium showed no such changes.

You can boost your chromium supplies by eating foods that provide it. One cup of broccoli contains 22 micrograms, 18 percent of the DV. A 2½-ounce waffle has almost 7 micrograms, 6 percent of the DV, and a 3-ounce serving of turkey ham has 10 micrograms, or 8 percent of the DV.

MAGNESIUM FOR GLUCOSE CONTROL

Experts estimate that 25 percent of people with diabetes are low in the mineral magnesium. The problem is even worse in those who have diabetes-related heart disease or a type of eye damage known as retinopathy. Since low levels of magnesium have been linked to damage to the retinas, it's likely that upping your intake of this mineral may help protect your eyes.

Good sources of magnesium include baked halibut, which contains 91 milligrams of magnesium per 3-ounce serving, 23 percent of the DV. Eastern steamed oysters are also good: 3 ounces contains 81 milligrams, 20 percent of the DV. And a half-cup serving of long-grain brown rice has 42 milligrams, 11 percent of the DV.

PUTTING IT ALL TOGETHER

Treating and preventing diabetes with foods involves more than just eating a few good foods. It's really a whole diet in which all the separate elements—fiber, vitamins, minerals, and so forth—are brought together in one good plan. You might consider working with a dietitian to develop a meal plan that promotes blood sugar control, coordinates with medications, and is tailored to your individual preferences and lifestyle.

The best place to start is by eating a variety of fiber-rich foods. Dr. James Anderson recommends that people with diabetes get 10 to 12 grams of soluble fiber or 35 grams of total dietary fiber a day. Soluble fiber is abundant in fruits, oats, barley, and legumes, while insoluble fiber is found primarily in wheat bran, cereals, and vegetables.

You don't have to be fanatical about counting fiber grams. You can easily get enough by eating 3 to 5 servings of vegetables, 2 to 4 servings of fruits, and 6 to 11 servings of breads, cereals, pasta, and rice a day, says Smith.

Two great sources of fiber are brussels sprouts and beans. A half-cup serving of brussels sprouts contains 4 grams of fiber, with 2 grams of soluble fiber. (That's more fiber than you'll get in a cup of pasta.) A half-cup of kidney beans contains nearly 7 grams of fiber, almost 3 grams of it soluble.

Even though vitamin C is essential for people with diabetes, this nutrient is readily destroyed during cooking. For example, boiled broccoli may retain only 45 percent of its vitamin C. Steaming, which can preserve 70 percent of the C, is better. Best of all is microwaving, which preserves as much as 85 percent.

Another way to increase your intake of vitamin C is to pick the ripest fruits. Scarlet tomatoes, garnet strawberries, and deep chartreuse kiwifruit are much more nutrient-dense than fruits that haven't yet hit their prime.

To get the most vitamin E, you need to occasionally use oils rich in polyunsaturated fats, like soybean oil, corn oil, and sunflower oil. Of course, these oils don't provide the benefits of the monounsaturated fats like olive oil. Used in moderation, however, they will help boost your vitamin E to healthy levels.

When you're trying to get more chromium, barley is a good choice. One animal study done in England found that barley can help keep blood sugar levels under control. This grain makes great soups and breads and is a nice addition to casseroles.

To help your body retain the most chromium, it's helpful to eat lots of complex carbohydrates, like pasta and bagels, says Dr. Richard Anderson. Eating lots of sugary foods, on the other hand, will cause your body to excrete chromium. So even though it's fine to enjoy an occasional sugary snack, the emphasis should really be on the healthier whole foods, he says.

Diarrhea
Foods for Relief

Television commercials often portray a poor guy with diarrhea dashing to the nearest restroom—again and again. When you're the one making the dash, however, it's not so entertaining, particularly when you're doubled over with the cramps and bloating that often accompany this miserable condition.

Diarrhea usually occurs when bacteria or viruses cause inflammation in the intestine. In addition, certain foods, among them honey, sugar substitutes, and dairy foods, aren't completely digested and cause fermentation in the intestine. The body responds by drawing water into the intestine, which is what causes loose stools.

Luckily, diarrhea usually lasts only a day or two and then disappears. When it lasts longer, however, it can remove large amounts of fluids from the body as well as essential minerals that control blood pressure, heart rate, and muscle movement. This is why doctors usually recommend drinking fruit juice, flat cola, or a diluted sports drink whenever you have diarrhea. These drinks quickly replace the sugars and minerals that diarrhea takes out of you.

Until diarrhea has run its course, it's a good idea to eat only the blandest of foods, such as noodles, white bread, bananas, and applesauce, because they won't irritate an already cranky colon, says Marvin M. Schuster, M.D., director of the Marvin M. Schuster Digestive and Motility Disorders Center at Johns Hopkins Bayview Medical Center in Baltimore. An added advantage is that these foods contain fiber, which acts like a water-absorbing sponge in the intestine and helps to dry things up a bit. "The skin of apples, for example, contains the fiber pectin, which is one of the ingredients in the pill form of Kaopectate," says Dr. Schuster.

There's not a lot you can do to avoid all contact with diarrhea-causing viruses or bacteria. But if you're one of the millions of people who are sensitive to certain foods, you can prevent problems simply by watching what you eat.

Problems with Lactose

For many people, having cheese, a glass of milk, or a milkshake can, well, shake things up. This is because adults often don't have enough of the enzyme (lactase) that's needed to fully digest the sugar (lactose) found in dairy foods. In fact, about half of the world's population has this problem to a certain degree.

"Lactose intolerance is a common cause of diarrhea," says Dr. Schuster. "It's a major problem because there are so many products that contain dairy, and people don't make the connection."

If you've been having diarrhea and suspect that dairy foods may be to blame, give yourself this test. Avoid all dairy foods for a week to let your system adjust. Then drink a couple of glasses of milk, says Dr. Schuster. If you're lactose intolerant, your digestive system will let you know within a few hours that it's unhappy.

Even if you have lactose intolerance, however, you probably don't have to forfeit dairy foods completely. Researchers at the University of Minnesota in St. Paul found that people were generally able to drink up to 8 ounces of milk a day without having problems. Small amounts of cheese or other dairy foods may also be safe, especially if you have them as part of a meal rather than by themselves.

In addition, many people with lactose intolerance can eat yogurt without having problems since yogurt is naturally lower in lactose than other dairy foods.

A Toast to Health

Long before there was Pepto-Bismol, the ancient Greeks sipped wine as a digestive aid. Scientists today are finding that it just might work for traveler's diarrhea as well.

In laboratory studies, researchers from Honolulu doused diarrhea-causing bacteria with either red wine, white wine, or bismuth salicylate, the active ingredient in Pepto-Bismol. They found that both types of wine wiped out bacteria just as well as the medication did. In fact, even diluted wine worked better than the diluted pink stuff.

Although the research is promising, it's too early to say for sure whether drinking wine will do the trick against the trots. (And it certainly won't take the place of antibiotics, which are essential for some kinds of infections.) But if you decide to give wine a try, one glass is probably enough. The researchers in the Honolulu study estimate that 6 ounces of wine is all it takes to get the benefits.

A Honey of a Problem

Hot tea and honey can warm a cold winter's day better than the noontime sun. But too much of the sweet stuff can send some people running for the warm security of the bathroom. This is because honey and fruit juices contain a natural sugar called fructose. When you eat a lot of fructose, some of the sugar can slip into the large intestine undigested. Over time it begins to ferment, often causing gas and diarrhea.

Even small amounts of fructose may cause problems. Some of the people

GLOBE-TROTTING

After months of planning for an exotic vacation, the last thing you want is to spend it in the bathroom. Unfortunately, that's exactly where a lot of people wind up. Studies show that 30 to 40 percent of people traveling to "exotic" areas, which don't always have the same sanitation standards as the United States, will have encounters with traveler's diarrhea.

It's wise not to drink the water in less-developed countries, since it often harbors large amounts of bacteria. Here are a few additional tips that will help keep you in the loop and out of the loo.

Leave the lasagna. A common cause of traveler's diarrhea is restaurant food that's prepared early in the day, then reheated later on. Foods such as lasagna, quiche, and casseroles are more likely to become contaminated than dishes that go straight from the stove to your plate. To be safe, order foods that are made fresh and served hot.

Be careful in the garden. Salad greens are a common cause of traveler's diarrhea because the leaves may be washed in bacteria-laden water. The same is true of fruits. You can reduce the risk of diarrhea by avoiding raw vegetables and peeling all fruits, even apples, before eating them.

Put dairy out to pasture. When traveling abroad, it's best to leave the dairy to the cows. Local milk, cheese, and other dairy foods may not be pasteurized and can contain large amounts of bacteria.

in one study had diarrhea after eating 3 tablespoons of honey (nature's greatest source of fructose). Others had problems from just half that amount. The same is true of fruit juices. For some folks, having several glasses of juice a day won't cause problems. For others, the same amount or less may cause diarrhea, says William Ruderman, M.D., a gastroenterologist in private practice in Orlando, Florida.

If you've been having diarrhea, try cutting down on honey and fruit juices or give them up entirely, Dr. Ruderman advises. Then gradually start adding them to your diet again. Eventually, you'll find an amount that you can enjoy without having discomfort.

ARTIFICIAL PROBLEMS

Sometimes diarrhea is caused not by what you ate but by what you chewed. Sugarless gums and candies sometimes contain sorbitol, a sweetener that the digestive system has trouble handling, says Dr. Ruderman. As with fructose, sorbitol tends to ferment in the intestine, causing diarrhea.

As little as 5 grams of sorbitol—about the amount you'd get by chewing 2½ sticks of sugarless gum—may cause diarrhea. If you suspect sugarless gum has been causing your problems, you may want to switch to the regular kind. Or simply chew smaller pieces, Dr. Ruderman says.

DIVERTICULOSIS
THE FACTS ABOUT FIBER

With the Industrial Revolution came a whole new way of living. We traded sailboats for steamboats, wagons for freight trains, and whole-wheat bread for white. While the first two innovations made life easier, the last did not. In fact, it was partly responsible for a "new" intestinal disease called diverticulosis.

In the late 1800s, manufacturers developed a process that made it easy to remove the tough fibrous shells from wheat and other grains. Although breads made from these refined grains were softer and smoother, they had considerably less fiber. And this caused a lot of problems.

When there's a lot of fiber in your diet, stools are large, soft, and easy to pass. Take away the fiber, and the stools get small and hard. This makes it harder for the intestines to move them along. When the colon has to strain to do its job, it can stretch out of shape, causing small pouches to form in the muscular wall. Doctors call this condition diverticulosis. While diverticulosis was uncommon before the 1900s, about a third of Americans over age 45 have it today.

This is unfortunate, and not only because diverticulosis can lead to cramping, infection, and other problems. It's because this condition is almost entirely preventable—if you eat the right foods.

THE COLON'S BEST FRIEND

Our ancestors didn't know it, but the fruits, vegetables, legumes, and whole grains that they ate every day were protecting them from diverticulosis. It's really that simple. High-fiber foods are the secret to keeping the colon healthy, says Marvin M. Schuster, M.D., director of the Marvin M. Schuster Digestive and Motility Disorders Center at Johns Hopkins Bayview Medical Center in Baltimore.

In a four-year study of nearly 48,000 men, researchers from Harvard University and Brigham and Women's Hospital in Boston found that those who got the most fiber in their diets were 42 percent less likely to have diverticulosis than those eating the least. And although any fiber is good fiber, the men who got most of their rough stuff from fruits and vegetables got the best results.

The Daily Value for fiber is 25 grams. Eating several servings a day of fruits, beans, vegetables, and whole-grain cereals and breads will provide all the

Is Popcorn a Problem?

For a long time, doctors advised people with diverticulosis to avoid rough foods like seeds and popcorn. It was believed that hard particles of undigested food would become lodged in pouches in the intestine, possibly causing inflammation.

"That recommendation used to be in all the medical textbooks," says Marvin Schuster, M.D., director of the Digestive and Motility Disorders Center at Johns Hopkins Bayview Medical Center in Baltimore. "But there was never any evidence that these foods ever caused problems for people with diverticulosis. It was all just speculation."

While it's possible, doctors say, for a piece of popcorn or some other particle to lodge where it shouldn't, this really isn't a big concern. What is important, Dr. Schuster says, is getting more fiber, and if eating popcorn helps you get it, then go ahead and munch away. Of course, if you do have discomfort after eating certain foods, you'll know what to avoid in the future, he adds.

fiber your insides need to stay healthy.

It's important, however, not to suddenly increase your fiber intake, as that can cause gas and bloating, says William Ruderman, M.D., a gastroenterologist in private practice in Orlando, Florida. He advises adding fiber slowly to your diet by having an extra piece of fruit one day, for example, and a bowl of high-fiber cereal the next, until your body adjusts to the changes.

It's also important to drink at least eight glasses of water a day, which will help the fiber move smoothly through your system rather than getting dry and hard, says Dr. Ruderman.

The Fat Foes

Although not getting enough fiber is clearly the number one cause of diverticulosis, researchers have found that eating too many red meats or other high-fat foods can also be a problem.

Researchers from the Harvard study found that people who ate a low-fiber diet and also ate high-fat foods or 4 ounces of red meats a day were significantly more likely to get diverticulosis than those who merely skimped on the fiber.

It's not entirely clear what it is about red meats and high-fat foods that gives us a propensity for intestinal pouches. What is clear is that meats contain no fiber and don't add bulk to stools the way fiber does, says Dr. Ruderman. "And often meats replace healthier fiber foods in people's diets, which adds to the problem," he says.

FATIGUE
WHAT TO EAT
WHEN YOU'RE FEELING BEAT

Every day is the same. You slap the snooze button five or six times, then crawl out of bed—no time for breakfast. Struggle through the morning, fueled by generous mugs of strong coffee. Drag yourself to lunch. Drag yourself back to your office and muscle through the afternoon. Then drag yourself back home, where all you want is takeout, TV, your quilt, and the couch.

You're exhausted just thinking about it.

Fatigue in this country is at near-epidemic proportions. Fully half of all adults who seek medical treatment complain of fatigue. But it doesn't have to be this way. Making even small changes in your diet, experts say, can have a substantial effect on your energy levels.

BRAIN FUEL

There are some foods that make us sleepy and droopy, while others give us energy to burn. It's only in recent years, however, that scientists have begun understanding why. The answer, as it so often does, begins in the brain.

To a large extent our feelings, moods, and energy levels are controlled by neurons—nerve cells in the brain that communicate with the help of chemical messengers called neurotransmitters. Studies have shown that changes in the levels of neurotransmitters such as dopamine and norepinephrine can dramatically affect energy levels, which is why they're sometimes called wake-up chemicals. Studies show that people tend to think more quickly and feel more motivated and energetic when their brains are producing large amounts of these chemicals.

Our diets provide the raw materials needed for the production of these neurotransmitters. What we eat—or don't—can play a large role in how we feel. "We're talking about a whole symphony of brain chemicals that ebb and flow throughout the day," says Elizabeth Somer, R.D., author of *Food and Mood* and *Nutrition for Women*.

The building block for dopamine and norepinephrine, for example, is the amino acid tyrosine. Tyrosine levels are elevated when you eat high-protein foods such as fish, chicken, or low-fat yogurt.

You don't have to bolt huge amounts of protein to get the energizing effects. Eating just 3 to 4 ounces of a protein-rich food, like a broiled chicken breast or a hard-boiled egg, "feeds" your brain enough tyrosine to get the dopamine and norepinephrine flowing.

Even though protein-rich foods can help boost energy, the fats that often come with them can drag you down. Digesting fats diverts blood from the brain, which can make you feel sluggish. So don't overload a turkey sandwich with high-fat cheese and mayonnaise; dress it with mustard, lettuce, and tomatoes instead, recommends Somer.

Back to Basics

While much research has focused on the intricacies of brain chemistry, eating for energy can also be as simple as getting more fruits and vegetables and essential minerals like iron.

A study of 411 dentists and their wives found that those who consumed at least 400 milligrams of vitamin C a day reported feeling less fatigue than those consuming less than 100 milligrams. In both cases, of course, the amount of vitamin C was considerably higher than the Daily Value (DV) of 60 milligrams.

It's easy to boost the amounts of vitamin C in your diet. An 8-ounce glass of orange juice, for example, contains 82 milligrams of vitamin C, about 132 percent of the DV. A half-cup of strawberries has 42 milligrams, 70 percent of the DV, and a half-cup of cooked chopped broccoli has 58 milligrams, 97 percent of the DV.

Iron is also essential for energy. This is particularly true among women, who can lose large amounts of iron as a result of menstruation. In fact, 39 percent of premenopausal women may be iron deficient. What's more, even small iron deficiencies can leave you weary.

Fortunately, iron is very easy to get in the diet. Eating a half-cup of quick-cooking Cream of Wheat, for example, provides 5 milligrams of iron, 10 percent of the Recommended Dietary Allowance (RDA) for women and 50 percent of the RDA for men. Red meats are another good source of iron. You don't need much, says Melvyn Werbach, M.D., assistant clinical professor of psychiatry at the University of California, Los Angeles, and author of *Healing through Nutrition* and *Nutritional Influences on Illness*. A 3-ounce serving of broiled flank steak, for example, contains 2 milligrams of iron, 13 percent of the RDA for women and 20 percent of the RDA for men.

THE UPS AND DOWNS OF CARBOHYDRATES

Whereas eating high-protein foods often leaves us feeling energized, eating starchy foods like pasta and potatoes, especially for lunch, often leaves us nodding. The explanation, once again, is found in brain chemistry.

Eating high-carbohydrate foods like potatoes or rice causes an amino acid called tryptophan to be delivered to the brain. This, in turn, jump-starts the production of serotonin, a "calm-down" chemical that regulates mood. The system is highly sensitive. Eating as little as 1 ounce of rice, for example, can get the serotonin flowing.

In one study, researchers in England gave people a variety of lunches to see how their energy levels fared. One lunch was low-fat, high-carbohydrate; another was medium-fat, medium-carbohydrate; and the third was high-fat, low-carbohydrate. As you might expect, the people eating the high-carbohydrate (and also the high-fat) lunches reported feeling more drowsy and muddled than those getting the lower-carbohydrate fare.

"What you want to do is balance your carbohydrate-protein mix so that the bulk of your diet comes from complex carbohydrates, laced with a bit of proteins," Somer says. "That's how most people will improve their energy levels."

Paradoxically, the opposite is true in people known as carbohydrate-cravers. Experts aren't sure why, but these people tend to get an energy boost after eating high-carbohydrate meals or snacks. Researchers at the Massachusetts Institute of Technology in Cambridge speculate that carbohydrate cravings are the body's attempt to boost low serotonin levels.

If you're one of those people who seem to get energy after eating starchy foods, don't fight it, advises Somer. Enjoy a baked potato, bread, pasta, or other starchy food at lunch. While you're at it, feel free to eat a starchy snack—like whole-wheat crackers or a banana—to stave off fatigue at midday.

Incidentally, it's generally better to eat several small meals a day instead of two or three large meals. Smaller meals will help keep blood sugar levels stable, which will help stave off fatigue, says Wahida Karmally, R.D., director of nutrition for Columbia–Presbyterian Medical Center in New York City.

Snooze Foods

It's 3:00 P.M. Do you know where your energy is?

Not at the coffee cart. While a cup or two of coffee early in the day has been shown to boost alertness and mental functioning, drinking large amounts day after day tends to lower energy levels. The same thing is true of sweet pick-me-ups like doughnuts. The quick surge of energy, for some people, is often followed by an equally quick—and longer-lasting—crash.

"Sugar can contribute to feelings of fatigue, particularly if you're sensitive to it," says Larry Christensen, Ph.D., chairman of the department of psychology at the University of South Alabama in Mobile and an expert on the effects of sugar and caffeine on mood.

Unlike starches, which gradually release their energy into the bloodstream, sugars (called glucose) careen in all at once, causing blood sugar to spike. To cope with the sugar surge, the body releases insulin, which quickly removes sugars from the blood and carries them into individual cells. The result, of course, is lower levels of blood sugar. And the lower the level of sugar in your blood, the more fatigued you become.

Sugar can also cause fatigue by indirectly stimulating the production of serotonin, which, as we've seen, is the brain chemical that plays a calming role. That's exactly what you don't need when you're fighting off fatigue.

Experts aren't sure why caffeine tends to sap your energy, says Dr. Christensen. They do know that the caffeine buzz caused by cup after cup of coffee—or cola, tea, or other caffeine-containing drinks—is often followed by the caffeine crash.

To get re-energized, many people simply drink more coffee. This creates a cycle that can leave you alternately jittery and heavy-lidded, says Dr. Werbach.

In one study, people with a history of fatigue, depression, and moodiness were put on a sugar- and caffeine-free diet for two weeks. Not surprisingly, many of them quickly improved on this diet. More interesting is what happened later. When they resumed getting caffeine and sugar in their diets, 44 percent got fatigued all over again.

Fat Substitutes
Better Than the Real Thing

There's nothing quite like the flavor of a tender, juicy burger, the aroma of freshly baked cookies, or the smooth sensation of ice cream on your tongue. The one ingredient that really makes these foods stand out—the one that delivers aroma, flavor, texture, and feelings of satisfaction like nothing else—is fat.

Unfortunately, fat is the "ultimate" in more ways than one. Nothing adds to our waistlines the way fat does. And nothing else puts us more at risk for obesity, high blood pressure, heart disease, stroke, diabetes, and even cancer.

Researchers think that fat is so bad, in fact, that even a taste of fatty foods may cause triglycerides, which are potentially dangerous fats in the bloodstream, to rise. In one study, researchers at Purdue University in West Lafayette, Indiana, gave people crackers topped with either regular or fat-free cream cheese and asked them to chew the food and spit it out. Those who nibbled the full-fat spread ended up with triglyceride levels almost twice as high as those of the people who had the nonfat spread.

It's little wonder, then, that manufacturers are working overtime to create foods using fat substitutes and that we're gobbling them up as quickly as they hit the shelves.

Using these foods is no substitute for a diet that's high in naturally low-fat foods such as fruits, vegetables, and grains. The substitutes, however, are a great way to reduce (or even eliminate) the fat in many common foods, like cheese and salad dressings, says Christina M. Stark, R.D., a nutrition specialist in the division of nutritional sciences at Cornell University in Ithaca, New York.

Making the Bad Better

There are many different kinds of fat substitutes. Some are simply made from carbohydrates or proteins that have been processed to mimic the mouthfeel and texture of fat. Others are made from actual fat molecules that have been chemically altered so that they can't get through the intestinal wall and into the bloodstream. These fat fill-ins aren't intended for home use but are used by food manufacturers to whittle calories from snack foods, desserts, and other high-fat favorites.

And the fat savings can be substantial. Using 2 tablespoons of fat-free

Italian salad dressing, for example, can save 11 grams of fat and more than 100 calories over the same amount of the regular kind. Similarly, you can slice off 5 grams of fat and 40 calories from a grilled cheese sandwich by using fat-free cheese instead of regular American.

Fat substitutes are good in yet another way. Because they're often made from carbohydrates or proteins, they can provide a few health benefits beyond their ability to cut calories. Here's a quick guide to the most-common faux fats.

Fiber Fillers

The original and possibly the best fat substitutes are those made from carbohydrates, which are listed on food labels as dextrins, maltodextrins, modified food starches, polydextrose, and gums. They contain between 0 and 4 calories per gram, instead of the 9 calories provided by fat. Since they can hold up to 24 times their weight in water, they're often used for adding moisture to low-fat baked goods.

The best thing about carbohydrate-based fat substitutes is that they're made from fiber, says Mark Kantor, Ph.D., associate professor of nutrition and food science at the University of Maryland in College Park. "They not only have fewer fat calories, but because they contain soluble fiber, they can help lower cholesterol levels as well as help control your weight," he says.

In one study, researchers found that when people with mildly high cholesterol ate large amounts of Oatrim, a carbohydrate-based fat substitute, for five weeks, their cholesterol went down 15 percent. In addition, their systolic blood pressure readings (which measured how hard their hearts worked to pump blood through their arteries) declined and their blood sugar levels were steadier.

Although you're not likely to eat as much Oatrim as the people in the study, who essentially had it with every meal, it's good to know that it provides at least a small benefit, says Dr. Kantor.

Ice Cream Clones

There's nothing quite like the smooth, creamy texture of ice cream, which traditionally comes from the high fat content. To duplicate the mouth-feel of full-fat ice cream, manufacturers use fat substitutes made from proteins such as milk or egg whites, which glide across your tongue in the same way that fat does.

Protein-based fat substitutes, such as Simplesse and Trailblazer, are listed on the label as microparticulated protein products (MPP). Providing 1 to 4 calories per gram, they're used mainly in ice cream, butter, sour cream, yogurt, mayonnaise, and other creamy foods.

Like their carbohydrate-based kin, protein fat substitutes have health benefits besides just cutting fat, says Dr. Kantor. "Although you shouldn't depend on these foods, they do contribute small amounts of protein, which is needed for building muscle, making hormones, and fighting infection, to your diet," he says.

Other protein-based fat substitutes, called protein blends, combine vegetable or animal proteins with gums or starches and are used in frozen desserts and baked goods. Although these fat substitutes do supply some protein, the amount is not significant.

INTO THE FRYING PAN

For a long time, one of the problems with fake fats was that they didn't melt and come to a boil, which meant that they couldn't be used for making fried foods such as potato chips and crackers. This changed with the introduction of a fat-based product called olestra (Olean)—the first fake fat that could stand up to the deep fryer.

Olestra is made from large molecules that are held together in such a way that they cannot be broken down by digestive enzymes, which is why it has no calories. But even though olestra can be a real boon for snackers, it simply isn't healthful in large amounts.

Because olestra is made from fats, it absorbs and eliminates fat-soluble nutrients from your body. People who eat a lot of olestra may lose vitamins A, D, E, and K as well as fat-soluble phytonutrients such as the beta-carotene in winter squash or the lycopene in carrots and sweet potatoes. One study found that even small amounts of olestra reduced beta-carotene levels by 34 percent and lycopene levels by 52 percent. This is a serious problem, because low levels of carotenoids and related plant compounds may increase the risk of heart disease, eye damage, and certain cancers, says Dr. Kantor.

Olestra is now fortifed, so it replaces many of the vitamins it takes out. What it doesn't replace, however, is the protective phytonutrients like beta-carotene. "Most people don't get enough of these nutrients to begin with, and olestra may take away some of what they do get," says Dr. Kantor. In addition, people who eat a lot of foods containing olestra may have loose stools, abdominal cramps, and other digestive complaints.

"The bottom line is that foods containing olestra, like the high-fat foods they replace, shouldn't be staples in your diet," Stark says. "If you eat them only as an occasional indulgence, you should be able to reap the fat-reducing benefits without facing the other consequences."

FIBER
The Ultimate Healer

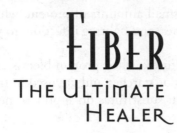

Healing Power
Can help:
Lower cholesterol

Reduce the risk
of heart disease
and cancer

Prevent constipation

Over a century ago, food manufac-
turers began stripping away the tough outer coatings of grains, leaving behind
pure white flour. Breads made with white flour had a lighter texture and more
delicate taste than whole-grain breads, and people preferred them. Other tech-
nological advances soon followed, and within a few years processed foods were
on every kitchen shelf. As a result, people began eating fewer fruits, vegetables,
legumes, and whole grains.

For the first time in history, dietary fiber was largely absent from our diets.
No one missed it very much. After all, fiber contains no nutrients. It isn't absorbed by the body, and it passes out of the digestive tract almost as quickly as
it goes in. It just didn't seem to do very much.

Fast-forward to the 1960s. Researchers began noticing that in the United
States, England, and other industrialized countries, serious conditions like diabetes, heart disease, and cancer seemed to be on the rise. But in parts of the
world where people still got a lot of fiber in their diets, these problems were
much less common. The reason, researchers guessed, was fiber. We simply
weren't getting enough of it. All of a sudden, those "advances" that took the fiber
out of foods didn't seem so great anymore.

Two-Way Protection

What is it about dietary fiber, which is simply the tough, structural parts
of fruits, vegetables, legumes, and grains, that makes it so good for our health?
The most important thing is this: Fiber isn't broken down during digestion.
Rather, it travels more or less intact from the stomach to the intestines and from
the intestines into the stool. This isn't a problem. In fact, it's precisely because
fiber isn't absorbed that it's such a powerful healer.

Although we often discuss fiber as if it were a single substance, there are actually two main types, soluble and insoluble, says Barbara Harland, Ph.D., professor of nutrition at Howard University in Washington, D.C. Most foods from plants contain both types, although they usually have more of one kind than the other. Apples, for example, contain mainly soluble fiber, while grains are high in the insoluble kind.

Even though both types of fiber pass through the intestine without being absorbed, that's where the similarity ends. They act in totally different ways inside the body, and as a result, they help protect against different conditions, says Dr. Harland. If you have high cholesterol, for example, your doctor may advise you to get slightly more soluble fiber in your diet, which can help lower the amounts of this dangerous substance in your bloodstream. People with a family history of colon cancer, however, may want to get more of the insoluble kind.

Don't worry too much about what kind of fiber you're getting, Dr. Harland adds. If you get a lot of fruits, vegetables, whole grains, and legumes, you'll automatically get healing amounts of both kinds.

Soluble Fiber: An Essential Barrier

Many of the things that cause disease, from chemicals in the environment to too much cholesterol in the diet, make their first assault inside the digestive tract. When you eat a steak, for example, molecules of fat and cholesterol pass through your intestinal wall and into your bloodstream. Or suppose there's a harmful substance inside the stool. As it rubs against the colon wall, it can damage sensitive cells, possibly increasing the risk of cancer.

It's here, inside the digestive tract, that soluble fiber provides the most protection. When it dissolves, it forms a sticky gel that acts like a protective coating, preventing harmful substances from doing damage, says Dr. Harland.

Remember the example of the steak? If you accompanied it with a bowl of beans, the soluble fiber in the beans would turn into a gel, trapping molecules of cholesterol and preventing them from getting into your body, explains Beth Kunkel, R.D., Ph.D., professor of food and nutrition at Clemson University in South Carolina. And because the soluble fiber itself isn't absorbed, it passes out of the body in the stool, taking the cholesterol with it.

Research has shown that people who get the most soluble fiber in their diets are the least at risk for heart disease. In one study, for example, researchers at the Harvard School of Public Health found that men who got 7 grams of soluble fiber a day were 40 percent less likely to die from heart disease than those getting only 4 grams.

Soluble fiber has other benefits as well. Because it causes nutrients to be absorbed more slowly, it helps people feel more satisfied after eating, so they snack less.

THE FIBER FAIR

If you asked your doctor to name the one thing you need to stay healthy, he'd probably say it was dietary fiber. Because fiber is found in so many foods, it's easy to get the Daily Value of 25 grams. To help you get started, here is a list of 42 top fiber foods.

Food	Portion	Soluble Fiber (g.)	Insoluble Fiber (g.)	Total Fiber (g.)
Cereals				
Kellogg's All-Bran	½ cup	1.0	12.8	13.8
Kellogg's Bran Buds	⅓ cup	3.0	7.0	10.0
Kellogg's 40% Bran Flakes	⅔ cup	0.4	3.9	4.3
Kellogg's Raisin Bran	1 cup	1.2	5.9	7.1
Post Grape-Nuts	¼ cup	0.8	2.0	2.8
Quaker Oat Bran, cooked	1 cup	3.0	2.3	5.3
Quaker Oat Bran, ready-to-eat	¼ cup	3.0	1.8	4.8
Quaker Oatmeal, cooked	1 cup	1.7	2.7	4.4
Fruits				
Apple	1 small	1.0	1.8	2.8
Avocado, pureed	½ cup	2.0	4.8	6.8
Blackberries	½ cup	0.7	1.8	2.5
Figs, dried	2	1.5	2.0	3.5
Gooseberries	½ cup	0.7	1.2	2.9
Guava	1	0.8	3.8	4.6
Kiwifruit	1 large	0.7	1.0	1.7
Mango	½	1.7	1.2	2.9
Prunes, pitted, dried, stewed	½ cup	2.3	1.8	4.1
Raspberries, red	½ cup	0.5	1.1	1.6

INSOLUBLE FIBER: AN INTESTINAL SPONGE

The remarkable thing about insoluble fiber is that it leaves the digestive system in very nearly the same condition in which it went in, which is why doctors once believed that "roughage" played little part in good nutrition.

Food	Portion	Soluble Fiber (g.)	Insoluble Fiber (g.)	Total Fiber (g.)
Grain Products				
Barley, pearl	³/₄ cup	1.8	2.7	4.5
Brown rice, long-grain	¹/₂ cup	0.2	1.6	1.8
Bulgur	¹/₂ cup	0.7	3.4	4.1
Rye flour	2¹/₂ Tbsp.	0.8	1.8	2.6
Wheat germ	4¹/₂ Tbsp.	1.0	4.2	5.2
Whole-wheat macaroni	¹/₂ cup	0.4	1.7	2.1
Whole-wheat spaghetti	¹/₂ cup	0.6	2.1	2.7
Legumes				
Black beans	¹/₂ cup	2.4	3.7	6.1
Butter beans	¹/₂ cup	2.7	4.2	6.9
Kidney beans	¹/₂ cup	2.8	4.1	6.9
Lentils	¹/₂ cup	0.6	4.6	5.2
Mung beans	¹/₂ cup	0.7	2.6	3.3
Navy beans	¹/₂ cup	2.2	4.3	6.5
Pinto beans	¹/₂ cup	1.9	4.0	5.9
Split peas	¹/₂ cup	1.1	2.0	3.1
Vegetables				
Artichoke	1 medium	2.2	4.3	6.5
Broccoli, chopped, cooked	¹/₂ cup	1.2	1.2	2.4
Brussels sprouts, fresh or frozen	¹/₂ cup	2.0	1.8	3.8
Carrots, sliced, cooked	¹/₂ cup	1.1	0.9	2.0
Celeriac (celery root)	¹/₂	1.9	1.2	3.1
Parsnips, sliced	¹/₂ cup	1.8	1.5	3.3
Sweet potato, mashed	¹/₂ cup	1.8	2.3	4.1
Turnips, sliced	¹/₂ cup	1.7	3.1	4.8

But insoluble fiber is more than just hardy. It's also incredibly absorbent. It can soak up many times its weight in water as it passes through the intestines. As a result, it causes stools to become larger, firmer, and easier to pass. This is why doctors recommend that people with constipation and other digestive complaints get more insoluble fiber in their diets.

Insoluble fiber helps in yet another way. Because it causes stools to become larger, the intestine is able to move them along more quickly. This is important because the more time stools and any harmful compounds they contain stay in the colon, the more likely they are to damage cells and kick off the cancer process, Dr. Kunkel says.

When researchers from the National Cancer Institute of Canada analyzed 13 studies involving more than 15,000 people, they found that people who ate the most fiber-rich foods were able to lower their risks of colon cancer by at least 26 percent. In fact, the researchers estimated that if people increased the fiber in their diets by only 13 grams a day, they might lower their risks for colon cancer by as much as 31 percent.

It's not only the colon that benefits from insoluble fiber. Evidence suggests that it may help reduce the risk of breast cancer as well.

The more estrogen women are exposed to during their lifetimes, the greater their risks of breast cancer. But insoluble fiber binds to estrogen in the digestive tract, leaving less estrogen in circulation in the body. A study by researchers at the University of Toronto and the National Cancer Institute of Canada found that women who ate 28 grams of fiber a day had about a 38 percent lower risk of developing breast cancer than those getting 14 grams a day.

Staying Lean

Even though soluble and insoluble fibers act in different ways, they combine their talents in the one area that Americans need them most: losing weight. Every year, more and more of us try to shed a few pounds, and every year we get a little heavier.

Fiber is an incredibly powerful tool for controlling weight, says Dr. Harland. Since foods that are high in fiber are very filling, you'll naturally eat a little less. Plus, when you're eating more fiber-rich foods, you'll automatically eat less of other more-fattening foods. "A very important way to lose weight and keep it off is to eat more fiber," Dr. Harland says.

Making the Change

People often think of high-fiber foods as being dry, heavy, or tasteless. But in fact, many of the foods we like best, such as fruits, freshly baked breads, or baked beans, are also high in fiber. So it's easy to get the Daily Value of 25 grams of fiber. Here are a few tips for getting started.

Start your day with cereal. Breakfast cereals have a reputation for being nutritional lightweights, but many cereals, both hot and cold, are very high in fiber. A serving of Wheaties, for example, has 3 grams of fiber in a 1-cup serving. Oat bran is also good, with 2 grams of fiber per serving.

Shop for whole grains. White bread, white rice, and other processed foods contain very little fiber. Whole grains, however, have the most. So when you're stocking up on high-fiber foods, look for breads, flour, and pasta that say "whole grain" on the label.

Mix them up. To get a good mix of soluble and insoluble fiber, it helps to eat a variety of grains, Dr. Harland says. Foods made with oats, for example, contain mostly soluble fiber, while wheat and rice contain higher amounts of the insoluble kind.

Take advantage of produce. Fruits and vegetables also contain healthy amounts of fiber, says Dr. Harland. Eating several servings of produce a day will provide much of the fiber you need. A half-cup of brussels sprouts, for example, has more than 3 grams of fiber, while a half-cup of raspberries has more than 4 grams.

Keep the peel. Much of the fiber in potatoes, fruits, and vegetables is found in the skins—the parts that many people throw away. To get the most benefit, whenever possible, serve them with their "coats" on, advises Dr. Harland.

Save the stems. When preparing vegetables like broccoli and asparagus, we often tend to throw away the stems, which are the most fiber-rich parts, Dr. Harland says. But even when the stems are too tough to munch on, you can salvage much of the fiber by cutting them into small pieces and adding them to casseroles, soups, or stews.

Stock up on beans. Regardless of whether you buy them canned or dry, beans are among the best fiber foods you can find. A half-cup of split peas, for example, has 8 grams of fiber, while a half-cup of lima beans has 7 grams.

CHICKPEAS WITH ONIONS AND RAISINS

1 tablespoon olive oil

1 cup diced red onions

2 tablespoons raisins

2 cans (15 ounces each) chickpeas, rinsed and drained

1 tablespoon chopped fresh cilantro

In a medium saucepan over medium heat, warm the oil. Add the onions and raisins. Cook for 4 to 5 minutes, or until the onions start to soften. Stir in the chickpeas. Cook, stirring, for 2 to 3 minutes, or until heated through. Remove from the heat. Sprinkle with the cilantro. Stir to mix.

Makes 6 side-dish servings

PER SERVING

calories	**159**
total fat	**4.8 g.**
saturated fat	**0.3 g.**
cholesterol	**0 mg.**
sodium	**281 mg.**
dietary fiber	**7.6 g.**

FIBROCYSTIC BREASTS
RELIEF FROM TENDERNESS

Nothing gives a woman more relief than learning that a lump in her breast is harmless. But relief can turn to frustration when the lump gets larger and more tender or when additional lumps begin appearing. Even though the discomfort eases after menstruation, it comes back month after month.

This condition, called fibrocystic breasts, occurs when tiny, fluid-filled sacs form in the milk-producing glands. For many women, making a few simple changes in their diets can help keep it under control, says Bruce H. Drukker, M.D., professor of obstetrics and gynecology at Michigan State University in East Lansing. In fact, by giving up a few foods, you may be able to eliminate the lumps entirely.

THE CAFFEINE CONNECTION

If you drink a lot of coffee, tea, or cola, your breasts may be paying the price. Beverages with caffeine contain compounds called methylxanthines, which can cause lumps in your breasts to become inflamed and tender. And the more caffeine you consume, the more tender your breasts are likely to be.

In a study at Ohio State University in Columbus, 45 women who drank an average of four cups of coffee a day quit cold turkey. After two months, 37 of the women—82 percent—reported that the lumps and tenderness were entirely gone.

Women who drink little or no coffee are much less likely to get fibrocystic breasts in the first place. Researchers at Yale University School of Medicine found that women who drank about two cups of coffee a day were 150 percent more likely to develop fibrocystic breasts than women getting no caffeine. Women who had four to five cups a day were 230 percent more likely to have the problem.

"I strongly advise women with fibrocystic breasts to eliminate caffeine from their diets," says Dr. Drukker. Just don't expect instant results, he adds. "You need to eliminate caffeine for two to three months to determine whether it makes any difference."

LEAN RELIEF

It's not only what you drink but also what you eat that can cause tender breasts. Research has shown that women who get a lot of fat in their diets—especially saturated fat, the kind found in meats and dairy foods—are more likely to develop fibrocystic breasts than women who eat leaner fare. This is probably because a high-fat diet increases the amount of estrogen in the body, which can fuel the growth of lumps in the breasts, says Dr. Drukker.

In one small study, 10 women with fibrocystic breasts reduced their intake of dietary fat to 20 percent of total calories. Three months later, all 10 said that their breast pain was gone.

"You need to eat a low-fat diet for about three months to see if it helps," says David P. Rose, M.D., Ph.D., chief of the division of nutrition and endocrinology at the Naylor Dana Institute of the American Health Foundation in Valhalla, New York, and the leader of the study. "That's how long it takes for the estrogen circulating in your blood to decrease."

To get the most protection, you should limit the amount of fat in your diet to 20 percent of total calories—the same amount used in the study, says Dr. Rose. There are many ways to reduce the amount of fat in your diet, he says. For example, you should avoid red meats, drink low-fat (1 percent) milk instead of whole milk, and eat more fruits, vegetables, legumes, and whole grains.

The Fiber Factor

Reducing fat isn't the only way to lower estrogen levels in your body. Eating more fruits and vegetables not only reduces fat but also provides more fiber in your diet "Fiber can help reduce swelling and tenderness of the breasts by absorbing excess estrogen and carrying it out of the body," Dr. Rose explains.

The Daily Value (DV) for fiber is 25 grams. That should be enough to reduce the estrogen and help ease the pain of fibrocystic breasts, Dr. Rose says. One of the easiest ways to get more fiber is to eat bran-containing cereals at breakfast, he says. Eating vegetables, fruits, legumes, and grains will also add fiber to your diet.

Get Ease with E

There isn't solid scientific evidence to prove that it works, but some women—and their doctors—say that getting more vitamin E can help reduce the pain of fibrocystic breasts. Since vitamin E helps stabilize fluctuations in a woman's hormones, it makes sense that it might help, Dr. Drukker says.

One way to get extra vitamin E is to take supplements. But getting more vitamin E in your diet can also help, Dr. Drukker says. Even though the best sources of vitamin E are vegetable oils like sunflower and safflower oils, you can get this nutrient from foods as well. A quarter-cup of toasted wheat germ, for example, has 8 international units of vitamin E, 27 percent of the DV. Almonds are also an excellent source, with 1 ounce of toasted, unblanched almonds containing 7 international units, 23 percent of the DV.

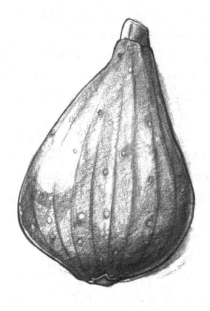

FIGS
A FABULOUS FIBER FIND

HEALING POWER
CAN HELP:
Lower high blood pressure

Relieve constipation

Control cholesterol

Prevent colon cancer

Best known in this country for its role in the ever-popular Fig Newton, the fig is perhaps the most significant fruit in history. The Assyrians used figs as sweeteners as far back as 3000 B.C. Figs were Cleopatra's favorite fruit. And some historians believe that figs, not apples, were the forbidden fruit of the Garden of Eden—a debate that may never be resolved, although certainly fig leaves were a convenient fashion accessory of the time.

Today, we know that the fig is a fabulous source of fiber and a significant source of potassium. Plus, figs can add some hard-to-come-by vitamin B_6 to your diet.

FIGS AND FIBER

The average American gets only about 11 to 12 grams of dietary fiber a day, far short of the 25 to 30 grams recommended by the American Dietetic Association. The Daily Value (DV) is 25 grams.

"Fiber is so good for so many things," says Diane Grabowski-Nepa, R.D., a dietitian and nutritional counselor at the Pritikin Longevity Center in Santa Monica, California. "Because fiber builds heavier stools, it helps you eliminate waste more quickly and efficiently, which studies show helps prevent constipation and colon cancer." Getting more fiber in your diet also helps lower cholesterol and thus the risk of heart disease.

Figs are an excellent source of fiber. Three figs, dried or fresh, provide about 5 grams of fiber, 20 percent of the DV. That 5 grams can go a long way. A Harvard University study of 43,757 men ages 40 to 75 found that those who got the most fiber had about half the risk of having heart attacks as those who got the least. Plus, men who added just 10 grams of fiber a day to their diets dropped their risks of heart disease by almost 30 percent.

"Figs are particularly good for people who are overweight, which is another risk for heart disease," says Grabowski-Nepa. Because they're so high in fiber, figs stay in the stomach longer, helping people eat less. "And they're very sweet, so they satisfy those sweet cravings," she adds.

HELP FOR HIGH BLOOD PRESSURE

Figs are a good source of potassium, a mineral that's crucial for controlling blood pressure. Studies have shown that people who eat plenty of potassium-rich foods not only tend to have lower blood pressures but also have less risk of related conditions like stroke.

Potassium helps pull down high blood pressure in a number of ways. For one thing, it helps prevent dangerous low-density lipoprotein cholesterol from building up on artery walls, says David B. Young, Ph.D., professor of physiology and biophysics at the University of Mississippi Medical Center in Jackson. Plus, it helps remove excess sodium from inside cells, keeping the body's fluid levels in balance and blood pressure in check.

Three fresh figs contain 348 milligrams of potassium, 10 percent of the DV. Dried figs are even better, with three figs providing 399 milligrams, 11 percent of the DV.

A Boost of B$_6$

Finally, figs can add some vitamin B$_6$ to your diet. While most of us get plenty of vitamin B$_6$, older people don't absorb it as efficiently as they once did. And since taking certain medications can also interfere with getting enough, getting extra amounts can be essential. Three fresh figs contain 0.18 milligram of B$_6$, 9 percent of the DV.

Getting the Most

Explore the sweetness. One reason that people in this country don't eat a lot of figs is that they're not sure what to do with them. An easy way to get more of this fiber-rich food in your diet is to add it to foods that need a touch of sweetness, like cereals, cakes, or oatmeal. You can also mash figs into foods such as mashed potatoes.

Figs Stuffed with Orange-Anise Cream

16	dried figs
4	ounces nonfat cream cheese, at room temperature
1	tablespoon fresh orange juice
2	teaspoons grated orange rind
1½	teaspoons honey
½	teaspoon aniseed, crushed

Per serving

calories	228
total fat	0.9 g.
saturated fat	0.2 g.
cholesterol	2 mg.
sodium	146 mg.
dietary fiber	7 g.

Trim and discard the stems from the figs. Cut down through the stem ends vertically and horizontally to make an X. Gently push each fig open. Place the figs on a platter, cut side up.

In a medium bowl, combine the cream cheese, orange juice, orange rind, honey, and aniseed. With electric beaters or a wooden spoon, beat until creamy. Spoon a dollop of the mixture into the center of each fig.

Serve immediately or cover with plastic wrap and refrigerate for up to 2 hours.

Makes 4 servings

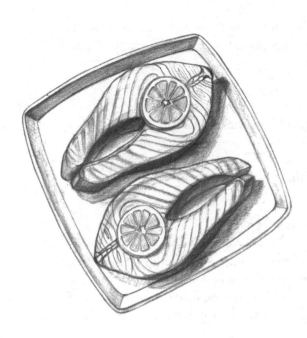

Fish
Health
from the Deep

Healing Power

Can help:
Reduce the risk
of heart disease

Prevent breast
and colon cancers

Promote larger-
birthweight babies

Reduce lung
inflammation in smokers

For years, Americans have wisely been reducing the amount of fat in their diets. But there's one fat you may want to get more of: the fat in fish. When it comes to healthy eating, fish swims to first place.

Cold-water fish contain a number of polyunsaturated fats, which are known collectively as omega-3 fatty acids. Omega-3's benefit the fish by helping them stay warm in chilly waters. In people, the same fats go a long way toward promoting better health.

Consider Greenland's Eskimos. They eat fish to their hearts' content, which may be why they have very low levels of heart disease. Similar benefits have been observed around the world. People are simply a lot less likely to die from heart disease when fish plays a role in their diets.

"While further research is needed, there is compelling research that the oils in fish may contribute to controlling several conditions," says Gary J. Nelson, Ph.D., research chemist at the U.S. Department of Agriculture Western Human Nutrition Research Center in San Francisco. A diet high in fish, which helps block the production of potentially harmful chemicals in the body, does more than reduce the risk of heart disease. It also has been shown to help fight colon and breast cancers, promote larger-birthweight babies, and reduce lung inflammation.

SWIM AWAY FROM HEART DISEASE

In the 1980s, a round of studies reported that a diet high in fish could help protect against heart disease, prompting many Americans to trade some of their red meat and poultry for a couple of fish meals each week.

They made the right choice. Research has shown that people who eat fish are less likely to die from heart disease than their non-fish-eating counterparts. What's more, you don't have to eat a lot of fish to get the benefits. Evidence suggests that two fish meals a week is all you need to help keep your arteries open and your heart working well.

The omega-3's in fish appear to put the brakes on the body's production of prostaglandins, leukotrienes, and thromboxane, naturally occurring compounds that, in large amounts, may cause blood vessels to constrict, elevating blood pressure. These compounds also may promote unwanted clotting in the bloodstream, which can lead to heart disease.

The ability of omega-3's to prevent clotting is particularly important, says James Kenney, R.D., Ph.D., nutrition research specialist at the Pritikin Longevity Center in Santa Monica, California. Clots that form in the bloodstream can block the flow of blood to the heart, possibly causing heart attacks. Further, the oil found in fish appears to raise levels of high-density lipoprotein (HDL) cholesterol, the "good" cholesterol that helps keep fatty sludge from depositing in the arteries.

Research shows that fish can offer particular benefits to people who have already had one heart attack. Having two fish meals (each including about 3 ounces of fish) a week may reduce the chances of suffering a second, fatal heart attack. It also appears that eating more cold-water fish such as salmon may help keep arteries from closing after angioplasty, a procedure used to unclog blocked blood vessels in the heart.

In addition to its favorable effects on clotting and cholesterol, the oil in fish appears to help keep the heart beating in a healthy rhythm. This is important because potentially serious heartbeat irregularities, called arrhythmias, may lead to cardiac arrest, in which the heart stops beating entirely. There is increasing evidence that the omega-3's in fish somehow fortify the heart muscle and keep it beating regularly. In one study, people getting nearly 6 grams of omega-3's a month—the equivalent of having a 3-ounce serving of salmon weekly—had half the risk of cardiac arrest as those who ate no omega-3's.

While the benefits of adding more fish to your diet are well-known, you don't want to overdo it. One study led by researchers at Northwestern University Medical School in Chicago found that those who ate more than 8 ounces of fish a week had higher stroke rates than those who ate less. This doesn't mean, however, that you should stop eating fish, says Dr. Kenney. Having small portions (2 to 3 ounces) twice a week will provide most of the benefits without the possible risks.

In the Kitchen

While fresh fish delivers some of the most delicate flavors imaginable, it goes bad in a hurry. One day may be all it takes to turn a beautiful, flavorful fish into a dish you'd rather forget. To get the best taste every time, here's what you can do.

Follow your nose. Fresh fish should smell just slightly briny. Off odors develop in the gut cavity first. When buying fish, always take a sniff in that area to make sure the fish is clean and fresh.

Incidentally, beware of fish that's prewrapped in plastic. Unless it's been frozen, it can go bad very quickly.

Look at the eyes. When buying whole fish, check the eyes to be sure they're clear, bright, and bulging. If the eyes are slightly milky or sunken, freshness is waning.

Check the gills. The gills should be moist and bright red, almost burgundy. If they are gray or brown, the fish is old, and you should pass it by.

Press the flesh. The flesh on fresh fish should be firm and springy. If you press it with your finger and the indentation remains, the fish is old and won't deliver the best flavor.

Stopping Cancer

Nutritionists have long advised us to eat less fat, especially the fats in meats and dairy products, to reduce the risk of certain types of cancer. But the fat in fish is a healthy exception. "There's excellent evidence that eating fish provides protection against breast and colorectal cancers," says Bandaru S. Reddy, Ph.D., chief of the division of nutritional carcinogenesis at the American Health Foundation in Valhalla, New York.

Fish protects against cancer in much the same way that it helps prevent heart disease—by reducing the body's production of prostaglandins. In large amounts, prostaglandins act as tumor promoters—that is, they encourage cancer tumors to grow, says Dr. Reddy.

In a study of people in 24 European countries, British researchers found that people who regularly included fish in their diets were much less likely to get cancer. Indeed, they estimated that having small servings of fish three times a week, in addition to decreasing intake of animal fats, would reduce the death rate from colon cancer in men by nearly one-third.

Better Breathing

You wouldn't think that eating fish could improve breathing difficulties caused by smoking, but that's exactly what researchers have found. People who smoke sometimes have a condition called chronic obstructive pulmonary disease, in which the ability to move oxygen in and out of the lungs is greatly reduced. There's some evidence that eating fish may help prevent this from occurring.

There's only so much that the occasional tuna steak can do to protect you from developing this disease if you smoke. But if you're trying to quit or if you live with someone who smokes, eating fish is one way to reduce the damage.

MULTIPLE PROTECTION

Here are two additional reasons to get more fish in your diet. In one study, researchers looked at the fish-eating habits of more than 1,000 expectant moms in the Faeroe Islands, an area north of the United Kingdom. They found that the more fish the women ate, the larger their babies were likely to be. In fact, babies whose moms frequently had fish were, on average, nearly a half-pound heavier than those whose moms had less. This is important because larger babies are usually healthier than those who are underweight.

Researchers speculate that the omega-3's in fish help promote blood flow through the placenta, allowing the fetus to get more nutrients. In addition, by blocking the effects of prostaglandins, which are responsible for initiating uterine contractions, omega-3's might help prevent early labors and deliveries.

Getting the Most

Shop for salmon. All fish provide some omega-3's, but salmon is perhaps the best choice, with a 3-ounce serving of Chinook salmon providing 3 grams.

Look for deep colors. The more deeply colored the salmon, the more omega-3's it provides. For example, Chinook salmon has the most oil, while the lighter pink salmon has a bit less. As a rule of thumb, the more expensive varieties of salmon generally have the most omega-3's.

Shop for variety. It's not only salmon that has omega-3's. Other good sources include mackerel, rainbow trout, tuna, whitefish (fresh, not smoked), and pickled Atlantic herring.

Enjoy it canned. One of the easiest way to get more omega-3's into your diet is to pick up a can of water-packed tuna. But if you're making tuna salad, be sure not to drown it in mayonnaise. The unhealthy fats in regular mayonnaise will more than offset the benefits of the healthy fats in the fish.

While you're in the canned food aisle, you may want to pick up a can of sardines, which also have good amounts of omega-3's.

Use your microwave. The high cooking temperatures used in conventional cooking methods such as broiling can destroy nearly half the omega-3's in fish. Microwaving has little effect on these beneficial oils, however, so it's a good cooking choice for getting the most benefits from your catch.

Microwave-Steamed Salmon with Leeks

4 **Chinook (king) salmon fillets (4 ounces each)**

1 **large leek**

1 **tablespoon grated fresh ginger**

1 **tablespoon dry sherry**

2 **teaspoons reduced-sodium soy sauce**

Per serving

calories	**229**
total fat	**11.9 g.**
saturated fat	**2.9 g.**
cholesterol	**75 mg.**
sodium	**232 mg**
dietary fiber	**0.9 g.**

Rinse the salmon with cold water. Pat dry with paper towels.

Trim both the tough green part and the root end from the leek and discard them. Cut the leek in half lengthwise. Rinse thoroughly with cold water, pulling apart the layers to remove all the grit.

Cut the leek into very thin slices. Spread two-thirds of the slices evenly over a large microwaveable plate. Cover loosely with wax paper and microwave on high power for 30 seconds.

In a small bowl, combine the ginger, sherry, soy sauce, and the remaining leeks.

Place the salmon on the plate, skin side down and with the pieces arranged in spoke-fashion so the thickest parts face outward. Pour the leek mixture evenly over the top. Cover loosely with wax paper.

Microwave on high power for 4 to 6 minutes, or until the salmon is opaque in the center. Test for doneness by inserting the tip of a sharp knife in the center of 1 fillet.

Let stand for 5 minutes before serving.

Makes 4 servings

FRENCH-STYLE TUNA SALAD

Dressing

3 tablespoons white-wine vinegar

1 tablespoon Dijon mustard

1 teaspoon dried tarragon

1 tablespoon olive oil

Tuna Salad

12 ounces green beans

2 tablespoons water

2 medium tomatoes, cut into wedges

2 cans (6 ounces each) water-packed albacore tuna, drained

Ground black pepper

PER SERVING

calories	**196**
total fat	**6.3 g.**
saturated fat	**1 g.**
cholesterol	**36 mg.**
sodium	**440 mg.**
dietary fiber	**3 g.**

To make the dressing: In a small bowl, combine the vinegar, mustard, and tarragon. Whisk to mix. Slowly whisk in the oil.

To make the salad: Combine the green beans and water in a medium microwaveable baking dish. Cover and microwave on high power for a total of 4 to 5 minutes, or until the beans are bright green and crisp-tender; stop and stir after 2 minutes. Drain in a colander; rinse with cold water to stop the cooking. Drain and pat dry with paper towels.

Arrange the beans on a platter. Arrange the tomatoes around the beans, then drizzle a little of the dressing over the beans and tomatoes. Mound the tuna on top of the beans, then drizzle the remaining dressing over the tuna. Season with the pepper.

Makes 4 servings

Cook's Note: This makes a great light lunch for 4 or a heartier dinner for 2.

FLAVONOIDS
THE HEALING PIGMENTS

HEALING POWER
CAN HELP:
Reduce the risk
of heart disease

Treat liver disorders

Inhibit the growth
of cancer

When tea first arrived on the shores of England, merchants sold it like snake oil. "Cure your migraines, drowsiness, lethargy, paralysis, vertigo, epilepsy, colic, gallstones, and consumption—guaranteed!" And the public bought it by the ton.

People didn't get the medical miracles they were hoping for, of course. And yet, they may have gotten something better. Tea, along with apples, onions, cranberries, broccoli, grapes, and other fruits and vegetables, contains tiny crystals called bioflavonoids, or flavonoids for short. These compounds, which give foods some of their colors, have been shown to help prevent a number of serious health threats, including heart and liver diseases.

What makes flavonoids so powerful is their antioxidant abilities. Antioxidants help neutralize dangerous oxygen molecules found naturally in the body, called free radicals, thus preventing them from damaging tissue and causing disease.

"We hear so much about the antioxidant capabilities of vitamins C and E and beta-carotene, but medical science is only beginning to catch on to the flavonoids," says Elliott Middleton Jr., M.D., professor emeritus of medicine and pediatrics at the State University of New York at Buffalo School of Medicine and Biomedical Sciences.

While vitamin C is found in the water inside and outside of cells, and vitamin E goes to work in fatty tissues, flavonoids do their job in both of those areas, which makes them particularly effective as antioxidants, explains Joe A. Vinson, Ph.D., professor of chemistry at the University of Scranton in Pennsylvania.

"There is a legion of things these compounds do, including boosting immunity, inhibiting cancer, preventing hardening of the arteries, and maybe even slowing down the aging process," says Dr. Middleton.

Help for the Heart

For years, researchers pondered how the French could pack away enough butter and lard to fill a Parisian pastry shop, have higher cholesterol levels than Americans, and smoke just as much as we do yet still have heart disease rates 2½ times lower than ours.

While the French may take delight in puffed pastries, they also eat a lot of fruits and vegetables. This is important because these foods, along with red wines, are good sources of flavonoids, which appear to help stop the process that allows cholesterol to stick to artery walls.

One Dutch study examined the eating habits of 805 men ages 65 to 84. They found that those who ate the most flavonoid-rich foods—the equivalent of about 4 cups of tea, an apple, and about ⅛ cup of onions a day—were half as likely to have heart disease and a third less likely to die from heart disease as those who ate the least.

In another study, Finnish researchers found that people with very low intakes of flavonoids during a 25-year period had higher risks of heart disease.

Much of the credit for these benefits goes to quercetin, one of the most powerful of the flavonoids. "Quercetin is a more powerful antioxidant than vitamin E, which is well-known for its role in heart disease prevention," says John D. Folts, Ph.D., professor of medicine and director of the coronary thrombosis laboratory at the University of Wisconsin Medical School in Madison.

It's not only the antioxidant action that makes flavonoids so protective, says Dr. Folts. Evidence suggests that these compounds may also act like a non-stick coating in the bloodstream, preventing platelets, the tiny discs in the blood that cause clotting, from sticking to artery walls and causing blockages.

In fact, flavonoids may prove better than aspirin at preventing excessive clotting, Dr. Folts adds. When people are under stress, their adrenaline levels rise, making aspirin less effective, but that's not the case with flavonoids. In one study, Dr. Folts and his co-workers gave a group of monkeys aspirin, then gave them a dose of the stress hormone adrenaline. Sure enough, the monkeys' blood started clotting. When the monkeys were given flavonoid supplements instead of aspirin, their blood continued to flow smoothly, even when they were under stress. Best of all, flavonoids don't upset your stomach the way that aspirin can, adds Dr. Folts.

Elixir for the Liver

In European countries, where natural plant compounds are commonly used for their curative qualities, flavonoids are long-time favorites. For example, European clinics commonly use silymarin, a flavonoid found in certain types of artichokes, to treat alcohol-related liver disorders. Researchers have found that in alcoholics with cirrhosis of the liver, high doses of silymarin can reduce mortality rates by about half.

In addition, scientists in the Netherlands have found that giving large doses of silymarin to animals prior to surgery can stem the liver damage that may result from oxygen deprivation during the operation.

Hope for Cancer

Just as free radicals in the body can damage blood vessels leading to the heart, they also can damage DNA, the genetic material inside cells that tells them how to function. This damage can lead to cancer. Since flavonoids help block free radicals, it would seem to make sense that they would help prevent cancer as well.

So far, a number of large studies have failed to establish a cancer-protective link. In part, this may be because researchers have concentrated on the major flavonoids, like quercetin, rather than on some of their lesser-known kin.

It appears that some flavonoids, like silymarin and tangeretin, which is found beneath the rind of oranges, lemons, and other citrus fruits, may, in fact, play a role in preventing cancer.

In studies on mice, for example, researchers at Case Western Reserve University in Cleveland found that, when applied to the skin, silymarin was able to stop tumors from forming. Other laboratory studies have found that tangeretin can help prevent the growth of human breast cancer cells. While these compounds clearly are protective, more research is needed to determine how effective they are when we get them in food.

Finding Flavonoids

It can be a bit tricky to get enough flavonoids in your diet. It's not because they're scarce but because they often hide in out-of-the-way places—in the white stuff beneath an orange rind, for example, or inside an apple's peel.

"People who eat a really good diet might get up to a gram of flavonoids a day," says Dr. Middleton. "That's good enough to provide a significant flavonoid concentration in the body, but you could do even better by consciously choosing some flavonoid-rich foods."

The richest sources of flavonoids include onions, kale, green beans, broccoli, endive, celery, cranberries, and citrus fruits (in the peel and white pulp). Also good are tea (green or black), red wines, lettuce, tomatoes, tomato juice, sweet red peppers, broad beans, strawberries, apples (with the skin), grapes, and grape juice.

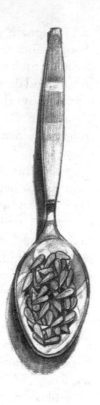

FLAXSEED

GOOD FOR THE HEART—AND MORE

HEALING POWER

CAN HELP:
Improve kidney function

Reduce the risk
of heart disease

Prevent cancer

For centuries, flaxseed (and the plant from which it comes) was used for just about everything except food. Flax is one of the oldest sources of textile fiber and is used in making linen. Its seed, also known as linseed, is used for making paint. In the modern world, the closest it ever came to being a food was its use as a livestock feed.

Until recently, that is.

Nowadays, because of its new-found fame as a "health food," Americans are enjoying the slightly sweet, nutty taste of flaxseed. And they're getting protection from heart disease and cancer as a reward.

CANCER CONTROL

Flaxseed is an incredibly rich source of a group of compounds called lignans. While many plant foods also contain lignans, flaxseed has the absolute most—at least 75 times more than any other plant food. (You'd have to eat about 60 cups of fresh broccoli or 100 slices of whole-wheat bread to get the same amount of lignans that are in ¼ cup of flaxseed.) This is important because lignans may have powerful antioxidant properties that can help block the damaging effects of harmful oxygen molecules called free radicals. These molecules are thought to cause changes in the body that can lead to cancer.

IN THE KITCHEN

Unlike pumpkin or sunflower seeds, which you can eat out-of-hand, flaxseed is usually used as an ingredient in other foods. Here are a few ways that you can prepare it.

Soften them up. Since flaxseed is protected by a tough outer shell, soaking a few tablespoons of seeds overnight in a little water will make them soft enough to eat. Then you can either eat them by the spoonful or add them to cereals or even a fruit shake.

Grind them fine. An easy way to get more flaxseed in your diet is to grind the seeds in a spice or coffee grinder and add the ground meal to muffins, breads, or other baked goods. You can replace several tablespoons of your usual flour with flax flour without noticeably changing the taste or texture of the food.

"Lignans subdue cancerous changes once they've occurred, rendering them less likely to race out of control and develop into full-blown cancer," says flax researcher Lilian Thompson, Ph.D., professor of nutritional sciences at the University of Toronto.

Lignans show particular promise for battling breast cancer. They do this by blocking the effects of estrogen, which, over time, seems to increase breast cancer risk in some women. Even when estrogen-sensitive tumors get a chance to grow, lignans exert a restraining influence that can slow or even halt their growth. In a laboratory study, breast tumors in animals given flaxseed shrank by 50 percent in seven weeks.

Flaxseed has two additional cancer-fighting secrets. It's a rich source of polyunsaturated fats, including omega-3 fatty acids, which appear to limit the body's production of chemicals called prostaglandins. This is important because prostaglandins, in large amounts, can "speed up tumor growth," says Bandaru S. Reddy, Ph.D., chief of the division of nutritional carcinogenesis at the American Health Foundation in Valhalla, New York.

In addition, flaxseed is very high in fiber. Three tablespoons of seeds contains 3 grams of fiber, about 12 percent of the Daily Value. Fiber in the diet is very important because it can help block the effects of harmful compounds in the body that over time may cause damage to cells in the intestine and lead to cancer. It also helps to move these compounds out of the intestine more quickly, making them less likely to do harm.

HEART AND KIDNEY HELPER

Some of the same compounds in flaxseed that help battle cancer also show promise for reducing the risk of heart disease. Studies show that the omega-3 fatty acids that flaxseed contains (which are also found in fish) appear to reduce the incidence of blood clotting that can increase the risk of heart disease and stroke.

Flaxseed also appears to lower levels of dangerous low-density lipoprotein (LDL) cholesterol, the kind that contributes to heart disease. In one small study, people who ate 50 grams (about 5 tablespoons) of flaxseed each day for four weeks were able to reduce their levels of harmful LDL cholesterol by as much as 8 percent.

In addition, flaxseed shows promise for reversing kidney damage caused by lupus, a condition in which the immune system produces harmful substances that attack and damage healthy tissues. When researchers at the University of Western Ontario gave flaxseed to nine people with lupus-related kidney disease, they discovered that several measurements of kidney function, including the ability to filter waste, quickly improved. The researchers speculate that the lignans and omega-3's in flaxseed fight inflammation in the tiny and very fragile arteries that supply blood to the kidneys, helping reduce the artery-clogging process that can lead to kidney damage.

Finally, laboratory research suggests that the lignans in flaxseed may have bacteria- and fungus-fighting abilities, which means that it could be an aid in fighting infections.

Getting the Most

Buy it processed. Many people sprinkle whole flaxseed on salads or fresh-baked breads. Flaxseed in this form provides little benefit, however, because the body is unable to crack open the hard little shells. So it's actually best to buy the cracked or milled forms, which readily give up the nutritious goodness that is packed inside.

Pass on the oil. Some manufacturers, in an attempt to capitalize on flaxseed's healthful reputation, are touting flaxseed oil as a source of omega-3's. Some are even offering high-lignan oil that contains some of the seed residue.

But you shouldn't spend your money just yet. There are good reasons to let the oil slide.

Most of the lignans found in flaxseed are in the meal, which is the non-oil part of the seed. While the oil may contain some lignans, it can't compete with the seeds. In addition, while flaxseed oil isn't without benefits, it doesn't provide as much of the other healthful compounds found in the seeds, like fiber, protein, and minerals.

"Even though you might get the same amount of one health-promoting substance from the oil, it's better to go for the whole food," says Cindy Moore, R.D., director of nutrition therapy at the Cleveland Clinic Foundation in Ohio. "Chances are, you'll be getting other substances that you need for good health that researchers haven't even discovered yet."

FLAX BANANA BREAD

½ cup packed light brown sugar
½ cup low-fat buttermilk
¼ cup fat-free egg substitute
3 tablespoons canola oil
¾ cup unbleached all-purpose flour
½ cup whole-wheat flour
¾ cup ground flaxseed
1 teaspoon baking powder
1 teaspoon baking soda
⅛ teaspoon salt
1 cup pureed bananas

PER SLICE

calories	**202**
total fat	**8.3 g.**
saturated fat	**0.4 g.**
cholesterol	**0 mg.**
sodium	**227 mg.**
dietary fiber	**2.4 g.**

Preheat the oven to 350°F. Coat a no-stick 8″ × 4″ loaf pan with no-stick spray.

In a large bowl, combine the sugar, buttermilk, egg substitute, and oil. Whisk until smooth.

In a medium bowl, combine the unbleached flour, whole-wheat flour, flaxseed, baking powder, baking soda, and salt. Whisk to mix. Add to the liquid ingredients. Stir just until blended; do not overmix. Add the bananas and stir to mix.

Pour into the prepared pan. Bake for 40 to 50 minutes, or until a knife inserted in the center comes out clean. Remove the pan to a wire rack and let the bread cool slightly. While it is still slightly warm, turn the bread out of the pan.

Makes 10 slices

Cook's Notes: For best results, choose very ripe bananas, place them in a blender or food processor, and puree until smooth.

Ground flaxseed is sold in natural food stores. Store any unused flaxseed in a tightly sealed container in the refrigerator or freezer.

Food Allergy
The Dangers of Dining

A man who is allergic to shellfish orders a hamburger and fries. Minutes after his meal, he's gasping for breath. He finds out later that the oil used for the french fries was also used to fry shrimp.

A woman with an allergy to mustard orders chicken. After finishing her meal, she begins feeling faint. It turns out that the chicken was coated in a batter containing mustard.

When it comes to food allergies, knowing which foods will trigger an attack isn't always enough, since the offenders can appear in the most unexpected places. That's the problem with food allergies: You have to be on guard literally all the time.

Confused Defenses

Food allergies occur when your body's immune system mistakenly identifies food proteins as enemies rather than friends. When you eat an offending food, your immune system launches an attack. The result may be congestion, digestive complaints, itchy skin, swelling of the mouth and hands, and even difficulty breathing. Even healthful foods such as low-fat milk or wheat are capable of triggering this assault.

Food allergies are most common in children. Usually they outgrow them, but some allergies, mainly those involving peanuts and shellfish, can last a lifetime, says Talal M. Nsouli, M.D., clinical associate professor of allergy and immunology at Georgetown University School of Medicine and director of the Watergate Allergy and Asthma Center, both in Washington, D.C. Foods that commonly cause allergies include eggs, soy, wheat, peanuts, and shellfish, although any food is capable of causing problems in some people, Dr. Nsouli says.

Food allergies usually run in families, says Sheah Rarback, R.D., spokesperson for the American Dietetic Association in Miami. In fact, if one of your parents has a food allergy, you have a 20 to 30 percent chance of developing one yourself. And if both of your parents have food allergies, your risk climbs to 40 to 50 percent.

It's not clear what causes food allergies. One theory, says Dr. Nsouli, is that infants and children who eat problem foods before their immune systems have

Earaches: The Food Connection

Ear infections are one of the most common reasons for office visits to pediatricians, and they're also the leading reason for surgery on children in the United States. They're frustrating to treat because, despite taking antibiotics, some children get the infections over and over again.

Food allergies may play a key role in ear infections, says Talal M. Nsouli, M.D., clinical associate professor of allergy and immunology at Georgetown University and director of the Watergate Allergy and Asthma Center, both in Washington, D.C. The reason is that children who are allergic to foods often have frequent congestion. As fluids and bacteria accumulate in the tube connecting the nose and middle ear, infections are much more likely to occur.

In a study done by Dr. Nsouli and his colleagues, 81 of 104 children with recurrent ear infections were found to have food allergies. In fact, when Dr. Nsouli put the children on diets without the offending foods, most had significant improvements. When the children who had improved were allowed to eat the foods again, 94 percent got another ear infection.

"Any child who has recurrent ear infections should go to an allergist," Dr. Nsouli says.

fully matured may develop life-long allergies to those foods. For this reason, doctors often recommend that infants should not be given solid food until they're six months old and that cow's milk should be avoided until after the first year. In addition, eggs should be avoided until after the second year and fish and peanuts until after the age of three. Another way to prevent food allergies in children is to breastfeed them as infants.

Little Tastes, Big Problems

People with mild allergies may be able to eat small portions of an offending food every once in a while. But for some people, the allergies are so severe that even a trace of the food can cause a potentially life-threatening condition called anaphylaxis. For those with serious allergies, the problem foods "should be avoided like poisons," Dr. Nsouli says.

Because it's often hard to know exactly what is in the foods you eat, doctors advise that people with severe food allergies should carry self-injecting syringes loaded with epinephrine. This medication can stop anaphylactic attacks almost instantly, says William Ziering, M.D., assistant clinical professor at the University of California School of Medicine and an allergist at the Ziering Allergy and Respiratory Center, both in Fresno.

Eating Safely

Even though there is no cure for food allergies, there are many things you can do to prevent attacks. For starters, always read labels carefully. You can't assume that a product doesn't contain the offending ingredient, Dr. Nsouli says. If you're allergic to peanuts, for example, it's obvious that peanut butter is *verboten*. But many other foods, including plain M&M's candies, also contain peanuts, in the form of peanut powder.

To make things more complicated, food companies may throw consumers a curveball by periodically changing ingredients in their products, Rarback says. Just because a food doesn't contain an offending ingredient today doesn't mean that it never will. "You can never rest," Rarback says. "You have to keep reading the labels."

If all food labels used everyday language, such as "milk," for example, or "wheat," avoiding certain foods would be easy. But in the complex world of food processing, it's not always easy to tell what you're getting. That's why people with food allergies often need a crash course in food vocabulary. If you're allergic to dairy foods, for example, you'll soon learn that ingredients such as casein and whey are just as dangerous as a glass of milk. Be sure to ask your doctor for a complete list of the products and ingredients that you'll need to avoid, Dr. Nsouli says.

Even when you know what foods to avoid, eating in restaurants can be tricky since you can't control what goes into each dish. Quiz the cook, Rarback advises. Ask about oils, spices, and any other ingredients that you may be concerned about.

One way to make sure your dinner doesn't take you by surprise is to tell people just how serious your food allergy is. Explain that it's not only certain ingredients that can make you ill but even what those ingredients have touched, like mixing bowls and spoons. "Warn them," Dr. Nsouli says. Once they understand how serious your condition really is, they'll pay closer attention to what goes on your plate.

Some foods are very easy to eliminate from your diet because there are so many substitutes available. People who are allergic to cow's milk, for example, often switch to soy or rice milk, says Dr. Nsouli. (These products are often fortified with calcium, so you get the benefits of milk without the problems.) Other foods are more difficult to replace. Even though you can make bread with rice flour, for instance, it doesn't have quite the taste or texture of bread made with wheat. You may want to try rye, millet, or barley flour instead. You'll just have to experiment to find foods that satisfy your taste buds without upsetting your system.

Food Supplements
When Diet Lets You Down

Try as you might to eat 2 to 3 servings of fruits, 3 to 5 servings of vegetables, and 6 to 11 servings of grains every day, sometimes all you can manage is a superburger accompanied by an equally large serving of fries.

We live fast-paced lives, and we spend too many lunch hours rushing through fast-food lines. So we head to the supermarket or pharmacy, where we load up on vitamins, minerals, and food extracts in the hope that the pills in these bottles will give us a little health insurance when our diets let us down.

But are they doing us any good?

"They certainly can," says Mary Ellen Camire, Ph.D., chair and associate professor in the department of food science and human nutrition at the University of Maine in Orono. "When you're running around and skipping meals, taking a multivitamin can help you get nutrients that you may be missing."

In fact, many doctors now believe that supplements do more than make up for shortfalls in nutrition. Evidence suggests that even when you're eating well, taking supplements will make you healthier, says Michael Janson, M.D., author of *The Vitamin Revolution in Health Care*.

"The scientific literature is clear that people who get certain nutrients, like vitamins C and E, in higher levels than you can get from foods are going to get additional benefits," says Dr. Janson.

Beyond the Minimum

For more than 50 years, the federal Food and Nutrition Board has been telling us how much of the various nutrients we should try to get from foods each day. The board's recommendations, called Recommended Dietary Allowances, are meant to serve as goals for basic good nutrition. (A shorthand version of these recommendations, called Daily Values, or DVs, are the numbers that you see on food labels.)

In recent years, however, scientists have begun finding connections between vitamins and a number of health threats, such as cancer and heart disease, that no one was aware of previously. Even though the DVs are high enough to prevent deficiency diseases such as rickets and scurvy, they may not be high enough to have an impact on preventing other diseases.

This is particularly true of the antioxidants like vitamins C and E. Antioxidants are essential for blocking the effects of free radicals, destructive oxygen molecules that damage healthy cells throughout the body and are thought to be a major contributor to heart disease, cancer, and other serious conditions. Because free radicals are created in enormous numbers every day, the amounts of antioxidants represented by the DVs may not be high enough to stop the damage.

In addition, it can be difficult to get enough of some nutrients from food alone. About the only place you can get large amounts of vitamin E, for example, is in vegetable oils and other high-fat foods. When people reduce the amount of fat in their diets, they may get smaller amounts of vitamin E as well. "A vitamin E supplement may help you reach your goal—without all the fat," says Joanne Curran-Celentano, R.D., Ph.D., associate professor of nutritional science at the University of New Hampshire in Durham.

How High Should You Go?

The research is still fairly new, so scientists aren't sure how far above the DV you should aim. But for some nutrients, such as vitamin C, evidence suggests that you need two to four times the DV to get maximum protection.

In a study of more than 1,500 middle-aged men, for example, researchers in Chicago found that those who got 138 milligrams of vitamin C a day (along with small amounts of beta-carotene) were 37 percent less likely to die from cancer than those getting 66 milligrams of vitamin C a day. (The DV is 60 milligrams.) Other studies have shown that getting amounts of vitamin C above and beyond the DV can boost immunity, improve lung function, and lower the risks of cancer, heart disease, and cataracts.

Vitamin E is a very powerful antioxidant. Studies show that it can block the process that causes cholesterol to stick to artery walls, while at the same time preventing platelets, the blood components that are responsible for clotting, from clumping together in the bloodstream and raising the risk of heart disease. Studies show that it's most effective, however, when you get far more than the DV of 30 international units. In fact, researchers at the University of New South Wales in Australia have found that the minimum amount of vitamin E you need to prevent heart disease is about 500 international units, which is more than 16 times the DV. It's almost impossible to get that much vitamin E from foods alone. "Most healthy people would benefit from getting additional vitamin E," says Dr. Janson.

While supplements make sense for some nutrients, the picture isn't quite so clear with beta-carotene. Even though foods rich in beta-carotene, such as carrots, spinach, and kale, have been shown to help prevent a variety of illnesses, including cancer, beta-carotene supplements haven't proven as useful. It appears that this nutrient works best when it's taken in combination with other protective plant compounds—in other words, when you get it in its natural form from foods.

Besides, the amount of beta-carotene that seems to be protective, which is somewhere between 6 and 10 milligrams a day, is easy to get from foods. One sweet potato, for example, contains almost 15 milligrams of beta-carotene. Other good sources include bright orange and dark green vegetables such as winter squash, collard greens, and broccoli and fruits such as cantaloupe and dried apricots.

Some people, however, simply don't get enough fruits and vegetables. That's when beta-carotene supplements may be helpful, says Dr. Janson.

The Incredible Shrinking Foods

The next time you're buying vitamins and minerals, check out the new-comers on the shelves. Unlike vitamin and mineral supplements, which contain isolated nutrients, the so-called nutraceutical supplements contain compounds extracted from whole foods, then concentrated and shrunk down into a Jetson-like pill. You'll find pills containing broccoli, spinach, tomatoes, mixed vegetables, and many other foods.

The advantage of nutraceuticals is that they contain not just one vitamin or mineral but all of the compounds that are naturally found in foods, in the same proportions that nature intended.

Can they take the place of the real thing?

Probably not. Most researchers feel that it's unrealistic to think that you can reduce foods down to pills and still get all the benefits. For one thing, even if the pills contain all of the health-protecting compounds that you'd get from fruits and vegetables, they may not contain the fiber, says Dr. Camire. Plus, the process of making the pills may damage some of the healthful chemicals they contain. "Mother Nature's chemicals are much more potent than the ones we make in our factories," she adds.

At the very least, however, vegetables-in-a-pill may provide a bit of a hedge for folks who aren't always able to eat the way they'd like to. "There are a lot of people out there who simply do not and will not eat vegetables," says Dr. Camire. "In that case, the pills might be somewhat beneficial."

It's important, however, to read labels carefully, she explains. Some products that are called nutraceuticals actually contain just one or a few isolated ex-tracts—of carotenoids, for example—and not the full complement of health-promoting compounds found in the real foods. When buying nutraceu-ticals, check the label to be sure they contain a variety of nutrients. "Scientists still don't know how all these chemicals work," she says. "In isolation, they may be worthless—or worse, harmful to your health."

Free Radicals
A Natural Danger

Oh, no!" shrieked Dorothy, as she, the Scarecrow, and the Cowardly Lion looked on in horror as their metallic friend stiffened in the rain. "The Tin Man is rusting!"

The wizard-bound bunch should have been more careful than to leave their iron-clad friend stranded in the rain. When moisture meets iron, it undergoes a chemical process called oxidation, causing the reddish coating that we know as rust.

Unlike the Tin Man, we don't have to worry about rusting in the rain. But the same oxidation that causes metal to rust is also at work inside our bodies.

As the word suggests, oxidation simply means that something has reacted with oxygen. More specifically, it means that oxygen molecules have lost an electron during their interactions with other molecules. These renegades become what scientists call free radicals—wounded, unstable oxygen molecules that are just as dangerous as their name sounds. In their quest to "heal" themselves, free radicals steal electrons from any healthy molecule they can grab, creating more free radicals in the process.

What does this have to do with us? Whenever oxygen mixes with other molecules, free radicals form. Slice a banana and the oxygen-exposed fruit turns brown from free radical damage. Inhale, and you too have been exposed. In fact, every breath we take generates free radicals, which, as they seek to stabilize themselves, damage our healthy cells.

The damage that free radicals do is staggering. More and more research is showing that free radical damage contributes to many major illnesses, including hardening of the arteries, degenerative eye diseases such as macular degeneration, certain cancers, and even aging itself.

Living with the Enemy

It's a mistake to think of free radicals as being foreign invaders like viruses or bacteria. Most free radicals are manufactured within your own body. "People often don't realize that free radicals occur naturally," says Balz Frei, Ph.D., director of the Linus Pauling Institute at Oregon State University in Corvallis.

Heavy Breathing: Is It Safe?

Breathe in. Breathe out. You've just generated hundreds of free radicals.

Breathe in. Breathe out. Pant. Pant. Pant. A couple of miles on your Nikes and now you've created thousands of free radicals. Is all this exercise really good for you?

Recently, there's been some concern that exercise, which is supposed to make us healthier, may speed the production of free radicals to potentially dangerous proportions. If free radicals are a by-product of energy production, scientists reason, then exercise must result in a free-radical overload.

"Because it turns up the metabolism, exercise does create more free radicals," says Balz Frei, Ph.D., associate professor of medicine and biochemistry at Boston University School of Medicine. "But remember, free radicals are only damaging when they're not balanced by neutralizing antioxidants. People who exercise also typically have healthier lifestyles, so they have more antioxidant stores. Plus, the benefits you get from exercise are enormous and very well established. People should not stop exercising because they're worried about free radicals," he says.

"The body produces them when it generates energy."

Normally, every cell in your body transforms the oxygen you breathe into water. But about 1 percent of the oxygen leaks from the production chain. It's this 1 percent that turns into free radicals, says Dr. Frei.

"White blood cells also generate free radicals purposely, in order to kill invading bacteria and microorganisms," he adds. "Unfortunately, these free radicals don't have very good aim, and they end up not just killing the foreign bacteria but also causing damage to healthy tissue."

Staying in Balance

So if every breath that we take creates a free radical free-for-all, what prevents us from deteriorating soon after we suck our first breaths of air? In keeping with the laws of nature, for every force there is a counterforce. And for every free radical that our bodies produce, there is an antioxidant to control it.

You've heard of antioxidants such as vitamins C and E and beta-carotene. Antioxidants literally come between free radicals and your body's healthy molecules. By offering up their own electrons, antioxidants stabilize free radicals and stop them from doing further damage.

Nature anticipated the danger from free radicals and made preparations.

As we've seen, certain foods are loaded with antioxidant vitamins. In addition, just as your body manufactures free radicals, it also manufactures antioxidants to block their effects.

"We have a whole orchestra of defense mechanisms to detoxify free radicals," explains Robert R. Jenkins, Ph.D., professor of biology at Ithaca College in New York. "As free radicals are being made, our bodies are detoxifying them, either with antioxidant enzymes or vitamins."

In addition to the free radicals generated within our bodies, we live in an environment that also creates them in huge numbers. Exposure to such things as pollution, ultraviolet light, radiation, and car exhaust vastly increases free radical production.

"Cigarette smoking, for example, is a significant external source of free radicals," says Dr. Frei. "When you're producing such an excess of free radicals, your antioxidants have a hard time keeping up." In fact, it takes 20 milligrams of vitamin C—one third of the Daily Value—to neutralize the effect of just one cigarette.

THE DAMAGE THEY DO

Once free radicals are running rampant, the damage they cause mostly depends upon where they launch their attacks. "The best example of the damage free radicals can cause is atherosclerosis, or hardening of the arteries," says Dr. Frei. "It's well-documented that free radicals contribute to this disease in a very important way."

Cardiovascular disease often occurs when the "bad" low-density lipoprotein (LDL) cholesterol in your bloodstream clumps together and sticks to your artery walls, causing hardening and blockages. Scientists have found that free radical damage is the reason that LDL cholesterol begins sticking to the artery walls.

Other times, free radicals may go for your DNA. When they damage those critical strands of genetic information, cells may undergo changes that cause them to replicate uncontrollably. In other words, they may become cancerous, says Dr. Frei.

Free radicals can also cause damage to your eyes. In a study that will send you searching for your Ray-Bans, researchers from Harvard Medical School found that there is a strong link between macular degeneration, which is the leading cause of irreversible vision loss in people over the age of 50, and free radical damage. Beautiful though it is, sunshine contains a tremendous amount of dangerous ultraviolet (UV) light, which is one of the leading producers of free radicals.

And your eyes aren't all that suffers under the sun's powerful rays. So does your skin. Free radical damage caused by UV rays is also believed to be the perpetrator responsible for wrinkles, skin thickening, and other signs of premature skin aging.

Although the research is still highly speculative, free radicals may also be one of the keys to unlocking mysterious neurological disorders like Alzheimer's and Parkinson's diseases. Some scientists believe that free radicals may poke holes in the barrier that usually shields the brain from outside invaders like viruses and bacteria. In response to the injury, the immune system produces more free radicals, which may cause damage that researchers believe leads to neurological disease.

"Very often, free radicals aren't involved in initiating the disease," Dr. Jenkins adds, "but the free radicals that result from the disease itself keep the damage going."

Such is the case with rheumatoid arthritis. The inflammation within joints creates free radicals, which seem to do more damage than the actual disease itself. The same can be said for many digestive diseases. Free radicals may not be the cause of inflammatory bowel diseases like Crohn's disease, but they certainly do contribute to the damage.

FIGHTING FREE RADICALS

If breathing and being in the sun are such risky propositions, how can you be sure that your body has sufficient antioxidant reserves to ward off free radical attacks? "Aside from avoiding things that you know generate excessive amounts of free radicals, like cigarette smoke, one of the best things that you can do for yourself is eat a plant-based diet that's rich in fruits and vegetables," advises Dr. Jenkins.

Fruits and vegetables contain an abundance of natural antioxidants, particularly vitamins C and E and beta-carotene as well as dozens of other free radical–fighting compounds. "When you look at long-term population studies, people eating vegetarian diets appear to gain protection from diseases that are believed to be related to free radical damage," says Dr. Jenkins. "They live longer, healthier lives."

For optimum antioxidant protection against free radicals, he suggests that people increase their intake of vitamin C to between 200 and 400 milligrams and increase their daily doses of vitamin E to between 100 and 400 international units.

In the Cambridge Heart Antioxidant Study, which followed 2,000 people with atherosclerosis, researchers found that those getting between 400 and 800 international units of vitamin E daily for a year could reduce their risk of heart attack by about 75 percent.

Research has also shown that people with the highest intakes of carotenoids—plant compounds that are powerful antioxidants—had a 43 percent lower risk of macular degeneration than those getting the lowest amounts.

Some of the best food sources of antioxidant compounds include vitamin C–packed citrus fruits, broccoli, green and sweet red peppers, and dark green leafy vegetables; beta-carotene–rich carrots, sweet potatoes, and spinach; and wheat germ and vegetable oils, which are loaded with vitamin E.

"You also need to keep things in perspective," adds Dr. Frei. "Even if it turns out that free radicals play a major role in disease, they are still only one player among many factors. You shouldn't get too panicky about them. Rather, live healthfully, eat sensibly, and exercise."

GALLSTONES
CLEANING UP THE CLUTTER

Even though your body needs some cholesterol, this thick, gummy substance has earned a reputation for being nothing but trouble—and with good reason. In large amounts, cholesterol not only contributes to heart disease, high blood pressure, and stroke but it also plays a role in the formation of gallstones, which are hard, compact little nuggets that can cause excruciating pain.

As the name suggests, gallstones form in the gallbladder, which is simply a storage area for bile (also known as gall) that the body uses to digest fats in the small intestine. This bile is normally in a liquid state, with small particles of cholesterol, protein, and fat mixed in.

But when you get too much fat and cholesterol in your diet, there's a tendency for these particles to come together and form gallstones, says Henry Pitt, M.D., director of the Gallstone and Biliary Disease Center at Johns Hopkins Hospital in Baltimore.

So it makes sense that the best advice for people who are prone to stones is to eat fewer red meats and whole-fat dairy foods and less of anything else that contains large amounts of fat and cholesterol, says Dr. Pitt.

Another way to help prevent gallstones is simply to eat more often. Since gallstones are caused by buildups of debris, making the gallbladder contract more often will help remove debris before it compacts into stones, says Robert Charm, M.D., assistant clinical professor of medicine at the University of California, Davis, School of Medicine and a gastroenterologist in Walnut Creek, California. The gallbladder contracts every time you eat, so having several small meals a day rather than two or three large ones will help keep it active and debris-free. Drinking a lot of water will also help keep stones from forming.

Fish may be an important part of an anti-gallstone plan. Fish and seafood contain a type of fat called omega-3 fatty acid, which has been shown to help lower cholesterol levels. Preliminary studies at Johns Hopkins University School of Medicine suggest that getting more of this fat in your diet may play a role in preventing gallstones as well. Salmon is a very good source of omega-3's, with a 6-ounce serving containing about 2,900 milligrams, which is roughly the amount that seems to be effective, says Dr. Pitt.

People who are overweight are much more likely to form gallstones than those who are lean, adds Michael D. Myers, M.D., a physician in private prac-

Ironing Out Gallstones

Not getting enough iron in the diet has been linked to conditions ranging from depression to fatigue. Now some researchers are wondering if it also causes gallstones.

There's a protein in blood called transferrin that transports iron in the body. People with low levels of iron produce more transferrin—the body's attempt to make what little iron it has go further. "There are some proteins that cause cholesterol crystals to form more rapidly, and transferrin is one," says Henry Pitt, M.D., director of the Gallstone and Biliary Disease Center at Johns Hopkins University in Baltimore. This cholesterol, in turn, can cause gallstones to form.

In laboratory studies, animals low in iron that were given a high-cholesterol diet produced more gallstones than those with normal iron levels, Dr. Pitt says. While similar studies haven't been done in humans, evidence suggests that a similar process occurs. For example, pregnant women, who tend to be low in iron, have a very high risk of developing gallstones, says Dr. Pitt.

While the results of the study are intriguing, they are still preliminary, Dr. Pitt adds. "It may be that treating iron deficiency will help prevent gallstones, but that's a big jump," he says. "This is a whole new concept."

tice in Los Alamitos, California. "For every pound of fat you have in your body, you produce 10 milligrams of cholesterol," Dr. Myers explains. So along with eating fewer high-fat foods, it's a good idea to add more fruits, vegetables, legumes, and whole grains to your diet since these foods are the cornerstone of any weight-loss plan.

Even though losing weight can help prevent gallstones, losing too much, too fast can have the opposite effect because it causes cholesterol levels in the gallbladder to rise, Dr. Myers says. What's more, if you seriously cut back on the amount of food you eat, your gallbladder will naturally be less active, permitting stone-forming sludge to accumulate.

According to the National Institutes of Health, a diet of fewer than 860 calories a day can increase your risk for gallstones. If you're counting calories, staying in the range of 1,000 to 1,200 calories a day will help you lose weight without making you more prone to stones, says Dominic Nompleggi, M.D., Ph.D., assistant professor of medicine and surgery and director of the nutrition support service at the University of Massachusetts Medical Center in Worcester.

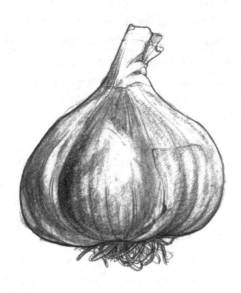

Garlic
Great Bulbs of Power

Healing Power
Can help:
Ease ear infections

Lower triglycerides
and cholesterol

Reduce the risk
of stomach
and colon cancers

Prevent heart disease
and stroke

Filmmaker Les Blank made a documentary in 1980 called *Garlic Is as Good as 10 Mothers*. If he were to make a sequel today, he might call it *Garlic Is as Good as 1,200 Studies*.

An enormous amount of research has been done on this pungent bulb, and the results have been, quite literally, amazing. Dozens of medical benefits have been linked to garlic.

- Studies show that garlic lowers cholesterol and thins the blood, which may help prevent high blood pressure, heart disease, and stroke.
- In the laboratory, garlic appears to block the growth of cancer cells. Population studies show that people who eat lots of garlic have fewer stomach and colon cancers than those who eat the least.
- In a study at Boston City Hospital, garlic was successfully used to kill 14 strains of bacteria taken from the noses and throats of children with ear infections.

In addition, research has shown that garlic can help boost immunity and reduce high levels of blood sugar. It may also relieve asthma and keep individual cells healthy and strong, perhaps delaying or preventing some of the conditions associated with aging.

Garlic's healing potential has been recognized for thousands of years. Historically, it's been used to treat everything from wounds and infections to digestion problems. In World War II, for example, when Russian soldiers ran out of penicillin for their wounds, they requisitioned garlic cloves. And today, in Germany, Japan, and other modern countries, garlic formulas are sold as over-the-counter drugs.

Good for the Heart

Thus far, researchers have identified two important ways in which garlic is good for the heart and circulation. First, it contains many sulfur compounds, including diallyl disulfide (DADS), which seem to help smooth blood flow by preventing platelets from sticking together and clotting. In a study at Brown University in providence, Rhode Isalnd, researchers gave 45 men with high cholesterol aged garlic extract—about the equivalent of five to six cloves of fresh garlic. When they examined the men's blood, they saw that the rate at which platelets clumped and stuck together had dropped anywhere from 10 to 58 percent.

"High platelet activity means that you're more likely to have arteriosclerosis or a heart attack or a stroke," says researcher Robert I. Lin, Ph.D., executive vice president of Nutrition International in Irvine, California. "But sulfur compounds are very potent. They thin the blood."

In the Kitchen

Unless you have taste buds made of asbestos, it's difficult to eat a lot of raw garlic at one sitting. But there is a way to substantially boost your garlic intake without hurting yourself in the process. It's called roasting.

Unlike eating raw garlic cloves, roasting gives the bulb a sweet, caramelized taste—garlic at its most polite. It delivers just a hint of heat rather than the full blast.

To roast garlic, cut the top from the garlic bulb to expose just the tips of the cloves. Rub the bulb lightly with a little olive oil and wrap in a piece of aluminum foil. Leave some air space around the bulb, but seal the edges tightly. Roast in a 350°F oven for about 45 minutes, or until very tender. (You can also "roast" garlic in the microwave; use the high setting and cook, uncovered and without oil, for about 10 minutes, turning twice during the cooking process.) Remove from the oven and let cool slightly.

To eat roasted garlic, simply squeeze the root end firmly to push the cloves out of their skins. You can spread the garlic on bread or toss it with cooked pasta or vegetables. If you're not eating it right away, you can refrigerate it in a tightly covered container for up to one week.

Garlic is also good for the heart because it lowers the levels of cholesterol and blood fats called triglycerides in the bloodstream. According to Yu-Yan Yeh,

Ph.D., professor of nutrition science at Pennsylvania State University in University Park, many of garlic's protective effects take place in the liver, where cholesterol is produced. In laboratory studies, rats given garlic extract produced 87 percent less cholesterol and 64 percent fewer trigylcerides.

"The liver is a primary place in the body for fat synthesis and for production of blood cholesterol," says Dr. Yeh. "When fewer of these substances are made in the liver, there are fewer of them in the blood."

In a review of 16 studies involving 952 people, British researchers found that eating garlic—whether fresh or in powdered form—lowered total cholesterol an average of 12 to 13 percent.

And according to a review by researchers at New York Medical College in Valhalla, scientific evidence suggests that eating one-half to one clove of garlic daily could reduce blood cholesterol levels by about 9 percent.

CANCER PROTECTION

There's increasing evidence that including garlic in the diet may play a role in preventing and treating cancer. Studies suggest that garlic can help block cancer in several ways: by preventing cell changes that lead to cancer, by stopping tumors from growing, or by killing the harmful cells outright.

• A compound in garlic called s-allylcysteine appears to stop the metabolic action that causes a healthy cell to become cancerous, says John Milner, Ph.D., professor and head of the department of nutrition at Pennsylvania State University.

• The substance called DADS, which we discussed earlier, appears to throttle the growth of cancer cells by interfering with their ability to divide and multiply. "DADS chokes cancer cells until their numbers are reduced and they start dying," says Dr. Milner.

• Another substance in garlic is diallyl trisulfide (DATS), which is 10 times more powerful than DADS at killing human lung cancer cells. "Its effectiveness is comparable to that of 5-fluorouracil, a widely used chemotherapy agent," Dr. Milner says. And since garlic is vastly less toxic to healthy cells than the chemotherapy drug, there's hope that some day garlic could form the basis for a gentler chemotherapy.

• Garlic contains compounds that help prevent nitrites—common substances found in some foods as well as a variety of everyday pollutants—from transforming themselves into nitrosamines, harmful compounds that can trigger cancerous changes in the body.

Garlic's benefits aren't seen only in the laboratory. For example, researchers have noted that people in Southern Italy, who eat a lot of garlic, develop less stomach cancer than the nongarlic-eaters to their north.

"In one province of northern China, people routinely eat four to seven cloves of garlic a day. For every 100 cases of stomach cancer in the neighboring province, where garlic intake isn't as high, the garlic-eating population will suffer eight or fewer cases," says Dr. Paxton.

Closer to home, a study of 41,837 women living in Iowa found that those who ate garlic at least once a week had a 35 percent lower risk of colon cancer than women who never ate garlic.

"If I had to take an educated guess, I'd say that eating three cloves of garlic a day might reduce your risk of many cancers by 20 percent," says Dr. Lin. "And eating six cloves could get you at least a 30 percent reduction," he adds.

WELCOME "GARLICILLIN"

A frightening trend in recent years has been antibiotic resistance—the ability of bacteria to shrug off the effects of once-effective drugs. Recent research suggests garlic may be effective where traditional drugs have failed or are too toxic.

In one study, researchers at Boston City Hospital swabbed 14 different strains of bacteria from the noses and throats of children with ear infections. Some of the infections had been impervious to treatment with antibiotics. In the laboratory, however, garlic extract effectively killed the resistant germs.

In another study, researchers at the University of New Mexico, Albuquerque, tested whether garlic could be used to treat otomycosis, or swimmer's ear. Swimmer's ear is caused, scientists think, by a fungus called aspergillus. And normal treatments for it are less than ideal. Topical drugs can be uncomfortable and cannot be used if the ear drum has already been broken.

In the laboratory study, researchers treated swimmer's ear fungi with a mixture of garlic extract and water. Even at very low concentrations, the garlic blocked the growth of fungi just as well as available drugs. And, in some cases, it proved even better.

Getting the Most

Enjoy it fresh. Crushed raw garlic contains allicin, a compound that breaks down quickly into a cascade of healthful compounds, like DADS and DATS. Of course, not everyone enjoys the bite of raw garlic. Try cutting a clove in half and rubbing it hard against the inside of a wooden salad bowl before putting in the salad. You'll get just a hint of garlic taste and more than a hint of garlic benefits.

But eat for convenience. You don't have to prepare fresh garlic to get the healing benefits; each form of garlic—raw, cooked, or powdered—has its own important compounds. By taking advantage of each of these forms, you can slip more garlic and its healing compounds into your menu.

Cut it fine. Whether you're cooking garlic or eating it raw, mincing, crushing, or pressing it vastly expands the surface area, maximizing the production and release of healthful compounds.

Cook it lightly. Overcooking garlic can destroy some of the delicate compounds. It's best to cook it lightly—stir-fried with vegetables, for example, or added to a long-cooking stew in the last few minutes of cooking time—suggests Dr. Lin. "The taste is much more gentle than raw garlic," he says.

GARLICKY SOUR CREAM TOPPING

3   medium cloves garlic

1   cup nonfat sour cream

2   tablespoons reduced-fat mayonnaise

1   tablespoon minced fresh parsley

PER ¼ CUP

calories	**91**
total fat	**2.5 g.**
saturated fat	**0.5 g.**
cholesterol	**3 mg.**
sodium	**45 mg.**
dietary fiber	**0.1 g.**

Place the garlic in a blender or food processor. Process to mince. Add the sour cream, mayonnaise, and parsley. Process for 1 minute, or until smooth.

Makes 1 cup

Cook's Note: Serve over baked or boiled potatoes, steamed vegetables, or fish.

GARLIC BREAD

1   whole-wheat French baguette (12 ounces)

2   tablespoons olive oil

4   cloves garlic, minced

1   teaspoon Italian herb seasoning

PER SERVING

calories	**126**
total fat	**4.1 g.**
saturated fat	**0.5 g.**
cholesterol	**0 mg.**
sodium	**231 mg.**
dietary fiber	**2.9 g.**

Preheat oven to 400°F.

Split the baguette in half lengthwise. Place directly on the oven rack. Bake for 10 minutes to toast.

In a small bowl, combine the oil, garlic, and Italian herb seasoning. Remove the bread from the oven and brush evenly with the garlic mixture. Return to the oven for 5 minutes.

Makes 8 servings

Cook's Note: If a whole-wheat French baguette is not available, a regular French baguette will work fine.

Gas
Eating to Stop the Wind

"It is universally well-known, that in digesting our common food, there is created or produced in the bowels of human creatures, a great quantity of wind."—Benjamin Franklin.

This was Dr. Franklin's way of saying that most us, like it or not, will have gas now and then. Gas, which is produced whenever food is broken down in the digestive tract, is a normal part of digestion.

Some foods, of course, produce more gas than others. Beans and other plant foods high in carbohydrates are notorious gas-producers. The reason for this is that these foods aren't entirely broken down during digestion. When small carbohydrate particles pass into the lower intestine, bacteria move in and begin feeding, producing a lot of gas in the process. This gas has to go somewhere—and out it goes, anywhere from 14 to 23 times a day.

It's not only plant foods that cause problems, of course. Almost anything you eat has the potential to cause gas, at least some of the time. Here are some of the usual culprits, along with tips for keeping gas under control.

A Problem with Enzymes

Most children can drink milk and eat cheese all day long, but many adults don't produce enough of the enzyme needed to fully digest the sugar (called lactose) found in dairy foods. When undigested lactose slips into the lower intestine, it begins to ferment, causing gas, says Marvin Schuster, M.D., director of the Marvin M. Schuster Digestive and Motility Disorders Center at Johns Hopkins Bayview Medical Center in Baltimore.

Even if you can't down two or three glasses of milk anymore, you can probably enjoy smaller amounts without having problems. In one study, researchers at the University of Minnesota in Minneapolis found that people were able to drink up to 8 ounces of milk a day without having gas. In addition, drinking milk with meals is much less likely to cause gas than having it alone.

Another way to enjoy milk without discomfort is to buy reduced-lactose milk, which has about 70 percent less lactose than regular milk. This way, you'll get the benefits of milk without the back talk. Or you can take lactase supplements, which make it easier for the body to digest the lactose in dairy foods.

Even people who can not handle milk are often able to enjoy live-culture yogurt. This type of yogurt contains bacteria that help break down the offending sugar. And the more help you get with digestion, the less likely you are to have gas.

FIBER FIREWORKS

We all know how important it is to get more fiber in your diet. Unfortunately, the same fiber that lowers cholesterol and protects against heart disease is also responsible for producing large amounts of gas. This is especially true when you've only recently started eating more fiber-rich foods.

"If you add fiber too quickly, the body can't cope with it properly," says Dr. Schuster. "The average American only eats about 12 grams of fiber a day. If you suddenly double that amount, it means a lot of gas."

To get the benefits of fiber without the gas, it's a good idea to add it slowly to your diet, says Marie Borum, M.D., assistant professor of medicine at George Washington University Medical Center in Washington, D.C. You might, for example, substitute whole-wheat spaghetti for your regular kind, which will provide an extra 2 grams of the rough stuff in a half-cup serving. A half-cup of cooked artichoke hearts will deliver more than 4 grams of fiber, and the same amount of lima beans will add almost 5 grams. If you gradually introduce fiber-rich foods to your diet each day over a period of four to six weeks, you're less likely to have a problem with gas, Dr. Borum says.

HOW SWEET IT ISN'T

Sometimes you're darned if you do and darned if you don't. Many people get gas when they eat sweet foods like cookies or ice cream. But when they try to curb those cravings by having sugar-free candies or chewing gum, they still get gas. Why?

As it turns out, sugarless gum and candies are gas-producers, says Dr. Borum. They contain artificial sweeteners like sorbitol, xylitol, or mannitol, which the body has trouble digesting. While this helps keep calories down, it can also result in large amounts of gas.

Mother Nature's own sweeteners aren't without problems. Fructose, for example, a sugar found in honey, fruits, and juices, frequently causes gas. It doesn't take a lot of fructose to cause problems, either. In one study, Greek researchers found that having as little as 1½ tablespoons of honey was enough to cause gas in some people.

You certainly don't want to cut fruits from your diet, Dr. Borum adds. If gas is a problem, however, you may want to avoid the more concentrated sources of fructose such as honey or juices.

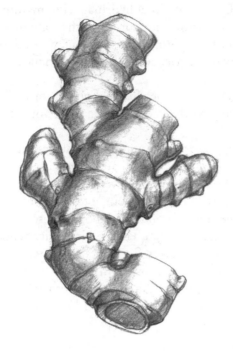

GINGER
THE PUNGENT HEALER

HEALING POWER
CAN HELP:
Prevent motion sickness

Soothe stomach upset

Relieve migraine
headaches

Reduce clotting in blood

Roman doctors kept it handy during military marches. Pythagoras, Greek philosopher and geometry whiz, touted it for digestive health. And King Henry VIII of England was convinced that it would protect against plague, although there's no evidence that ginger is that good. But there's plenty of evidence that this gnarled, piquant root can help relieve dozens of conditions, from motion sickness and other digestive complaints to migraines, arthritis, high cholesterol, and even dangerous blood clots. This is why millions of people worldwide swear by ginger as a potent healing food.

HELP FOR THE HEAVES

As anyone who has experienced motion sickness knows, even a mild bout can derail the best-laid vacation plans. That's why nearly every travel checklist, along with reminders to buy sunscreen and feed the cat, includes the notation, "Buy Dramamine."

The next time you travel, you may want to stop at the supermarket instead of the pharmacy. As it turns out, ginger is one of the best motion sickness remedies you can buy.

In a classic study conducted by Daniel B. Mowrey, Ph.D., director of the American Phytotherapy Research Laboratory in Salt Lake City, 36 motion sickness–prone students were strapped into tilted rotating chairs and spun until they felt ill. Those who were given 100 milligrams of dimenhydrinate (Dramamine) beforehand couldn't take the stomach-churning ride for more than about 4½ minutes, and most gave up sooner. Half of those given ginger, however, were able to withstand the ride for the full 6 minutes, with less nausea and dizziness than the drug-treated group.

In another study, Dutch researchers testing the effects of ginger on seasick naval cadets found that ginger pills reduced the cadets' nausea and vomiting, providing relief for as long as 4 hours.

Experts aren't sure why ginger suppresses a queasy stomach. But researchers in Japan have suggested that gingerols, one of the ingredients in ginger, may be indirectly responsible for blocking the body's vomiting reflex.

To use ginger for combating motion sickness, take about ¼ teaspoon of fresh or powdered ginger 20 minutes before getting in a car or on a boat, advises Varro E. Tyler, Ph.D., professor emeritus of pharmacognosy at Purdue University School of Pharmacy in West Lafayette, Indiana. Repeat every few hours as needed.

You can also use ginger to help relieve a run-of-the-mill upset stomach. Prepare a cup of ginger tea by adding three or four thin slices of fresh ginger to a cup of boiling water, and sip as needed, advises Charles Lo, M.D., a doctor of Chinese medicine in private practice in Chicago.

RELIEF FOR MIGRAINES

If you're one of the millions of Americans who suffer from migraine headaches, ginger may help keep the pain and nausea away. In a small study, researchers at Odense University in Denmark found that ginger may short-circuit impending migraines without the bothersome side effects of some migraine-relieving drugs. It appears that ginger blocks the action of prostaglandins, substances that cause pain and inflammation in blood vessels in the brain.

Research is still very preliminary, so experts are reluctant to recommend specific treatment plans for using ginger to fight migraines. If you feel a headache coming on, you may want to try taking ⅓ teaspoon of fresh or powdered ginger, which is the amount suggested by the Danish researchers.

AID FOR ARTHRITIS

Are the joints in your fingers so stiff and sore that you can't fumble the childproof cap off the aspirin bottle? You may want to add ginger to your medicine chest.

In one study, Danish researchers studied 56 people who had rheumatoid arthritis or osteoarthritis and who treated themselves with fresh or powdered ginger. They found that ginger produced relief in 55 percent of people with osteoarthritis and 74 percent of those with rheumatoid arthritis.

Some experts speculate that ginger may ease arthritis pain the same way it helps block migraines, by blocking the formation of inflammation-causing prostaglandins that cause pain and swelling.

To soothe arthritis pain, Dr. Lo recommends brewing a mild tea, again, by putting three or four slices of fresh ginger in a cup of boiling water. You can also try taking ½ teaspoon of powdered ginger or up to an ounce (about 6 teaspoons) of fresh ginger once a day.

Help for the Blood

Blood clots can be a good thing. When you cut your finger, for example, platelets—components in blood that help it clot—help "stick" the wound together so that it can heal.

But these sticky platelets can also cling to artery walls and to each other. When that happens, clots stop being beneficial and become some-

In the Kitchen

If you've never used it, fresh ginger can look a mite mysterious. But don't let its brown, knobby appearance throw you. Fresh ginger is more user-friendly than it looks. Here's what you need to know.

Wrap and refrigerate. Fresh, unpeeled ginger will last for up to two weeks, as long as you wrap it tightly in plastic wrap. In the freezer, it will keep for up to two months.

Pare away the skin. There's no flavor worth having in the tough, light brown skin. So before using ginger, peel away the skin with a vegetable peeler or sharp paring knife.

Cut it fine. To get the most flavor from fresh ginger, you want to cut (or grate or mash) it as fine as possible. Perhaps the easiest way to extract the juice is to cut a small piece of ginger and press it in a garlic press.

thing to worry about. Many people routinely take aspirin to help keep their blood clear of clots that could lead to strokes or heart attacks.

The gingerol in ginger has a chemical structure somewhat similar to that of aspirin. Research suggests that getting ginger in the diet—although at this point, experts aren't sure how much—may inhibit the production of a chemical called thromboxane, which plays a key role in the clotting process.

Getting the Most

Use it fresh. Ginger comes in a variety of forms, including fresh, dried, crystallized, and powdered. It's best to use it fresh, advises Dr. Lo. "Fresh ginger is more active than dried," he says. Crystallized ginger is almost as good, he adds.

Try to buy the freshest ginger to get the most healing compounds. "Avoid ginger with soft spots, mold, or dry, wrinkled skin," Dr. Lo advises.

Use a grater. Grating fresh ginger releases more of its potent juice than slicing or chopping, says Dr. Lo. Using a garlic press will also extract the maximum amount of juice from the root.

Enjoy it often. To squeeze the most health benefits from ginger, consume it as often as possible, says Dr. Lo. But you don't need to go ginger-crazy to get the healing benefits. Less than an ounce a day will do. "Drinking a few cups of ginger tea or adding a small amount of fresh ginger to a stir-fry should be enough."

Choose the right root. Whenever possible, buy ginger grown in Africa or India, says Stephen Fulder, Ph.D., a private research consultant and author of *The Ginger Book*. Studies show that these varieties are more potent than the common Jamaican kind.

You can't tell the difference in gingers just by looking, though. Ask the produce manager at the supermarket or health food store. He should be able to tell you which variety he's selling.

GINGER CHICKEN AND SNOW PEAS

1 **pound skinless, boneless chicken breasts**
2 **teaspoons cornstarch**
1/3 **cup defatted reduced-sodium chicken broth**
2 **teaspoons reduced-sodium soy sauce**
2 **teaspoons canola oil**
2 **cloves garlic, minced**
1 **tablespoon grated fresh ginger**
1 **cup snow peas**

PER SERVING

calories	**170**
total fat	**5 g.**
saturated fat	**0.9 g.**
cholesterol	**63 mg.**
sodium	**150 mg.**
dietary fiber	**1 g.**

Cut the chicken crosswise into thin slices.

Place the cornstarch in a small bowl. Add the broth and stir to dissolve the cornstarch. Stir in the soy sauce. Set aside.

In a wok or large frying pan, warm the oil over high heat. Add the chicken and stir-fry for 2 to 3 minutes, or until the chicken is no longer pink. Add the garlic and ginger. Stir-fry for 30 seconds, or until fragrant. Add the snow peas and toss.

Add the broth mixture. Cook, stirring constantly, for 1 to 2 minutes, or until the sauce thickens and becomes translucent.

Makes 4 servings

Cook's Note: Serve over hot cooked rice or noodles.

DOUBLE-GINGER GINGERBREAD

¾ **cup unsweetened applesauce**

½ **cup molasses**

¼ **cup fat-free egg substitute**

3 **tablespoons canola oil**

1½ **cups unbleached all-purpose flour**

1 **teaspoon baking soda**

1 **teaspoon ground ginger**

1 **teaspoon ground cinnamon**

⅛ **teaspoon salt**

⅓ **cup finely diced candied ginger**

PER SERVING

calories	**211**
total fat	**4.8 g.**
saturated fat	**0.4 g.**
cholesterol	**0 mg.**
sodium	**192 mg.**
dietary fiber	**1 g.**

Preheat the oven to 350°F.

In a large bowl, combine the applesauce, molasses, egg substitute, and oil. Stir to mix well.

In a medium bowl, combine the flour, baking soda, ground ginger, cinnamon, and salt. Stir to mix. Add to the applesauce mixture and stir until just mixed.

Mix in all but 1 tablespoon of the candied ginger.

Pour into an 8″ × 8″ no-stick baking dish. Bake for 25 to 30 minutes, or until a knife inserted in the center comes out clean.

Cool on a wire rack. Cut into squares. Sprinkle each piece with the remaining candied ginger just before serving.

Makes 9 servings

Cook's Note: A dollop of nonfat sour cream makes a delicious garnish for the gingerbread.

GOUT
PROTECTION AGAINST PURINES

If you're reading this, you likely either have gout, suspect that you might have it, or know someone who does. It's a big fraternity that nobody wants to be in.

Gout is a form of arthritis in which glasslike shards of uric acid jab into joints, causing searing pain. For some, the mere weight of a blanket on an inflamed toe is too much to bear. Fever and chills can be part of the package, too, as the immune system attempts to fight off the assault.

Gout afflicts about one million Americans, and doctors say that it's on the rise as the population ages. Most of the people with gout are overweight men over 40, but women get it as well.

TOO MUCH OF A BAD THING

The uric acid that causes gout is a normal part of our metabolisms. Our bodies make uric acid when they break down protein by-products called purines.

Normally, uric acid dissolves in the blood, is filtered out by the kidneys and is sent packing in the urine. Not so in those with gout who, perhaps through some metabolic glitch, either produce too much uric acid or have trouble getting rid of it. Over time, the excess acid condenses into sharp little crystals that lodge in joints and the connective tissue around them, resulting in inflammation and pain, says Doyt Conn, M.D., senior vice-president of medical affairs at the Arthritis Foundation in Atlanta. The big toe is a favorite target of gout attacks, but the ankles, knees, hands, and shoulders have been known to take the first blow, too.

Gout is deceiving because attacks can be separated by long periods with no apparent symptoms. When it does strike, it usually hits at night and, without medication, the pain can go for days or weeks. If you get hit, count on getting hit again. Half of those with a first attack have a second one within a year; three-quarters within five years.

Pain isn't the only thing you have to worry about. Without treatment, gout attacks often become more frequent and severe. After about 10 years, lumps of uric acid crystals, called tophi, may begin building up around a joint and in cartilage elsewhere in the body. Tophi are sometimes visible under the skin, particularly when they occur in the outer ear. Left untreated, these deposits gradually grow bigger and can irreversibly cripple a joint. In addition, people with gout are more likely than others to develop uric acid kidney stones.

There isn't a cure for gout. Drugs can keep it under control, but people with the disease have other weapons, too. Slimming down, eating right, cutting back on alcohol, and drinking plenty of water all help lower uric acid levels and decrease the risk of attacks, says Dr. Conn.

WEIGHING THE RISKS

Weight control is especially important for people with gout because obesity has been linked to high uric acid levels in the blood. Crash diets and fasting aren't the answer, however, since they can actually raise uric acid levels. Slow and steady weight loss is not only better for you generally but also more likely to keep gout under control, says Dr. Conn.

In a study at Johns Hopkins University in Baltimore, researchers

CRASHING THE CLUB

What was long thought to be a men's club is now increasingly open to women. But you won't hear any cheers from the ladies.

About 20 percent of the people in the United States who have gout are women, the vast majority of whom are past menopause. Why?

Doctors suspect that estrogen helps prevent a buildup of uric acid in the blood, says Doyt Conn, M.D., senior vice-president of medical affairs at the Arthritis Foundation in Atlanta. But this shield slips at menopause, when a woman's estrogen levels fall. As the vast numbers of women in the baby boom generation age, the incidence of gout is sure to increase.

"Women who have attacks of gout tend to be overweight, and many times they have high blood pressure and are on diuretics," adds Dr. Conn.

followed 1,200 medical students for more than 30 years. They found that those who gained the most weight during early adulthood (a time when most people let out the belt a bit) were the ones at highest risk to develop gout later in life. Even a slight weight gain—6 to 10 pounds—between the ages of 25 and 35 has been shown to nearly double a person's risk of developing gout.

As you know, it's a lot easier to keep weight off than to take it off later on. Keeping your weight in control now will go a long way toward preventing gout in the future.

EATING FOR RELIEF

In the past, the only thing to do for gout was to cut out purine from the diet. The therapy didn't work very well and often made for boring meals, says

FRUITFUL RELIEF

The recorded use of cherries to treat gout dates at least to the 1950s, to a Texan named Ludwig W. Blau, Ph.D., who was crippled by a gouty big toe and forced to use a wheelchair. Dr. Blau reported in a Texas medical journal that a diet including six cherries a day soon had him up and walking. Further, he noted that his physician tried the cherry diet on 12 patients and had equally good results.

Do cherries work? While there's no scientific evidence to suggest that they do, some people swear by them. In a survey by *Prevention* magazine, about 700 respondents said that they had tried cherries for gout, and about 67 percent of them said that the cherries made them feel better.

Black cherry juice reportedly has the same effect, says Steve Schumacher, a kinesiologist in Louisville, Kentucky. "I must say that of all the remedies I have ever used for people with various health problems, this has been a hit with everyone," he says.

In his book *Natural Prescriptions*, Robert M. Giller, M.D., notes that cherries (and other dark red and blue berries) are rich in compounds that help prevent the destruction of collagen. The body uses collagen to form connective tissue, which is damaged by gout.

For some people, he writes, eating a half-pound of cherries (about 34) daily for a week will help relieve the symptoms.

Donna Weihofen, R.D., a clinical dietitian at the University of Wisconsin Hospital and Clinics in Madison.

"Just eliminate those foods highest in purines," Weihofen says. "It will enhance the effects of the drugs and perhaps prevent some of the severe symptoms." Some of the foods highest in purines include organ meats—such as liver, kidney, and sweetbreads—and sardines, anchovies, mackerel, asparagus, mushrooms, and beans.

While you're cutting back on purine-rich foods, it's also a good idea to make sure that if you drink, you do so only in moderation. Beer, wine, and other alcoholic beverages increase the risk for gout attacks in two ways. They increase the body's production of uric acid and also impair the kidneys' ability to get rid of it. It's also a good idea to skip the heavy red wines, such as port and Madeira, because they have the most purines.

Getting more water in your system, however, will dilute the uric acid in the bloodstream and help prevent crystals from forming, Weihofen says. Both soda and fruit juices can help, but water is really the best choice because it passes through the body quickly without adding unnecessary sugars. She recommends drinking at least 10 to 12 glasses of water a day.

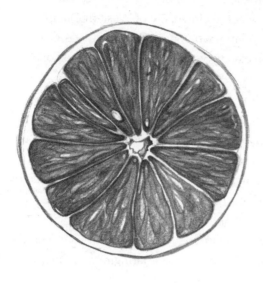

GRAPEFRUIT
THE POWER OF PECTIN

HEALING POWER
CAN HELP:

Relieve cold symptoms

Prevent cancer

Reduce bruising

Prevent heart disease and stroke

Grapefruit may be the biggest fruit on the breakfast block, but in terms of popularity, it sometimes gets rolled aside. Its sour taste just isn't as appealing to some people as its sweeter citrus kin.

But in the health game, grapefruit, particularly the red variety, shines. It contains a number of antioxidant compounds—not just vitamin C but also such things as lycopene, limonoids, and naringin. Together, these compounds can help reduce cold symptoms and also help decrease the risks of heart disease and cancer.

What these substances have in common is their ability to mop up excess dangerous oxygen molecules in the body called free radicals. While free radicals are a natural part of metabolism, they can have dangerous effects as well. When you eat grapefruit, you're essentially getting a chemical "mop" that helps clean up problems before they occur.

In addition, grapefruit contains large amounts of pectin, a type of fiber that has been shown to substantially lower cholesterol, thus reducing the risks of heart disease, high blood pressure, and stroke.

RED WITH HEALTH

One of the compounds in grapefruit that gives them their distinctly pinkish hue is lycopene. Also found in tomatoes and sweet red peppers, lycopene "is a very important, very potent antioxidant and free radical scavenger," says Paul Lachance, Ph.D., professor of nutrition and chairman of the department of food science at Rutgers University in New Brunswick, New Jersey. "Our cancer and heart disease situations would be a lot worse if not for the lycopene in our foods."

Grapefruit is also an excellent source of limonoids, which, like vitamin C, have been shown to have anti-cancer properties. In laboratory studies, researchers at the U.S. Department of Agriculture Fruit and Vegetable Chemistry Laboratory in Pasadena, California, found that limonoids increase the level of certain enzymes that help detoxify cancer-causing agents and aid in their excretion from the body.

"Grapefruit is probably your best source of limonoids," says Antonio Montanari, Ph.D., research scientist with the Florida Department of Citrus Research Center in Lake Alfred. A 6-ounce glass of grapefruit juice, for example, contains over 100 milligrams of various limonoid compounds.

Grapefruit is rich in an additional compound, naringin, which doesn't appear to be present in other fruits. In laboratory studies, naringin has been shown to stop the growth of some kinds of breast cancer cells.

Finally, grapefruit is an excellent source of vitamin C. It's one of the few foods that can provide more than the entire Daily Value (DV) in one serving. A cup of grapefruit sections contains 88 milligrams of vitamin C, 146 percent of the DV.

While vitamin C is a powerful antioxidant vitamin, it also is part of the recipe for collagen, the "glue" that binds skin cells together. If you don't get enough vitamin C, cuts will be slow to heal and your gums may bleed. Vitamin C has also been shown to help relieve cold symptoms by reducing levels of histamine, a naturally occurring chemical that makes your nose run.

PECTIN POWER

Grapefruit has received a lot of attention in recent years due to its generous supply of pectin, a type of soluble fiber that can help lower cholesterol to healthy levels. It does this by forming a gel in the intestine that helps block the absorption of fats into the bloodstream.

In animal studies, James Cerda, M.D., professor of medicine at the University of Florida College of Medicine in Gainesville, found that pectin could produce a drop in cholesterol of 21 percent. At the same time, it helped prevent sticky components in blood, called platelets, from forming clots in the bloodstream and increasing the risk of heart disease and stroke. Dr. Cerda found that animals given a diet containing 3 percent grapefruit

IN THE KITCHEN

While many people truly enjoy the bittersweet bite of grapefruit, others prefer a slightly sweeter taste. To find fruit with a mellower taste, here's what to do.

Buy it at its peak. While grapefruit is available in supermarkets all year long, the peak season is between January and June. That's when the fruit will be most mature and sweetest.

Shop for hybrids. There are a number of "almost-grapefruits" that are much sweeter than the real thing. Grapefruit hybrids such as oroblancos and melogolds taste like grapefruit but with the sugar already sprinkled on top.

Another grapefruit alternative is the pummelo. Sold in specialty markets, "it's a bit drier and sweeter than grapefruit and it's always less bitter and acidic," says Andrea S. Boyle, manager of consumer affairs for the Sunkist Growers' fresh-fruit division.

Add your own sweetener. Sprinkling a little sugar or honey on grapefruit is a tasty way to take off the sour edge. Or try sprinkling it with a little brown sugar, then broil the fruit for a few minutes, or until the sugar bubbles.

pectin for nine months had more than 5 percent of their artery walls covered with plaque. In animals not given pectin, plaque covered 14 percent of the artery walls.

A 4-ounce serving (about ½ cup) of grapefruit provides 1 gram of pectin. It's found not only in the flesh but also in the peel and the thin white layer just beneath the peel.

Getting the Most

Eat the sections. When you eat grapefruit halves, scooping out the flesh with a spoon, you leave about half the pectin behind. To get the most fiber, experts say, peel the grapefruit and eat the entire section.

Sip your juice. Compared to the flesh, grapefruit juice is a concentrated source of naringin. You can make your own juice, but ready-made may be better since, during commercial processing, parts of the healthful peel go into the juice.

Buy it red. Red grapefruits contain more lycopene than the white varieties. Good choices include Ruby Red, Flame, and Star Ruby, says Bill Widmer, Ph.D., research scientist with the Florida Department of Citrus Research Center in Lake Alfred.

HONEY-MARINATED GRAPEFRUIT

4   **ruby grapefruit**

2   **tablespoons honey**

1   **tablespoon minced fresh mint**

PER SERVING

calories	**110**
total fat	**0.3 g.**
saturated fat	**0 g.**
cholesterol	**0 mg.**
sodium	**5 mg.**
dietary fiber	**3.8 g.**

Grate about 1 teaspoon of the rind from 1 grapefruit. Cut that grapefruit in half through the middle and squeeze the juice; set aside.

Place the honey in a small microwaveable bowl. Microwave on medium power (50 percent) for 20 to 30 seconds, or until warm. Add the juice and the grated rind. Mix well.

Peel the remaining 3 grapefruit with a sharp paring knife, cutting away most but not all of the white pith below the peel. Carefully separate the grapefruit into sections. Remove any seeds and pierce each section in 1 or 2 places with the tip of the knife so the marinade can permeate the grapefruit.

Arrange the grapefruit sections on dessert plates. Pour the honey mixture over the sections. Let stand for at least 15 minutes to let the flavors to blend. Chill, if desired. Sprinkle with the mint before serving.

Makes 4 servings

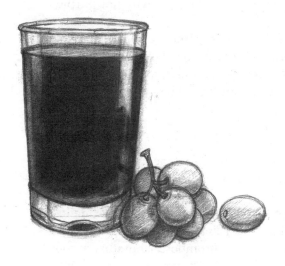

GRAPE JUICE
A DRINK FOR THE HEART

HEALING POWER
CAN HELP:
Lower cholesterol

Decrease the risk
of heart disease

Lower high blood
pressure

Grape juice got its start in this country toward the end of the nineteenth century, when certain teetotaling churches decided that they needed a nonalcoholic substitute for wine to serve for Communion.

Today, abstainers from alcohol are still toasting that innovation. They can receive similar benefits to those enjoyed by their wine-drinking counterparts (both wine and grape juice contain powerful compounds that can help lower cholesterol, prevent hardening of the arteries, and fight heart disease) without the unwanted effects of alcohol.

GIVING YOUR HEART SOME JUICE

Researchers might never have stumbled across the health benefits of grape juice and its spirited sibling, wine, had it not been for the heart-healthy folks from the country that also brought us croissants, berets, and Brigitte Bardot.

A few years back, scientists discovered a phenomenon that they dubbed the French Paradox. Specifically, they found that while the French ate almost four times as much butter and three times as much lard, had higher cholesterol and blood pressure, and smoked just as much as Americans, they fell victim to heart attacks 2½ times less often.

At least part of the French secret to heart health, researchers believe, is red wine, which contains compounds called flavonoids. These compounds have been linked to lower rates of heart disease.

If red wine confers protection, the researchers thought, why not purple grape juice?

As it turns out, grape juice contains some of the same flavonoids that are found in wine. Studies suggest that these compounds may help lower cholesterol, prevent cholesterol from sticking to artery walls, and keep blood platelets from sticking together and forming dangerous clots in the bloodstream.

GREAT GRAPES

Scientists are still unraveling the mysteries of how grape juice helps protect against heart disease. One thing they do know is that it appears to help in more than one way.

The flavonoids in grape juice are among the most powerful antioxidants around—maybe even better than vitamins C or E, says John D. Folts, Ph.D., professor of medicine and director of the coronary thrombosis laboratory at the University of Wisconsin Medical School in Madison. In your body, they help prevent low-density lipoprotein (LDL) cholesterol from oxidizing—the process that enables cholesterol to stick to your artery walls and create blockages.

Keeping LDL cholesterol in check is a good start against heart disease. But you also need to keep the platelets, components in blood that cause it to clot, from sticking together unnecessarily. The flavonoids in grape juice do that too, Dr. Folts says. A study at the University of Wisconsin found that when grape juice was given to laboratory animals, abnormal clotting was significantly reduced. So drinking grape juice gives you two benefits for the price of one.

Actually, it's more than two. Grape juice is also a fair source of potassium, with 8 ounces providing 334 milligrams, 10 percent of the Daily Value. This is important because potassium helps control high blood pressure and protects against stroke.

THE MISSING LINK

While grape juice does contain powerful compounds, it doesn't contain a lot of them. In fact, you need three times as much grape juice as wine to get the same protective effects, says Dr. Folts.

All of a grape's protective flavonoids are in the "must," a chunky mixture of grape skins, pulp, seeds, and stems that is used to make wine and grape juice, says Dr. Folts. When must is fermented to make wine, a lot of the flavonoids are drawn into the liquid, he explains. Since grape juice isn't fermented, you get only the flavonoids that are drawn into the juice during the heating and processing stages.

The compounds that end up in the drink are still plenty strong, he adds. You just need more juice to get them.

Getting the Most

Pour a big glass. Since you need to drink more grape juice than wine to get the same health benefits, you'll want to down up to 12 ounces a day, Dr. Folts says.

Drink it dark. "Since flavonoids are what give juice its rich purple hue, if you're looking for the grape juice with the most flavonoids, pick the darkest of the bunch," advises Dr. Folts.

Drink juice, not drink. Grape drink is nothing but a watered-down, sugared imitation of the original article. Nutritionally, it doesn't compare. So when you want the benefits of grape juice, be sure to buy the real thing.

GRAPE SLUSH

3 **cups dark grape juice**

1 **tablespoon sugar**

1 **teaspoon vanilla**

PER SERVING

calories	**130**
total fat	**0.2 g.**
saturated fat	**0 g.**
cholesterol	**0 mg.**
sodium	**6 mg.**
dietary fiber	**0.2 g.**

Pour the grape juice into a medium saucepan. Add the sugar and stir to mix. Bring to a boil over high heat, then reduce the heat to medium and cook for 6 to 8 minutes, or until reduced to 2 cups. Stir in the vanilla. Pour into a 9" or 10" freezerproof glass pie plate and set aside to cool.

Place in the freezer for 1 to 1 1/2 hours, or until the edges are mostly solid and the middle is still liquid. Mash with a fork to break up any large ice crystals.

Return to the freezer for 1 hour, or until frozen through but not hard. Break up the crystals with a fork before serving.

Makes 4 servings

Cook's Note: After the second freezing, the slush can be stored in a covered container in the freezer for up to 1 day before serving. Remove from the freezer and let stand at room temperature for 5 to 10 minutes before serving.

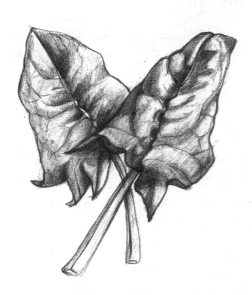

GREENS
NATURE'S BEST PROTECTION

HEALING POWER
CAN HELP:
Control blood pressure

Reduce the risk
of heart disease

Reduce the risk of cancer

Protect against vision loss

Double coupons, good gas mileage, blue-light specials—if there's one thing that Americans appreciate, it's getting more for less.

That is why we really ought to love leafy green vegetables. They deliver more nutrients for fewer calories than virtually any food out there.

"You get so many important nutrients from leafy green vegetables—magnesium, iron, calcium, folate, vitamin C, and vitamin B_6, plus all the heart disease– and cancer-fighting phytochemicals," says Michael Liebman, Ph.D., professor of human nutrition at the University of Wyoming in Laramie. "These are the most nutrient-dense foods that we have available."

Experts are quick to note, however, that American's favorite "salad starter"—the bland-tasting iceberg lettuce—doesn't count as a "leafy green" vegetable. Of all the foods in this powerhouse family, iceberg is the runt. Far better are such things as kale, Swiss chard, dandelion greens, beet greens, mustard greens, turnip greens, spinach, and chicory greens.

LEAVES FOR THE HEART

To some extent, the difference between people who have heart attacks and those who don't may be how many trips they make to the salad bar.

IN THE KITCHEN

With the exception of residents of the Southern states, Americans as a rule aren't familiar with cooking greens. We throw them in salads and maybe put them on sandwiches. But why limit yourself? Greens are very easy to cook once you know a few tricks.

Trim the stems. While the leaves are often surprisingly tender, the stems on leafy greens can be unpleasantly tough and should often be discarded. Before cooking greens, run a sharp knife alongside the stem and center rib, separating the leaf from the stem.

Clean them well. Since the leafy greens grow close to the ground and the frilly leaves readily capture dirt and grit, it's important to wash them thoroughly. The easiest way is to fill the sink or a large bowl with cold water and swish the greens around, allowing any dirt or sand to sink to the bottom. When the greens are clean, transfer them to a colander to drain.

Cut them to ribbons. When cooking thick greens like kale or Swiss chard, it's helpful to cut them into ribbons or small pieces. This will help them cook quickly and become tender.

Boil them quickly. The easiest way to prepare greens is to submerge them in boiling water. Start with a cup of boiling water, drop in the greens, cover, and cook for about 4 minutes, or until tender.

Researchers from the Jean Mayer USDA Human Nutrition Research Center on Aging at Tufts University in Boston and the Framingham Heart Study in Massachusetts studied more than 1,000 people between the ages of 67 and 95 to learn what dietary factors affect heart health. In this, as in so many issues touching on food, the answer boiled down to chemistry—specifically, to an amino acid called homocysteine.

Homocysteine is a natural compound that is harmless as long as the body keeps it in check. When it reaches high levels, however, it becomes toxic and may contribute to clogged arteries and heart disease. The researchers found that among people with the most clogged arteries, 43 percent of men and 34 percent of women had high levels of homocysteine in their blood.

What's the connection with greens? The body uses folate and vitamins B_{12} and B_6 to keep homocysteine under control. Many of the people in the study were falling short of these vital nutrients—especially folate and vitamin B_6. As it turns out, leafy greens are outstanding sources of folate, and they also provide vitamin B_6. That's why experts advise adding plenty of leafy green vegetables to your diet to counteract homocysteine levels.

Boiled spinach is probably your best bet for managing homocysteine. A half-cup of Popeye's favorite snack delivers 131 micrograms of folate, 33 percent of the Daily Value (DV). It also contains 0.2 milligram of vitamin B_6, 10 percent of the DV.

In addition to these important B vitamins, certain greens—particularly beet greens, chicory, and spinach—provide the heart-healthy minerals magnesium, potassium, and calcium. These minerals, along with sodium, help regulate the amount of fluid that your body retains. All too often, researchers say, people have too much sodium and too little of the other three, leading to high blood pressure.

Even though eating leafy greens is an excellent way to help regulate blood pressure, it's important to note that the calcium from spinach and beet greens isn't well-absorbed by the body. Be sure to eat a wide variety of greens to meet all your mineral needs.

MEAT OF THE DIET

Large studies overwhelmingly show that many cancers occur least often in countries where people regard leafy greens, along with a wide variety of fruits and vegetables, as the "meats" of their meals.

In one study, researchers compared 61 men with lung cancer in Chile with 61 men of similar age and smoking habits who were cancer-free. The one difference they found was that men with cancer consumed significantly fewer carotenoid-rich foods, especially Swiss chard, chicory, and spinach as well as beets and cabbage, than those without the disease.

The carotenoids, which are found in large amounts in most leafy greens, are like bodyguards against cancer-causing agents, explains Frederick Khachik, Ph.D., research chemist at the Food Composition Laboratory at the U.S. Department of Agriculture in Beltsville, Maryland. Scientists believe that certain cancers are brought on by the constant onslaught of free radicals—harmful oxygen molecules made by our bodies and also found in air pollution and tobacco smoke—which attack our bodies' healthy cells. Carotenoids counteract free radicals by acting as antioxidants, meaning that they step between the free radicals and our bodies' cells, neutralizing them before they can do damage, he explains.

"There is also plenty of evidence that carotenoids may fight cancer by activating the body's detoxification enzymes—called phase II enzymes—which are responsible for ridding the body of harmful, often cancer-causing chemicals," says Dr. Khachik.

"Dark green, leafy vegetables are among the best sources of some very important carotenoids, like lutein, alpha-carotene, and the one that everyone's familiar with, beta-carotene," he says. While all leafy greens are rich in carotenoids, the granddaddy is spinach, with a half-cup providing 1 milligram of beta-carotene.

Seeing Green

Carrots must be good for your eyes, the old joke has it, since you never see a rabbit wearing glasses. According to research, it's probably not only carrots that are good for the eyes but also all the leafy greens that Peter and his cotton-tailed friends munch.

In one study, scientists from the Massachusetts Eye and Ear Infirmary in Boston compared the diets of more than 350 people with advanced age-related macular degeneration—the leading cause of irreversible vision loss among older adults—with the diets of more than 500 people without the disease. They found that people who ate the most leafy green vegetables—particularly spinach and collard greens—were 43 percent less likely to get macular degeneration than those who ate them less frequently.

Experts believe that carotenoids protect the eyes in much the same way as they work against cancer, by acting as antioxidants and neutralizing tissue-damaging free radicals before they harm the body—in this case, the macular region of the eye.

Smile and Say "Greens"

In some parts of the world, like rural China, where vegetarianism is a way of life, people meet their daily calcium needs not by drinking milk but by eating greens.

In fact, 1 cup of turnip or dandelion greens can deliver about 172 milligrams of calcium, 17 percent of the DV. That's more than you'd get from a half-cup of skim milk.

The only problem with getting calcium from leafy green vegetables is that some of them contain high amounts of oxalates—compounds that block calcium absorption, says Dr. Liebman. "Spinach, Swiss chard, collards, and beet greens have the most oxalates, so don't consider these a source of calcium," he says. "The others are fine. Research has shown that the calcium in kale is particularly well-absorbed."

Pumping Up at the Salad Bar

If you're among the many folks cutting back on meats these days, you may be cutting down on a very important mineral—iron—as well. Here again, the leafy greens can help. Many vegetables, especially spinach and Swiss chard, are good sources of iron, a mineral your body needs to produce red blood cells and transport oxygen.

A half-cup of boiled spinach has 3 milligrams of iron, 20 percent of the Recommended Dietary Allowance (RDA) for women and 30 percent of the

Popeye probably never had kidney stones, because if he had, he wouldn't have kept downing all those cans of spinach.

Spinach, along with Swiss chard and beet greens, contains high amounts of oxalates, acids that the body cannot process and that are passed through the urine. For people who are sensitive to oxalates, eating too many of these greens can cause painful kidney stones to form. So if you're prone to stones, says Michael Liebman, Ph.D., professor of human nutrition at the University of Wyoming in Laramie, forget the chard, spinach, and beet greens, and choose among other leafy greens instead.

RDA for men. The same amount of Swiss chard provides 2 milligrams, which is 13 percent of the RDA for women and 30 percent of the RDA for men.

Unfortunately, the iron found in plants isn't as readily absorbed by the body as the iron found in meats—unless it's accompanied in the same meal by vitamin C. Good news again. Along with their high doses of iron, leafy green vegetables also contain ample amounts of vitamin C, which substantially improves iron absorption.

All the leafy greens provide ample amounts of this important nutrient, but the green giants of vitamin C are chicory (a half-cup serving has 22 milligrams, 37 percent of the DV) and beet and mustard greens, which both provide almost 18 milligrams, 30 percent of the DV.

In addition, beet greens and spinach are rich sources of riboflavin—a B vitamin that is essential for tissue growth and repair as well as helping your body convert other nutrients into usable forms. A half-cup of cooked spinach or beet greens provides 0.2 milligram of riboflavin, 12 percent of the DV.

Getting the Most

Cook them quickly. To cook or not to cook? That's often the question asked by people who want to maintain high levels of nutrients in vegetables. The answer with leafy greens, experts say, is yes, no, and maybe a little.

"It's always a trade-off between increasing the digestibility of nutrients when you cook foods and losing some nutrients in the cooking process," says Dr. Liebman. "But while it's great to eat them raw, you're more likely to eat more of certain vegetables if they're cooked. Just watch your cooking method. You don't want to boil them to death. Any quick-cooking method, such as blanching, is fine. One of the best cooking methods for retaining nutrients seems to be the microwave," he says.

CREAMED SWISS CHARD WITH ONIONS

1 teaspoon olive oil

1 medium onion, sliced

1 pound Swiss chard, cut into bite-size pieces

1 tablespoon unbleached all-purpose flour

1 cup canned evaporated skim milk

2 teaspoons grated Parmesan cheese

1/8 teaspoon ground nutmeg

In a large no-stick skillet over medium heat, warm the oil. Add the onions. Reduce the heat to low. Cook, stirring frequently, for 5 to 6 minutes, or until softened. Add the chard. Cover and cook for 3 to 4 minutes, or until the chard starts to wilt.

Sprinkle with the flour and stir. Gradually add the milk, stirring constantly. Cook, stirring, for 2 to 3 minutes, or until the sauce thickens. Add the Parmesan and nutmeg. Stir to mix.

Makes 4 servings

PER SERVING
calories **102**
total fat **1.8 g.**
saturated fat **0.5 g.**
cholesterol **3 mg.**
sodium **316 mg.**
dietary fiber **2.2 g.**

MUSTARD GREENS WITH SMOKED TURKEY

2 pounds mustard greens

1 cup finely chopped onions

2 cloves garlic, minced

3/4 cup diced smoked turkey breast

1 tablespoon white-wine vinegar

Hot-pepper sauce

Tear the leaves of the greens away from the stems and discard the stems. Tear the greens into bite-size pieces.

Coat a large no-stick skillet with no-stick spray. Scatter the onions, garlic, and turkey evenly in the skillet. Warm over medium heat. As soon as the skillet starts to heat up, add as much of the greens as the skillet will hold. (If necessary, add the remainder after the first batch cooks down enough to make room for them.) Cover tightly and cook for 7 to 8 minutes, or until the greens wilt and soften.

Stir to combine. Sprinkle with the vinegar. Add hot-pepper sauce to taste.

Makes 4 servings

PER SERVING
calories **62**
total fat **1.2 g.**
saturated fat **0.3 g.**
cholesterol **14 mg.**
sodium **304 mg.**
dietary fiber **2.6 g.**

Spinach-Mushroom Salad

Salad

1 bag (6 ounces) spinach, washed and trimmed

1 cup sliced button mushrooms

1 cup bean sprouts, rinsed

1 orange, peeled and sectioned

Dressing

3 tablespoons nonfat plain yogurt

1 tablespoon reduced-fat mayonnaise

1 tablespoon fresh orange juice

2 teaspoons reduced-sodium soy sauce

¼ teaspoon dark sesame oil

To make the salad: In a large bowl, combine the spinach, mushrooms, bean sprouts, and orange. Toss to combine.

To make the dressing: In a small bowl, combine the yogurt, mayonnaise, orange juice, soy sauce, and sesame oil. Whisk until smooth.

Pour over the spinach salad. Toss to coat.

Makes 4 servings

Per serving

calories	**62**
total fat	**1.9 g.**
saturated fat	**0.4 g.**
cholesterol	**2 mg.**
sodium	**129 mg.**
dietary fiber	**2.5 g.**

Hay Fever
The Kitchen Connection

While the usual treatment for hay fever is to stay inside and take antihistamines, there's some evidence that the foods you eat while hiding from the pollen outside could make you feel even worse. So before shutting all the windows, take a look in your kitchen. There may be a few foods that you'll want to, well, sneeze at.

Doctors aren't sure why, but for many people with hay fever, the immune system responds not only to pollen but also to certain fruits and vegetables, especially melons and bananas, says John Anderson, M.D., head of the division of allergy and clinical immunology at Henry Ford Hospital in Detroit.

If you're allergic to ragweed, for example, having a slice of watermelon or cantaloupe or eating a banana could cause your mouth to itch and swell, or you might experience additional stuffiness, says Dr. Anderson. If you're allergic to tree and grass pollens, eating apples, cherries, peaches, carrots, or potatoes might make your symptoms worse.

People with this type of multiple allergy (doctors call it cross-reactivity) may be sensitive to these foods all year long. In most cases, however, they suffer more in the spring, when pollen counts (and the body's level of histamine) are already high. There's no real solution, except the obvious one. You may have to give up those fruits and vegetables that are causing your symptoms to flare up. Cooking the offending foods, however, will often eliminate their allergy-causing potential.

Some people with hay fever are sensitive to the pollen in honey. "If you have honey that's loaded with a specific pollen that you're sensitive to, you may have a reaction," says Dr. Anderson.

You probably don't have to give up honey entirely, he adds. Different kinds of honey contain different kinds of pollen. By switching brands a few times, you'll eventually find one that doesn't make your hay fever symptoms worse.

Finally, Austrian researchers have found that for some people with hay fever, having a glass of wine may cause problems. A small study found that red wine often contains histamine, the same chemical that makes people with hay fever so miserable. Pouring additional histamine into a system that's already loaded with the stuff may cause the bronchial tubes to constrict, making breathing difficult.

HEADACHES
FEED YOUR HEAD RIGHT

In some ways, headaches are an unavoidable consequence of modern life. There's nothing quite like late nights, traffic jams, or daily office politics to start your head pounding.

Yet stress and noise aren't the only things causing heads to throb. Many of the foods we eat, from hot dogs and cheese to chocolate brownies, can cause headaches. Not eating certain foods can also cause problems. This may explain, in part, why Americans spend more than $8 billion on over-the-counter and prescription pain relief. That's a lot of extra-strength aspirin, acetaminophen, and ibuprofen.

While changing your diet won't eliminate headaches entirely, it can make a big difference in reducing their frequency and keeping the pain under control. Best of all, relief won't come from a safety-sealed bottle but from your own refrigerator.

TWO TYPES OF PAIN

Before considering specific foods, it's helpful to understand the main types of headaches. The most common type, called muscle-contraction or tension headache, is often caused by kinked-up neck and scalp muscles.

The second type, which includes migraines, is called vascular headache. Headaches of this type are caused by the expansion and contraction of blood vessels in the face, head, and neck. Vascular headaches can be extremely painful or even disabling, as anyone who gets migraines can attest.

Both types can be caused by almost anything—stress, fluctuating hormone levels, or even changes in the weather. But substances found in foods—natural compounds as well as chemicals added during processing—are frequently to blame, says Melvyn Werbach, M.D., assistant clinical professor of psychiatry at the University of California, Los Angeles, and author of *Healing through Nutrition* and *Nutritional Influences on Illness*.

COMMON TRIGGERS

Although experts aren't sure what causes migraines, they have identified a number of foods and additives that can set the process in motion.

One of the most common migraine triggers is tyramine. Found in such things as chocolate, red wine, and aged cheese, tyramine is an amino acid that causes the body to release hormones that cause blood vessels to constrict. At some point the blood vessels rebound and dilate, setting off the familiar throb.

Another common cause of headache pain is nitrites. Used to preserve foods such as bologna, hot dogs, and canned meats, nitrites often cause blood vessels in the head and body to dilate painfully.

Monosodium glutamate (MSG), a flavor enhancer used in a variety of foods, including lunch meats, canned and dry soups, and frozen dinners, can be a problem. It's also a common additive in Chinese cooking. The term *Chinese restaurant syndrome* was coined to describe MSG-related headaches.

There's no easy way to avoid all of these substances or to be sure which one is causing the problem or if there is more than one culprit. About the only thing you can do is keep a headache diary, says Alan M. Rapoport, M.D., co-founder and director of the New England Center for Headache in Stamford, Connecticut, and assistant clinical professor of neurology at Yale University School of Medicine. When you feel a headache coming on, make a list of everything you ate in the last 24 hours. Eventually, you'll gain a better understanding of which foods may be to blame and which you'll need to avoid in the future.

The Carbohydrate Connection

Central to the headache-food equation is a brain chemical called serotonin, which transmits messages from one nerve cell to another. Falling levels of serotonin in the brain are often associated with headaches, says Dr. Rapoport. Raising the levels of serotonin can ease headaches or even prevent them entirely.

One way to boost serotonin in the brain is to increase the amount of carbohydrates in your diet. "There's no doubt that following a diet high in complex carbohydrates and low in fat can be very helpful for some people with migraine, although we don't know exactly why," says Dr. Rapoport.

If you're prone to headaches, it might be a good idea to eat more foods that are high in fiber and complex carbohydrates, like fresh vegetables, whole grains, and dried beans, Dr. Werbach advises.

But even though a high-carbohyrate diet can often be helpful, there are some people for whom it can actually make things worse. If you have low blood sugar, or hypoglycemia, for example, you may find that you do better if you consume fewer carbohydrates. "Having low levels of sugar in the brain can set off a headache," Dr. Werbach says. "These people may do well on a so-called hypoglycemic diet, which is usually a low-carbohydrate diet."

If you've noticed that your headaches often occur after you eat a lot of carbohydrates, says Dr. Werbach, try eating slightly more protein in the form of tofu, lean meats, eggs, or low-fat cheese.

The Benefits of B₆

Vitamin B_6 has been shown to keep the nervous system healthy, relieve pre-menstrual discomfort, and shore up the immune system. Studies suggest that it may help relieve migraines as well. Vitamin B_6 is used in the brain to increase serotonin levels, explains Dr. Rapoport, "so a good intake of B_6 might help relieve migraines, even if you're not deficient in it."

The Daily Value (DV) for vitamin B_6 is 2 milligrams. One medium potato or one banana contains 0.7 milligram of B_6, 35 percent of the DV. A 3-ounce serving of baked or broiled swordfish has 0.3 milligram, 15 percent of the DV.

While increasing your consumption of dietary B_6 is a good idea if you're headache-prone, your doctor may advise getting larger amounts (up to 150 milligrams) through a multiple vitamin. But you shouldn't take B_6 supplements unless prescribed by a doctor, as too much can cause damage to the nervous system.

Minerals for Relief

While the underlying reasons aren't yet clear, certain minerals, particularly magnesium, calcium, and iron, appear to play a role in both preventing and easing migraine and tension headaches.

People who suffer from migraine often have low levels of magnesium in their brain cells. Studies suggest that correcting a magnesium deficiency may help relieve migraine, says Dr. Rapoport.

Ready-to-eat breakfast cereals are good sources of magnesium, with some brands containing more than 100 milligrams of magnesium, 25 percent of the DV, in a 1-ounce serving. Nuts, seeds, and leafy green vegetables are also rich in magnesium. Nuts are also loaded with fat, however, so you'll want to eat them in moderation and get most of your magnesium elsewhere.

Calcium is another mineral that has been linked to headache relief. One study found that women who consumed 200 milligrams of calcium a day (20 percent of the DV) had fewer headaches than women who consumed less.

Dairy foods are the best sources of calcium. Topping the list is milk, with 1 cup of skim containing 302 milligrams, or 30 percent of the DV. Other good sources of calcium include ice milk, with 176 milligrams per cup, 18 percent of the DV, and low-fat fruit yogurt, with 312 milligrams per cup, 31 percent of the DV. There are many nondairy sources of calcium as well, among them broccoli, with 48 milligrams, and Swiss chard, with 101 milligrams in 1 cup.

Last on the list of minerals that may head off headaches is iron. As you know, not getting enough iron in the diet can lead to anemia, a condition in which the body doesn't get enough oxygen. To compensate, blood vessels dilate to admit more blood, says Dr. Rapoport. "This dilation compresses the nerves in the walls of the vessels, causing head pain," he explains. "Consuming more dietary iron may indirectly relieve headaches by treating the anemia."

It's generally easy to meet the DV of 18 milligrams of iron. A large baked potato, for example, has 7 milligrams, while 1 cup of Swiss chard has nearly 4 milligrams. Meats are even better sources, since the type of iron they contain (heme iron) is more readily absorbed by the body than the nonheme iron in vegetables. A 3-ounce serving of broiled top round steak has 3 milligrams of iron, and the same amount of roasted white turkey meat has 1 milligram.

SPICY RELIEF

When you're searching for a drug-free form of migraine relief, you might want to try a spoonful of the popular spice ginger. Researchers at Odense University in Denmark believe that ginger blocks the action of prostaglandins, substances that cause pain and inflammation in blood vessels. It might help prevent impending migraines without the side effects of some migraine-relieving drugs.

Research is still preliminary, so experts are reluctant to recommend specific amounts of ginger for fighting migraine. If you feel a migraine coming on, however, you might try taking ⅓ teaspoon of powdered ginger, the amount suggested by the Danish researchers.

When taking ginger, it's even better to use fresh rather than powdered because it's more active, says Charles Lo, M.D., a doctor of Chinese medicine in private practice in Chicago. He advises grating the ginger or pushing it through a garlic press. Either of these methods releases more of the potent juices than slicing or chopping. You can make a spicy ginger tea by steeping a teaspoon of the grated root in a cup of boiling water for at least five minutes, says Dr. Lo.

THE COFFEE CURE

For some people, sipping a cup of their favorite aromatic brew may work as well as popping an over-the-counter painkiller. The caffeine in coffee can counter a headache by temporarily constricting dilated blood vessels, which may be causing the pain, says Fred Sheftell, M.D., co-founder and co-director of the New England Center for Headache in Stamford, Connecticut. "Caffeine is an ingredient in some pain relievers," he says.

But overdo it. Too much coffee will eventually cause the blood vessels to dilate painfully again. Dr. Sheftell recommends that people who are headache-prone drink no more than two cups (5 ounces each) a day, which together contain about 200 milligrams of caffeine, depending on the strength of the brew.

HEARTBURN
PUTTING OUT THE FIRE

If you've ever had heartburn, you know the name is appropriate. It feels as though a fire is raging in your chest. The pain can be so intense, in fact, that some people rush to the doctor because they think they're having a heart attack.

But in fact, heartburn has nothing to do with the heart. It occurs when acid-laden digestive juices in the stomach surge upward into the esophagus, the tube that connects the mouth with the stomach. Normally, a tight little muscle at the base of the esophagus, called the lower esophageal sphincter (LES), prevents juices from escaping. But when the muscle relaxes at the wrong times, juices splash upward, literally scorching tender tissue in the esophagus. This is what causes the burn in heartburn.

As it turns out, many of the foods we eat every day and the times that we eat them are the main causes of heartburn. In addition, there are some foods that will quickly put the fire out. So before you rush to the pharmacy for an antacid, make a pit stop in your kitchen.

"Modifying the diet remains the first line of treatment for people with heartburn," says Suzanne Rose, M.D., a gastroenterologist and director of the esophageal and swallowing disorders center at New York Hospital–Cornell Medical Center in New York City.

INSIDE HEALING

One food that can help control heartburn is ginger, says John Hibbs, a naturopathic doctor and associate professor of clinical medicine at Bastyr University in Seattle. Ginger helps strengthen the holding power of the LES, which can help keep acid where it belongs. Since fresh ginger is quite spicy, a better strategy is to make ginger tea by adding ½ to 1 teaspoon of freshly grated ginger (or ¼ to ½ teaspoon of powdered ginger) to a cup of hot water. Let it steep for 10 minutes, strain out the ginger, and drink it down.

Another strategy for stopping heartburn is to eat pasta, rice, potatoes, or other foods high in complex carbohydrates, which absorb acid in the stomach, says Ara H. DerMarderosian, Ph.D., professor of pharmacognosy and medicinal chemistry at Philadelphia College of Pharmacy and Science.

Finally, it's a good idea not to lie down soon after eating, Dr. Rose says.

When your stomach is full, it's very easy for acid to rise up into the esophagus, especially when you lie down and gravity is working against you. Staying upright, whether on your feet or sitting in a chair, will help keep the acid down, she says.

COMMON OFFENDERS

Researchers estimate that up to 25 million Americans get heartburn every day. What's more, Americans get more calories from fat than just about anyone else on the planet. A coincidence? Researchers don't think so.

Studies have shown that a number of foods, particularly those that are high in fat, like butter and red meat, can temporarily reduce the holding power of the LES. In one study, for example, researchers at Bowman Gray School of Medicine of Wake Forest University in Winston-Salem, North Carolina, found that people who ate high-fat meals were exposed to acid about four times longer than those eating leaner fare.

Chocolate is another common offender, Dr. Rose adds. Not only is chocolate high in fat, it may contain other compounds that can relax the LES even more. In another study at Bowman Gray, researchers found that when people ate chocolate, stomach acid splashed into the esophagus for up to an hour afterward.

It's not only high-fat foods that can be a problem. Onions, for example, can bring on heartburn in some people. Researchers aren't exactly sure what it is about onions that can light the fire, but for some people, having even one slice of onion can cause heartburn to flare up.

Peppermint, which is often added to baked goods, ice cream, and candy, frequently causes heartburn, Dr. Rose adds. In one study, researchers at the State University of New York at Buffalo found that when people ate peppermint, the esophageal muscle lost some of its holding power within just a few minutes.

Finally, be careful about eating spicy foods until your heartburn has a chance to heal, says Dr. Rose. Many people don't think twice about dousing tender tissues in the esophagus with a meal of hot peppers or a swig of orange juice. You don't have to give up your favorite foods entirely, she adds. Just put them aside for a few days until you're feeling better.

HEART DISEASE
PRIMING YOUR PUMP

Doctors haven't always known what was best for our hearts. Only a few decades ago, little attention was paid to diet, and even smoking was thought to be acceptable.

Everything has changed.

After almost 40 years of investigating what makes heart disease our worst public-health enemy, scientists have come up with some pretty simple answers. Regular exercise is important, of course, as is giving up smoking. But most important of all is having a healthy diet. Reaching for the right foods is the best way to lower cholesterol and high blood pressure, two of the biggest risk factors for the heart.

All too often, however, we reach for the wrong ones. Let's take a look at the best—and worst—foods for preventing heart disease, starting with fats. While there are some fats that we'd be better off avoiding, others aren't so bad, and some might even be healthful.

THE BAD FATS

We all know that saturated fat, the kind found primarily in red meats, butter, and other animal foods, is incredibly bad for the heart. Study after study has shown that the more saturated fat people get in their diets, the higher their risks for heart disease.

Foods high in saturated fat raise levels of artery-clogging low-density lipoprotein (LDL) cholesterol, says Michael Gaziano, M.D., director of cardio-vascular epidemiology at Brigham and Women's Hospital in Boston. What's more, foods high in saturated fat are often high in cholesterol as well.

The danger is so great that the American Heart Association recommends that we get no more (and preferably less) than 10 percent of our calories from saturated fat. Suppose, for example, that you normally get 2,000 calories in a day. This means your daily limit for saturated fat is 22 grams. So in addition to having fruits, vegetables, and other low-fat foods, you could have 3 ounces of extra-lean ground beef (5 grams of saturated fat), a serving of macaroni and cheese (6 grams), and six onion rings (10 grams).

But even this modest amount of saturated fat isn't ideal. "Your best bet for lowering heart disease risk is to reduce the amount of saturated fat in your diet to less than 10 percent of your total calories," says Dr. Gaziano.

Another type of problem fat, called trans-fatty acids, has been shown to dramatically increase the amount of cholesterol in the bloodstream, says Dr. Gaziano.

Ironically, trans-fatty acids, which are found mainly in margarine, were meant to be a healthful alternative to the saturated fat in butter. Some studies have shown, however, that it may not be the best choice. In fact, trans-fatty acids may be just as bad as the saturated fat in butter, says Christopher Gardner, Ph.D., research fellow at the Stanford University Center for Research in Disease Prevention in Palo Alto, California. So you don't want to eat a lot of them. And it's not only margarine that may be a problem. Many cookies, cakes, and other snack foods contain partially hydrogenated oil, which is also high in trans-fatty acids.

SOME BETTER FATS

Unlike saturated fat and trans-fatty acids, some fats are relatively healthful. Here's an easy way to recognize them. Look for the prefix un-, as in polyunsaturated and monounsaturated fats. While these "un-fats" are still high in calories, in small amounts they play several beneficial roles.

Both monounsaturated fat (the kind found in olive and canola oils and most nuts) and polyunsaturated fat (found in corn, safflower, and sunflower oils) have been shown to lower levels of dangerous LDL cholesterol without lowering levels of beneficial high-density lipoprotein (HDL) cholesterol. This is important because you need HDL cholesterol to flush the bad cholesterol from your body.

Monounsaturated and polyunsaturated fats aren't exactly the same, however. Since monounsaturated fats aren't damaged by oxidation, they're less likely to cause buildups of cholesterol in the arteries. Polyunsaturated fats help keep blood pressure healthy and keep blood from clotting excessively. "Picking either of these fats over saturated fat or trans-fatty acids is a winning choice," says Dr. Gardner.

Nuts are particularly good sources of these healthful fats. In a study of Seventh Day Adventists, researchers found that those who consumed nuts at least four times a week had almost half the risk of fatal heart attacks of those who rarely ate them. "I tell people to aim for getting about 20 to 25 percent of total calories from fat, most of which should be in the form of monounsaturated and polyunsaturated fat," says Dr. Gaziano.

There's yet another kind of healthful fat, called omega-3 fatty acids. Found in most fish and also in flaxseed, omega-3's can help prevent clots from forming in the bloodstream. In addition, they help lower triglycerides, a type of blood fat that, in large amounts, may raise the risk for heart disease.

Studies show that eating fish once or twice a week (salmon is a good choice, because it contains high levels of omega-3's) can help keep your arteries clear and your heart working well.

Feast on Folate

Almost 30 years ago, a Harvard pathologist suggested that a vitamin deficiency could be a major cause of heart disease. The theory sounded so wacky that nobody listened. Now, instead of laughing, scientists are researching because evidence suggests that folate, a B vitamin abundant in beans and dark green, leafy vegetables, may play a major role in preventing heart attacks.

Folate is responsible for lowering levels of an amino acid called homocysteine. While the body needs homocysteine to produce muscle and bone tissue, in large amounts it can injure blood vessels, causing hardening of the arteries.

"High homocysteine levels are an important contributor to heart disease," says Dr. Gardner. "And it appears that homocysteine levels can be brought down easily with modest amounts of folate in the diet."

You don't need a lot of folate to get the benefits. The Daily Value (DV) of 400 micrograms may be plenty, Dr. Gardner says. Spinach is a good source of folate, with 1 cup containing 109 micrograms, nearly 28 percent of the DV. Lentils are even better, with a half-cup containing 179 micrograms, 45 percent of the DV. Even a 6-ounce glass of orange juice contains 34 micrograms of folate, 8 percent of the DV.

Aiming for Antioxidants

Doctors have known for years that the body's LDL cholesterol is bad news, but it wasn't until recently that they understood why.

Every day, your body produces harmful oxygen molecules called free radicals, which damage cholesterol. This process, called oxidation, is what causes cholesterol to stick to artery walls.

Fruits, vegetables, and other foods containing antioxidants such as beta-carotene and vitamins C and E are your best protection against oxidation and heart disease. In fact, one group of antioxidants, called flavonoids, is thought to be the reason that the Dutch and French have such healthy hearts, despite some decidedly unhealthy eating habits.

A study in the Netherlands, for example, found that men who ate the most flavonoid-rich foods, particularly apples, tea, and onions, were half as likely to have heart disease as those who ate the least. Flavonoids may also explain why the French, who eat more fat and cholesterol than we do, have heart disease death rates 2½ times lower than ours.

Doctors still aren't sure which foods—or which compounds found in foods—are the most effective. The National Cancer Institute calls for eating five to nine servings a day of a large variety of fruits and vegetables.

"You just can't lose by eating plenty of fruits and vegetables," says Dr. Gardner. "Study after study shows that people who eat the most of these healthful foods have the lowest rates of heart disease."

FORTIFY YOUR HEART WITH FIBER

Your grandmother called it roughage. Today, we call it fiber. But whatever it's called, it's an important part of any heart protection plan.

Fiber, especially the soluble kind found in beans, fruits, and grains, binds with cholesterol in the body and helps remove it along with the waste, says Diane Grabowski-Nepa, R.D., a dietitian and nutritional counselor at the Pritikin Longevity Center in Santa Monica, California.

Fiber is so effective, in fact, that a Harvard research team found that men who added just 10 grams of fiber a day to their diets were able to decrease their risks of heart attack by almost 30 percent.

The DV for fiber is 25 grams. Super sources of the rough stuff include whole grains, beans such as chickpeas, kidney beans, and lima beans, and dried fruits like figs, apples, and peaches.

SIP A LITTLE HEALTH

It's a tradition in many countries to raise a glass of wine and give a toast to good health. As it turns out, what's in that glass can make the toasts come true.

Studies have shown that drinking moderate amounts of alcohol raises levels of beneficial HDL cholesterol. Plus, alcohol acts like motor oil in the blood. It makes platelets, the tiny disks that aid in clotting, a little more slippery, so they're less likely to stick together and cause heart-damaging clots in the bloodstream.

All alcohol can help boost HDL cholesterol and reduce the tendency of blood to clot. But red wine is particularly good because it also contains heart-healthy flavonoids.

To get the benefits of alcohol without the problems, doctors advise drinking in moderation. For men, this means having no more than two drinks a day. Women, who are more susceptible to alcohol's effects, should limit themselves to one drink a day. (A drink is defined as 12 ounces of beer, 5 ounces of wine, or 1½ ounces of liquor.)

Hemorrhoids
No More Strained Veins

Sometimes the call of nature feels anything but natural. You have to go, but it takes more effort than you'd like. So you strain. And strain. This puts a lot of stress on tiny veins in the anus and rectum, which can cause them to swell and stretch out of shape. The result is a potentially painful but very common condition known as hemorrhoids. Since most hemorrhoids are caused by straining to have a bowel movement, the best way to prevent them is by making stools easier to pass, says Marvin Schuster, M.D., director of the Marvin M. Schuster Digestive and Motility Disorders Center at Johns Hopkins Bayview Medical Center in Baltimore. And the best way to do this is by eating the right foods.

Bulk for Your Bowels

The reason so many Americans have hemorrhoids is that the average fiber consumption in this country is 12 grams a day, a lot less than the Daily Value of 25 grams, says Dr. Schuster. Fiber is important because it adds bulk and weight to stools so they pass more easily. Studies have shown, in fact, that folks who eat a lot of fiber-rich foods have considerably fewer hemorrhoids than those who eat less fiber.

It's not difficult to get more fiber in your diet, Dr. Schuster adds. Eating five or more servings a day of fruits and vegetables and six servings of whole-grain breads, cereals, or legumes will provide all the fiber your digestive tract needs to work smoothly.

More Fluid Movements

Imagine eating a mouthful of saltines without drinking a little water. Hard to swallow, right? Well, a similar problem occurs when the digestive tract attempts to process food without getting enough liquid, says Marie Borum, M.D. assistant professor of medicine at George Washington University Medical Center in Washington, D.C. The stools become dry and difficult to pass—and this, as we've seen, is what causes hemorrhoids.

Water does more than aid digestion. Because it's absorbed by the stools, it makes them heavier and easier to pass. This is especially true when you're adding more fiber to your diet, because fiber absorbs water like a sponge, says Dr. Borum.

She recommends drinking six to eight glasses of water a day. This sounds like a lot, and it would be if you tried to drink it all at once. But keeping water handy and sipping it throughout the day—by having a glassful at your bedside, for example, or a plastic sipping bottle at your desk—makes it easy to get the necessary amounts.

BERRY GOOD FOR YOU

Even people who eat bushels of fiber and drink water by the pitcherful will occasionally have a problem with constipation and hemorrhoids. This is why some doctors believe that you should do everything possible to strengthen the anal veins, just in case.

Cherries, blackberries, and blueberries contain compounds called proanthocyanidins, which help strengthen the walls of capillaries and veins in the anus, making them less likely to stretch under pressure, says Andrew Weil, M.D., associate director of the division of social perspective in medicine at the University of Arizona College of Medicine in Tucson. Getting more of these berries in your diet could help prevent hemorrhoids, says Dr. Weil.

EASE THE PAIN

When hemorrhoids swell, they press against tender nerves, which is why they're often so painful. In addition, eating certain foods can make the pain even worse. So the next time hemorrhoids make an appearance, here are a few foods that you may want to avoid.

Say nada to java. Drinking coffee causes the intestines to contract, which can irritate an already tender hemorrhoid, says Marvin Schuster, M.D., director of the Digestive and Motility Disorders Center at Johns Hopkins Bayview Medical Center in Baltimore. Also, coffee is a diuretic, meaning that it causes the body to lose valuable water—and you need more, not less, water when hemorrhoids flare.

Take a break from alcohol. Like coffee, alcohol is a diuretic and can cause constipation. When you have hemorrhoids, it's a good idea to abstain from drinking until they go away.

Be a little bland. The same chemicals that give spicy foods their fire can burn you in the bathroom. So when hemorrhoids are hurting, put away the peppers and stick with blander foods instead.

While you can get the benefits of these compounds by eating whole berries, juices provide a more concentrated form to keep the veins strong. Doctors who specialize in nutritional healing recommend drinking 4 ounces of berry juice mixed with an equal amount of apple juice every day.

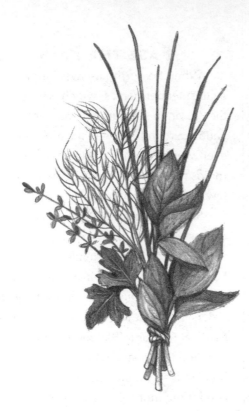

HERBS
HEALING THE NATURAL WAY

HEALING POWER
CAN HELP:
Prevent infections

Ease pain and swelling

Relieve menopausal discomfort

Lower cholesterol

Imagine marinara sauce without garlic. Gingerbread minus the ginger. Baked potatoes without chives. No one who enjoys food would want to live in a world without herbs.

But herbs do more than add depth to sauces or a tangy zip to potatoes and tofu. For millions of people worldwide, herbs are the medicines they depend on to stay healthy.

"Before the discovery of modern pharmaceuticals, both Europeans and Americans relied on herbs," says William J. Keller, Ph.D., professor and chair of the department of pharmaceutical sciences at Samford University School of Pharmacy in Birmingham, Alabama. Even today, people in Germany, France, and other European nations use herbal medicines nearly every day. "In this country, however, we've pretty much cast them aside—until now," says Dr. Keller.

Doctors are discovering that many herbs work as well as drugs for relieving common conditions, and for a very simple reason. The active ingredients in herbs may be virtually identical to the chemicals found in drugs. When you take an aspirin, for example, you get the benefit of a compound called acetylsalicylic acid, which eases pain, lowers fever, and reduces inflammation. But before there was aspirin, people made tea from willow bark. Willow contains a compound called salicin, which has many of the same effects as aspirin.

It's not only "simple" drugs that have herbal counterparts. Many prescription drugs also resemble (or are actually made from) herbs. The cancer drug etoposide, for example, is extracted from the root of the Mayapple plant, and the heart drug digitalis contains compounds similar to those found in purple foxglove. Researchers estimate, in fact, that up to 30 percent of the drugs we use today contain ingredients that are very similar to compounds found in plants.

From Plants to Penicillin

Researchers today use sophisticated equipment and expensive tests to discover which herbs are most effective. For the original herbalists, however, "research" often meant watching animals in the wild to see which leaves, bark, or berries they turned to whenever they were ill. Over the years, herbalists (and doctors) became pretty knowledgeable about which herbs were best—for easing a headache, for example, or stopping an infection.

By the middle of the twentieth century, however, scientists were less interested in the herbs themselves than in what the herbs contained. "With the advancement of laboratory chemistry, it became possible to isolate and purify the chemical compounds from plants to make pharmaceutical drugs," says Mark Blumenthal, executive director of the American Botanical Council in Austin, Texas, and editor of the journal *HerbalGram*.

The new drugs offered a lot of advantages over their leafy predecessors.

In the Kitchen

Most herbs are easy to grow, either in backyard gardens or simply in flowerpots on the windowsill. But to preserve their healing powers, you have to dry and store them properly. Here's how.

- When drying leaves or flowers, tie small bunches of herbs together and hang them upside down in a dry, well-ventilated area such as an attic or large pantry. To prevent them from getting dusty, you can hang the herbs inside paper bags with holes punched in the sides to allow air to circulate. Be careful not to crush the herbs, since this will cause the precious oils to dissipate.
- When drying roots, cut them into thin pieces, thread them on a length of string, and hang them to dry.
- When drying seeds, hang the entire plant upside down in a paper bag and allow to dry. As the plant dries, the seeds will fall to the bottom of the bag.
- To keep dried herbs fresh, store them in tightly sealed jars in a cool, dark place. When properly stored, dried herbs will retain their potency for about a year or more.

With laboratory precision, it was possible to make thousands (or millions) of pills, each with exactly the same strength. Drugs were also convenient. It was no longer necessary to spend hours searching for and preparing herbs—hanging them to dry, extracting their oils, or brewing them into tea—since it was possible to pop a pill that did the same thing.

"It wasn't because herbs were ineffective that people quit using them but because there were reliable, cheaper, sexier drugs, like the sulfa drugs and later, penicillin," Blumenthal says. "So herbs fell into a kind of twilight zone."

Back to Basics

Today, of course, it's much easier to find over-the-counter drugs than herbal remedies that do the same thing. But more and more Americans are putting drugs back on the shelves in favor of a more natural way of healing.

One advantage of using herbs is that they tend to cause fewer side effects than modern drugs. Drugs are highly concentrated, which is why taking one tiny pill or capsule can have such dramatic results. Since herbs are much less concentrated, you don't get as much of the active ingredient in your body at one time, so you're less likely to have uncomfortable reactions.

But the main reason that people are using herbs such as garlic, echinacea, and feverfew is that they work—which is why, in just one year, German physicians wrote 5.4 million prescriptions for ginkgo, an herb that has been shown to improve blood flow to the brain. They also wrote over 2 million prescriptions for echinacea, an immunity-boosting herb that's often used for treating colds and flu.

"Studies have shown that taking echinacea as soon as you start feeling ill shortens the duration of the infection," says Donald J. Brown, a naturopathic doctor and instructor at Bastyr University in Seattle and author of *Herbal Prescriptions for Better Health*.

Of all the healing herbs, garlic is perhaps the best-studied, and with good reason. This pungent bulb contains compounds that have been shown to lower cholesterol and high blood pressure, two of the leading risk factors for heart disease. In a landmark study, for example, people in two groups were given 2½ ounces of butter for several weeks, which raised their cholesterol levels. Half of the people were also given an extract containing the equivalent of seven cloves of garlic every day. Not surprisingly, people in both groups had increases in cholesterol. The garlic-eaters, however, showed less of an increase than those who did not eat garlic. What's more, they actually had a 16 percent decrease in triglycerides, another type of blood fat that has been linked to heart disease.

Feverfew is an herb that has received scientific attention because it appears to help prevent migraines. In one study, for example, researchers at University Hospital in Nottingham, England, gave migraine-prone people capsules of feverfew every day for four months. At the end of the study, the number of migraines in the group had dropped 24 percent.

Licorice root is a perfect example of an herb that may work as well or even better than its chemical counterparts. Licorice root contains compounds called phytoestrogens, which enhance the effects of the estrogen a woman produces naturally. As a result, it can be very helpful for treating a variety of women's problems, such as hot flashes and mood swings caused by menopause, says Mary Bove, a naturopathic doctor and director of the Brattleboro Naturopathic Clinic in Vermont.

For some women, in fact, licorice root may work just as well as the powerful drugs used in hormone-replacement therapy, Dr. Bove adds. Better yet, it doesn't appear to increase the risk of breast and uterine cancers the way the medications do. If you'd like to try licorice root, check with your doctor to see if it might work for you.

Putting Them to Work

When you're used to opening a bottle and popping a pill into your mouth, getting used to herbs can take a little time. Apothecaries and natural food stores often stock hundreds of healing herbs—packed into capsules, dissolved in oils, or lying loose in covered glass jars. It's not always easy to know which form to choose or how to prepare herbs once you get them home. Here are a few tips for getting started.

Choose the right form. Many herbal remedies come in three forms: as pills or capsules, as liquids (called extracts and tinctures), and in their natural form as leaves, bark, roots, and flowers. Each form provides healing benefits, but they act in slightly different ways, says Debra Brammer, a naturopathic doctor and clinical faculty member at Bastyr University Natural Health Clinic in Seattle.

When you're sick and want fast relief, herbal extracts are usually best because they're absorbed very quickly by the body, Dr. Brammer says. While they're not as convenient as taking a pill—you have to measure them, using a dropper or a teaspoon, into a glass of water or juice—they go to work almost instantly, she says.

When you're using herbs for long-term protection—to strengthen the immune system, for example—it doesn't matter how quickly they work. What does count is convenience, since you're going to be using them almost every day. Nothing's easier than taking herbs in pill or capsule form. Just be sure to check the label before buying them, Dr. Keller adds. Herbal pills should be standardized, which means that they contain a precise amount of the healing herb. Products that aren't standardized may contain little or none of the herb's active compounds.

You can also buy herbs in their natural form or ground into a powder. These are used for making teas, says Dr. Brammer. While herbal teas work somewhat more slowly than extracts, they're absorbed by the body faster than pills or capsules. Plus, many people enjoy the taste of freshly brewed herbal teas. "The

(continued on page 286)

THE HEALING HERBS

There are literally thousands of herbs that are used for healing around the world. Most herbs can be taken in capsule, tablet, or liquid forms, as well as in teas. Here are some of the most popular healing herbs and instructions for using them. Of course, if you are pregnant or have serious health problems, be sure to talk to your doctor before using medicinal herbs.

Herb	Benefits	How to Use
Anise	Eases hot flashes and other menopausal problems. Helps relieve gas.	Crush 1 tsp. seeds and steep in boiling water to make a tea.
Chamomile	Good for indigestion and gas and for easing sore throat.	Pour boiling water over 1–2 Tbsp. herb and steep to make a tea.
Echinacea	Strengthens the immune system.	Take 1/2 tsp. tincture 3 times a day at the first sign of a cold. Or pour boiling water over 1/2 tsp. coarsely powdered dried herb and steep to make a tea.
Fennel	Eases hot flashes and other menopausal problems. Helps settle the stomach.	Crush 1–2 tsp. seeds and steep in boiling water to make a tea.
Feverfew	Helps prevent and relieve migraines.	Eat 2–3 fresh leaves a day.
Garlic	Helps lower cholesterol and high blood pressure and reduces the risk for heart disease.	Eat 1–6 cloves a day.
Gentian	Stimulates appetite and improves digestion.	Pour boiling water over 1/2 tsp. finely cut or coarsely powdered herb and steep to make a tea.
Ginkgo	Helps prevent blood clots and increases blood flow to the brain. Eases anxiety.	Take a 40-milligram capsule 3 times a day for 1–2 months.
Horehound	A mild expectorant that's good for coughs.	Pour boiling water over 1 1/2 tsp. finely cut leaves and steep to make a tea.
Lemon balm	A calming herb that also helps ease cold sores.	Pour boiling water over 1–2 tsp. finely chopped leaves and steep to make a tea.
Licorice root	Relieves menopausal problems such as mood swings and hot flashes. Helps heal sore throat and ulcers.	Pour boiling water over 1/2 tsp. finely chopped root and steep to make a tea. Do not use for more than 4–6 weeks at a time. Avoid if you have high blood pressure.

Herb	Benefits	How to Use
Lovage	Relieves gas and fluid retention.	Pour boiling water over $1/2$–1 tsp. finely cut root and steep to make a tea. Repeat 3 times a day when using as a diuretic.
Milk thistle	Good for liver problems such as hepatitis and cirrhosis.	Take a 200-milligram capsule once a day.
Nettle	Helps relieve fluid retention.	Pour boiling water over 2 tsp. finely cut leaves and steep to make a tea.
Oregano	Good for parasitic infections and for blocking the effects of carcinogens in cooked meats.	Add generous amounts of whole leaves or powdered herb during cooking.
Parsley	A digestive aid and mild diuretic.	Add generous amounts of leaves and stems during cooking.
Peppermint	Eases upset stomach and reduces gas.	Pour boiling water over 1 Tbsp. dried leaves and steep to make a tea.
Rosemary	Eases digestion and helps stimulate appetite.	Pour boiling water over 1 tsp. finely chopped leaves and steep to make a tea.
St.-John's-wort	Eases nervousness and anxiety, improves memory and concentration, and has anti-viral and anti-inflammatory effects.	Take a 250-milligram capsule once a day.
Savory	Relieves gas and diarrhea and stimulates appetite.	Add generous amounts of crushed leaves during cooking.
Thyme	Eases cough and upper respiratory infections.	Pour boiling water over 1 tsp. dried herb and steep to make a tea.
Uva ursi (bearberry)	Helps relieve fluid retention and fights inflammation in the urinary tract.	Pour cold water over 1 tsp. coarsely powdered leaves and let stand for 12–24 hours to make a tea.
Valerian	Good for insomnia.	Pour boiling water over 2 tsp. finely cut root and steep to make a tea.
Willow bark	Helps ease pain, fever, and headaches.	Pour boiling water over 1–2 tsp. finely chopped bark and steep to make a tea.
Yarrow	Good for indigestion and for stimulating the appetite.	Pour boiling water over 1 heaping tsp. finely chopped herb and steep to make a tea.

ritual of brewing the tea and sipping it slowly is so relaxing that it often makes people feel better," Dr. Brammer adds.

Shop for freshness. The one problem with using fresh herbs is that they give up their benefits over time. "It's a bad sign if the herbs are lying in bins in the store's front window, with the sun pouring in, since herbs lose their potency when exposed to light and air," says Dr. Keller.

Before buying herbs, put your nose to work, Dr. Keller advises. Fresh herbs should smell, well, fresh. "Don't buy herbs that smell musty or look moldy, very dry, or discolored," he says. And once you get them home, be sure to store them in an airtight container in a cool, dark place, such as a kitchen cupboard away from the stove.

Shop often. Even though it's convenient to buy in bulk, dried herbs won't keep indefinitely, says Dr. Brammer. To get the most healing power, she says, it's best to buy herbs in small amounts and to replenish the supply a bit more frequently.

Treat them with respect. Even though herbs are often gentler than modern medicines, they can cause side effects, such as upset stomach, says Dr. Keller. It's a good idea to take healing herbs with meals rather than on an empty stomach. And because herbs are medicine, be sure to check with your doctor before taking them, especially if you're taking other medications for serious conditions such as diabetes or heart disease, says Dr. Keller.

Minty Pears

1   cup water
3   tablespoons sugar
1   tablespoon fresh lemon juice
½   cup tightly packed fresh peppermint or spearmint leaves, coarsely chopped
4   medium red Bartlett pears, ripe but firm

Per serving

calories	**153**
total fat	**0.8 g.**
saturated fat	**0 g.**
cholesterol	**0 mg.**
sodium	**19 mg.**
dietary fiber	**5.6 g.**

In a Dutch oven, combine the water, sugar, and lemon juice. Bring to a boil over medium heat. Add all but about 2 tablespoons of the mint leaves. Stir to mix. Cook for 1 to 2 minutes, or until the syrup starts to simmer.

Quarter the pears lengthwise and remove the cores. Add to the pot, skin side up. Cover and cook for 5 to 6 minutes, or until just tender. Test for doneness by inserting the tip of a sharp knife in a pear.

Divide the pears among serving dishes. Pour the mint syrup over them. Sprinkle with the reserved fresh mint. Serve warm.

Makes 4 servings

HERPES
THE POWER OF PROTEINS

The herpes simplex virus is a master of ambush. It spends most of its life dormant, hidden deep within the nerves and waiting for the immune system to drop its guard. When the coast is clear, it rushes to the skin, causing ugly, painful sores that can last a week or more. Then it retreats back into the nerves, waiting weeks, months, or even years before rearing its ugly head once more.

There is no cure for herpes, which can cause sores anywhere on the surface of the skin, so the last thing you want is to be infected with it. But if you already have herpes, there is some evidence that suggests that eating more of some types of foods and less of others can make the virus weaker and less likely to launch its attacks.

TAKE AWAY ITS STRENGTH

You wouldn't think that an egg or a bowl of baked beans would have much stopping power against the herpes virus. But these foods, along with meat, milk, and cheese, contain large amounts of lysine, an amino acid that can help prevent the virus from thriving.

"The herpes virus uses certain amino acids to build the protein sheath that surrounds it," explains Mark McCune, M.D., a dermatologist in private practice in Overland Park, Kansas. "Lysine inhibits the growth of the shield, so the virus can't flourish."

Doctors aren't sure how much lysine is needed to control herpes, but Dr. McCune recommends getting between 1,000 and 2,000 milligrams a day. In one study, researchers found that people who got 500 to 1,000 milligrams of lysine a day above their normal intake rarely had outbreaks. Even when they did have outbreaks, the sores were smaller than before and in some cases lasted only half as long.

It's easy to get large amounts of lysine in your diet. An ounce and a half of provolone cheese, for example, has 1,110 milligrams. Two eggs provide 900 milligrams, and 1 cup of baked beans has 960 milligrams. Pork is a lysine powerhouse, with one broiled, center-cut loin chop providing almost 2,000 milligrams.

Cut Off Its Supplies

Just as foods high in lysine can inhibit the herpes virus from building its protective coat, foods high in arginine may strengthen its defenses. "Arginine is an amino acid that herpes relies on for building its protein coating," says Dr. McCune. "If your diet is very high in arginine, this might help the virus grow aggressively."

High-arginine foods include chocolate, peas, nuts, and beer. You don't have to give up these foods entirely if you have herpes, Dr. McCune explains. What you should do, however, is balance them by eating other foods that are high in lysine.

"The whole lysine-arginine system doesn't work for everybody," Dr. McCune adds. "But I've seen lots of folks have success with it. And it doesn't have the side effects of drugs."

A Vitamin for Immunity

Vitamin C is well-known for its immunity-boosting, virus-fighting abilities. And while there aren't any studies to prove that it works against herpes, there is some evidence that vitamin C in combination with related compounds in foods, called bioflavonoids, may help block the virus, says Craig Zunka, D.D.S., past president of the Holistic Dental Association and a dentist in Front Royal, Virginia.

It's easy to get more vitamin C and bioflavonoids in your diet simply by eating several servings a day of fruits and vegetables. One guava, for example, has 165 milligrams of vitamin C, nearly three times the Daily Value (DV). Orange juice is also good, with a 6-ounce glass providing 93 milligrams, over 150 percent of the DV. Broccoli serves up 41 milligrams of vitamin C in a half-cup, 68 percent of the DV.

The Magic of Milk

Once a herpes sore forms, it can seem like an eternity before it goes away. But there is one way to hurry it along, and it's probably in your refrigerator right now. Doctors aren't sure why, but it appears that applying a milk compress to a cold sore may help it heal more quickly.

Just dip a washcloth or handkerchief in milk, apply it to the sore for 5 seconds, then remove it for another 5. Continue the process for 5 minutes, and repeat it every 3 or 4 hours, rinsing your skin between treatments.

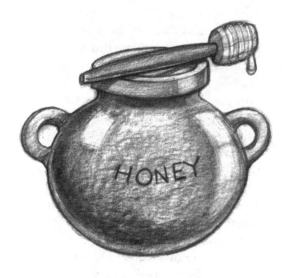

HONEY
THE BEST FROM THE BEES

HEALING POWER
CAN HELP:
Speed wound healing

Ease ulcer pain

Relieve constipation
and diarrhea

In Greek mythology, the infant Zeus was kept alive by bees that fed him honey while he was hidden away in a cave, and he was so grateful that he rewarded the bees by giving them high intelligence.

Even today, when sugary foods are hardly in short supply, there's something special about honey. Not only is it sweeter, ounce for ounce, than table sugar, but its wonderfully thick, liquid texture makes it a natural for spreading on cakes, crackers, and breads.

Although honey contains trace amounts of minerals and B vitamins, it's really not much more nutritious than plain table sugar. Yet honey does several things that sugar doesn't. Research suggests that honey can relieve constipation, speed healing, and prevent infections. "Some people have called honey a remedy rediscovered," says Peter Molan, Ph.D., professor of biochemistry and director of the Honey Research Unit at the University of Waikato in Hamilton, New Zealand, who has been studying the healing properties of honey for 15 years.

QUICKER HEALING

If you saw a jar of honey in your doctor's black bag, you'd just assume that he packed in the dark. But as it turns out, doctors have been using honey

In the Kitchen

Even though honey and sugar can be used interchangeably in most recipes, you may have to make some adjustments. For example:

- Honey is sweeter than sugar, so you can substitute 1 cup of honey for 1 1/4 cups of sugar, reducing liquid in the recipe by 1/4 cup.
- When using honey for baking, add a pinch of baking soda. This will neutralize honey's acidity and help the food to rise. (If the recipe contains sour cream or sour milk, however, you can forgo the baking soda.)
- When using honey instead of sugar in jams, jellies, or candies, increase the cooking temperature just a bit to allow the extra liquid to evaporate.

There are many different flavors of honey, and it's important to match the type to the recipe. Orange blossom honey, for example, has a light, delicate flavor and is best used for foods with mild tastes, like a honey nut cake. Honey produced from buckwheat flowers, however, has a considerably stronger flavor. It's often used for spreading on bread or when making whole-grain desserts.

for centuries. "Up until World War II, honey was used commonly to treat skin wounds," says Dr. Molan.

With the introduction of antibiotics in the 1940s, honey was taken out of doctors' bags and returned to the kitchen. But today, some doctors are trying to bring it back again. "We're finding that doctors are starting to use honey when modern medicines have been tried—and have failed—to cure skin wounds," Dr. Molan says.

Honey contains three ingredients that make it ideal for treating wounds. Because it's very high in sugar, it absorbs much of the moisture inside wounds, making it hard for bacteria to survive, Dr. Molan explains. In addition, many honeys contain large amounts of hydrogen peroxide, the same medicine you use at home to disinfect cuts and scrapes. Finally, some honeys contain propolis, a compound in nectar that can kill bacteria.

In a laboratory study, Dr. Molan smeared honey on seven types of bacteria that often cause wound infections. "It very effectively killed all seven types," he says.

Sweetness Within

Just as honey can stop infections on the outside of your body, it also can help to keep your body healthy on the inside.

A type of honey called Manuka, for example, which is produced when bees feed on a type of flowering shrub in New Zealand, appears to kill the bacteria that cause stomach ulcers. In one small study, people with ulcers were given 1 tablespoon of Manuka honey four times a day. "The honey relieved ulcer symptoms in all the people who took it," Dr. Molan says.

Honey also shows promise for treating diarrhea. In children particularly, diarrhea can be dangerous because it removes large amounts of water from the body. To replace fluids and essential minerals, doctors have traditionally treated diarrhea with a sugar solution. But a honey solution may be even better because honey can kill intestinal bacterial that may be causing the problem. In fact, researchers at the University of Natal in South Africa found that when children with diarrhea caused by a bacterial infection were given a honey solution, they got better in almost half the time of those who were given a traditional sugar solution.

Honey may work against constipation as well. It contains large amounts of fructose, a sugar that sometimes arrives in the large intestine undigested. When bacteria in the intestine begin the process of fermentation, water is drawn into the bowel, which acts as a laxative, explains Marvin Schuster, M.D., director of the Marvin M. Schuster Digestive and Motility Disorders Center at Johns Hopkins Bayview Medical Center in Baltimore. Honey is higher in fructose than just about any other food, he adds.

Getting the Most

Shop for raw honey. The high heats used in making processed honey will disable some of the protective compounds, says Dr. Molan. To get the most antibacterial power, raw honey is your best bet.

Make it Manuka. While most raw honeys contain some active ingredients, Manuka honey contains the most. This is particularly important when you're taking honey as a treatment for relieving ulcers, Dr. Molan says. You can often find Manuka honey in health food stores. It's important, however, to read the label to make sure that you're getting "active Manuka honey." If it doesn't contain the active compounds, the honey won't be effective for ulcers, Dr. Molan explains.

Citrus Honey

1 strip (1″ × ½″) orange rind
1 strip (1″ × ½″) lemon rind
1 tablespoon fresh orange juice
2 teaspoons fresh lemon juice
1 cup honey

Per 2 tablespoons

calories	**130**
total fat	**0 g.**
saturated fat	**0 g.**
cholesterol	**0 mg.**
sodium	**2 mg.**
dietary fiber	**0 g.**

In a small saucepan, combine the orange rind, lemon rind, orange juice, and lemon juice. Bring to a simmer over medium heat. Remove from the heat and strain through a fine sieve; discard the rinds.

In a separate pan, heat the honey until just warm. Stir the juice into the warmed honey and serve immediately.

Makes 1 cup

Cook's Note: Citrus Honey can be stored in a capped jar in the refrigerator for up to 2 weeks. Reheat gently in the microwave or on the stovetop before serving over pancakes, waffles, or French toast.

Immunity
Eating for Resistance

A co-worker sneezes and a cloud of viruses fills the air. Pick up a pen or a pair of socks and you're exposed to thousands, possibly millions of bacteria. Walk barefoot across the lawn and you're picking up fungi, parasites, and still more bacteria.

A dangerous world? It would be if you didn't have your immune system to protect you.

"Our bodies are constantly bombarded with bacteria, viruses, and other organisms trying to gain entry," says Thomas Petro, Ph.D., associate professor of microbiology and immunology at the University of Nebraska Medical Center in Lincoln. "The immune system is the one defense we have against this takeover."

It's truly a battle for survival. A single inch of freshly washed skin may be home to more than 1 million bacteria. Without strong immunity, microbes in and on our bodies would quickly multiply to unimaginable numbers. Yet every minute of every day, our immune systems keep these microscopic marauders in check.

To a large extent, your ability to maintain a healthy immune system depends directly on what you eat, says Dr. Petro. Research has shown, for example, that in parts of the world where healthy, nutritious foods are in short supply, people frequently have weak immune systems, and they are much more prone to developing infections. Similarly, in people with serious illnesses such as cancer, who often have trouble eating well, immunity can take a downturn.

Having a low level of even a single nutrient may cause the immune system to pay the price. In one small study, for example, researchers at Tufts University School of Nutrition in Medford, Massachusetts, put eight people on diets that were very low in vitamin B_6. Within three weeks, their levels of disease-fighting white blood cells plummeted. Then, when the people were allowed to eat foods high in vitamin B_6 once again, their immune systems quickly regained strength.

"Food is powerful medicine," says Keith Block, M.D., medical director of the Cancer Institute at Edgewater Hospital in Chicago. In fact, eating more of certain foods and less of others can substantially boost the body's ability to fight most illnesses, from colds to cancer.

A Magnificent System

Even though people talk about the immune system, it actually consists of two very different parts. One part of the immune system is nonspecific. That is, it attacks—or simply resists—just about everything it comes into contact with. Your skin, for example, provides a barrier against bacteria, viruses, and other invaders. It also secretes sweat and oil, which, because they are acidic, help prevent the growth of harmful bacteria. Your stomach secretes germ-killing acids and enzymes. Your saliva and tears contain an enzyme that destroys bacteria. Even the hairs in your nose keep germs from entering your body.

Should a microbe be lucky enough to breach the nonspecific part of the immune system, it's met by the next level of defense, the specific system. This part of the immune system is extremely selective. Depending on the type of invader it encounters, it launches customized weapons called antibodies, which are proteins designed to kill one particular invader and no other.

The immune system is capable of making more than 100 billion types of antibodies, so it can recognize and attack just about anything it comes into contact with. What's more, it has a long memory. Once you've been exposed to a germ, the immune system will remember. If that same germ ever comes back—months, years, or decades later—the appropriate antibodies will quickly go into action.

Foods for Defense

The most powerful protection you can give your immune system is to eat a well-balanced diet containing a variety of fruits, vegetables, whole grains, seeds and nuts, and seafood, says Michelle S. Santos, Ph.D., a research associate at the Jean Mayer USDA Human Nutrition Research Center on Aging at Tufts University in Boston. These foods are high in nutrients that can help keep your immune system healthy. What's more, some of these nutrients are antioxidants, which may help give the immune system an added boost.

Here's why antioxidants are so important. Every second, immune cells in your body are hit by a barrage of free radicals, harmful oxygen molecules that are created in enormous numbers every day. Since free radicals are missing an electron, they rush through your body, stealing electrons wherever they can find them. And every time they make a grab, another cell is damaged.

The antioxidants in foods, however, literally come between free radicals and healthy immune cells, offering up their own electrons. This neutralizes the free radicals, stopping them from doing further harm. In the process, your body's immune cells stay protected and strong.

In a study at Memorial University of Newfoundland in Canada, researchers found that people who got the most of a variety of nutrients, including antioxidants such as beta-carotene and vitamins C and E, in their diets were able to produce greater numbers of natural killer cells—immune cells that search out and destroy bacteria and other invaders—than folks getting the least. Another study found that people who got large amounts of a variety of antioxidants typically got sick about 23 days a year, while those getting smaller amounts got sick more than twice as often—about 48 days a year.

Some of the best foods for boosting immunity are those that contain beta-carotene, a plant pigment found in foods such as spinach and winter squash. Research has shown that getting 15 to 30 milligrams of beta-carotene a day—the amount in one or two large carrots—can have a significant impact on immunity. In one study, for example, researchers at the University of Arizona in Tucson found that people getting 30 milligrams or more of beta-carotene a day made more natural killer cells and virus-killing lymphocytes than folks getting smaller amounts.

Carrots, sweet potatoes, and spinach are excellent sources of beta-carotene. In fact, eating just one sweet potato and one large carrot a day will provide almost 30 milligrams of beta-carotene—the amount that appears to maximize immunity. You can also get a lot of beta-carotene from leafy green vegetables such as broccoli and kale.

Even though vitamin C is a powerful antioxidant, it helps the immune system in yet another way. The body uses vitamin C to make interferon, a protein that helps destroy viruses in the body. Plus, vitamin C may increase levels of a compound called glutathione, which has also been shown to keep the immune system strong.

In one large study, researchers at the University of Helsinki in Finland reviewed 21 smaller studies that looked at how well vitamin C was able to beat colds. They found that people getting 1,000 milligrams of vitamin C a day were able to shorten the duration of their illnesss and reduce their symptoms by 23 percent.

The Daily Value (DV) for vitamin C is 60 milligrams, but many researchers say that 200 milligrams is probably the minimum amount you need to maximize immunity. It's easy to get this much vitamin C in your diet, Dr. Block adds. Half a cantaloupe, for example, has 113 milligrams of vitamin C, almost twice the DV, while a half-cup of brussels sprouts has 48 milligrams, 80 percent of the DV. Of course, you can also get a lot of vitamin C in citrus fruits, broccoli, rutabagas, radishes, and rose hips tea.

Vitamin E has also gotten a lot of a attention for its role in boosting immunity. The body uses vitamin E to produce a powerful immune protein called interleukin-2, which has been shown to tackle everything from bacteria and viruses to cancer cells. In one study, researchers at the Jean Mayer research center at Tufts found that people taking large amounts (800 international units) of vitamin E a day were able to increase their levels of interleukin-2 by 69 percent.

Since the DV for vitamin E is 30 international units, there's simply no way to get amounts this large from foods alone, which is why some doctors recommend taking vitamin E supplements. But even when you get vitamin E just from foods, it does appear to provide some protection, says Dr. Block.

REDUCE FAT, RAISE IMMUNITY

Just as eating the right foods can help the immune system stay strong, eating the wrong ones—specifically, those that are high in fat—put it at a disadvantage. "A high-fat diet speeds up the aging of the immune system, although we don't know why," says Dr. Petro. "But we do know that it results in the production of more cell-damaging free radicals."

Studies have shown, in fact, that people who cut back on fat in their diets have a rapid increase in natural killer cell activity, which is a sign of immune-system strength. In one study, researchers at the University of Massachusetts Medical School in Worcester put men on low-fat diets for three months. For every 1 percent the men were able to reduce the amounts of fat in their diets, the activity of their natural killer cells went up nearly 1 percent.

It isn't necessary to go on an extremely low fat diet to boost immunity, Dr. Petro adds. For most people, getting no more than 30 percent of calories from fat—and preferably getting between 20 and 25 percent—is probably ideal.

A lot has been written about strategies for cutting fat, but in fact it's quite simple. Eat fewer processed foods, such as those that come in cans, packets, and boxes. With the exception of canned fruits, beans, and vegetables, many processed foods are often high in fat. Eat more fresh fruits and vegetables, beans, whole-grain breads, and cereals. In addition, switching from whole-fat dairy products to skim milk and low-fat yogurt and cheese and eating less red meat will help bring your fat levels into the safety zone.

INFECTIONS
Bacteria-Fighting Foods

There's no way to avoid germs entirely. What you can do, however, is eat your way to better health. "Eating the right foods not only helps prevent infections, but can also help fight them," says Frances Tyus, R.D., a consultant to the wound team at the Cleveland Clinic Foundation in Ohio.

A number of plant foods, such as apples, tea, onions, and kale, contain substances called flavonoids, which can prevent germs from taking hold, says Joseph V. Formica, Ph.D., professor of microbiology at Virginia Commonwealth University, Medical College of Virginia School of Medicine in Richmond. It may be the flavonoids in tea that make it an effective remedy for colds and flu.

One of the most powerful flavonoids is a compound called quercetin. Found in large amounts in onions and kale, quercetin has been shown to damage genetic material inside viruses, preventing them from multiplying.

Quercetin appears to be effective at blocking the herpes virus as well as one of the viruses that cause flu. The research is preliminary, so doctors can't say for sure how much quercetin (or other flavonoids) you need to block infections. For now, having several servings a day of flavonoid-rich foods will help keep germs in check, giving your immune system a fighting chance, says Dr. Formica.

A Spicy Healer

The next time you have an infection, reach for the garlic. Research has shown that these cloves contain compounds that can stop infections.

Researchers at the Medical College of Virginia School of Medicine found that water extracted from garlic was able to block a fungus that can cause a type of meningitis, a serious brain infection. In laboratory studies, garlic has wiped out *Candida albicans*, the fungus that can cause yeast infections.

"It's very clear that garlic has antiviral, antifungal, and antibacterial power," says John Hibbs, a naturopathic doctor and associate professor of clinical medicine at Bastyr University in Seattle. "For people with infections who enjoy eating garlic, we recommend that they chew as much fresh garlic as they can tolerate. Freeze-dried or other forms of garlic may also help."

You probably need to eat about a bulb of garlic a day to get the maximum healing benefits, says Elson Haas, M.D., director of the Preventive Medical

Center of Marin in San Rafael, California, and author of *Staying Healthy with Nutrition*. If the very idea of eating that much raw garlic makes your mouth hurt, you may want to try cooking it first. Baking a bulb of garlic until the cloves are soft will take away some of the garlic sting without taking away the benefits.

Eating for Immunity

If you think of your immune system as an army that battles infections, then two vitamins are its main generals. Vitamin A helps strengthen your body's defenses, while vitamin C helps the immune system go on the attack. This two-pronged approach provides powerful protection against incoming germs.

The body uses vitamin A, which you get in the form of beta-carotene from foods such as carrots, spinach, mustard greens, kale, and yellow and orange squash, to keep mucous membranes soft and moist. This is important, because these membranes, which line the nose, mouth, throat, and other parts of the body, are your first line of defense against infection. As long as they're moist, they're able to trap viruses and other germs before they get into your system.

As a form of double protection, the body also uses vitamin A to manufacture special enzymes that seek out and destroy bacteria that manage to get inside the body. "Vitamin A is critical for preventing infections," Tyus says.

While vitamin A's role is mainly defensive, vitamin C helps the body take the offensive. Eating oranges, broccoli, and other foods high in vitamin C strengthens the "gobbling power" of the body's germ-killing cells. In a study of people with respiratory infections, for example, English researchers found that those getting 200 milligrams of vitamin C a day—about the amount in three oranges—got better significantly faster than folks getting smaller amounts.

A Mine of Health

Of all the minerals, zinc is probably the most important for keeping immunity strong. Too little zinc can lead to a drop in infection-fighting white blood cells, which can increase your risk of getting sick.

In one study, for example, researchers from Tufts University School of Medicine in Boston found that children getting 10 milligrams of zinc for 60 days were much less likely to get respiratory infections than children getting less. In fact, the children who got enough zinc were 70 percent less likely to have fevers, 48 percent less likely to have coughs, and 28 percent less likely to have buildups of mucus.

Despite the proven powers of zinc, many Americans don't get enough of it. This is unfortunate because zinc is very easy to get in your diet. One Alaska king crab leg, for example, has 10 milligrams of zinc, 67 percent of the DV. A 3-ounce serving of lean top sirloin has 6 milligrams, 40 percent of the DV, and 1 cup of lentils has 3 milligrams, 20 percent of the DV.

INFERTILITY
EATING FOR THREE

Having a baby is one of life's most exciting moments. But for as many as 15 percent of couples trying to conceive, just getting pregnant can be a long, difficult process. While there are many physical problems that can lead to infertility, for some couples just changing what's on the menu may put them back on the baby track.

Research has shown, for example, that a man's sperm may not be up to the job if he doesn't get enough of a few key nutrients. And for a woman, starting the day with the usual pick-me-up—or ending it with the traditional calm-me-down—can make it much harder to get pregnant. So before you start picking out baby clothes, you might want to make a few changes in the kitchen.

TROUBLE BREWING

Morning in America means the buzzing of alarm clocks, followed by the chugging of electric coffeemakers. But when it's your biological clock that's doing the buzzing, you may want to unplug the Mr. Coffee.

Drinking coffee, tea, cola, or other beverages containing caffeine can significantly reduce a woman's chances of getting pregnant, says John Jarrett, M.D., a reproductive endocrinologist in private practice in Indianapolis.

In a study of over 1,400 women, researchers at Johns Hopkins University School of Hygiene and Public Health in Baltimore found that nonsmoking women who consumed at least 300 milligrams of caffeine a day (the equivalent of about five cups of coffee) were 2½ times more likely to have delayed conception than women consuming less.

Researchers aren't sure why caffeine puts the stork on the slow train. They speculate, however, that caffeine could change the balance of hormones in the body, interfering with a woman's ability to ovulate. "Reducing the amount of caffeine you drink may help at least a little bit," says Elizabeth E. Hatch, Ph.D., of the department of epidemiology and public health at Yale University.

A SIP OF PROBLEMS

Light the scented candles, pop in a Luther Vandross CD...and put the cork back in the burgundy. While a glass or two of wine may put you in the mood for love, it won't do much for your chances of making a baby.

Harvard researchers found that women who had more than one drink a day—not just wine, but also beer or liquor—were 60 percent more likely to be infertile than women who abstained. Even women who had one drink or less a day were 30 percent less likely to get pregnant than the nondrinkers.

Incidentally, it's not only women who should think twice about raising a glass. Even small amounts of alcohol can lower men's testosterone levels, making their sperm less hardy, says Dr. Jarrett.

THE ZINC LINK

Casanova, the legendary lover, always ate oysters before amour. History doesn't tell how many children he fathered, but he certainly had the right idea. Oysters are extremely high in zinc, a mineral that's essential for male fertility.

"Men need zinc to produce sperm and also to make those sperm healthy," says John Hibbs, a naturopathic doctor and associate professor of clinical medicine at Bastyr University in Seattle. "Zinc also affects sperm motility—how quickly and well sperm swim." In addition, low levels of zinc can reduce the body's production of testosterone, which can interfere with fertility.

Even though the Daily Value (DV) for zinc is only 15 milligrams, most men don't get enough, says Dr. Hibbs. By following Casanova's example, however, you'll get all the zinc you need, and then some. Oysters are an incredible source of zinc, with 12 cooked oysters supplying up to 152 milligrams, over 10 times the DV. Beef is also good, with 3 ounces of lean ground beef containing 4 milligrams, 27 percent of the DV.

WINNING THE RACE

When you look at sperm under a microscope, they resemble supercharged tadpoles, all racing in the do-or-die rush to get upstream.

At least, that's what they're supposed to do. In men who don't get enough vitamin C, however, sperm lose some of their forward momentum. In fact, they get sticky and start clumping together, a problem doctors call agglutination, says Earl Dawson, Ph.D., associate professor of obstetrics and gynecology at the University of Texas Medical School in Galveston. Once men start getting more vitamin C, however, sperm increase in number and quickly pick up speed. In one study, for example, infertile men took 1,000 milligrams of vitamin C a day. After three weeks, the percentage of sperm still clumping together had dropped from an average of 20 percent down to 11 percent.

Getting more vitamin C is particularly important for men who smoke, Dr. Dawson adds. Studies have shown that smokers who get extra vitamin C in their diets will have healthier, more active sperm than those who don't.

INSOMNIA
RESTFUL FOODS

When life gets hectic, we've all found ourselves wishing that there were more hours in the day. Sometimes, unfortunately, we get our wish—at the expense of our sleep.

Few things are more miserable than lying awake, frustrated and tired, when everyone else is sleeping soundly. Insomnia is usually temporary, of course, caused by too much coffee, perhaps, or anxiety about tomorrow's work. But sometimes insomnia really sticks around—not just for days but for weeks, months, or even years. After a few nights spent staring at the ceiling, you may feel as if you'll never be rested again.

Get out of bed, put on your slippers, and head for the kitchen. There's good evidence that what you eat before going to bed can help turn out the lights on insomnia.

NOSH TO NOD

Remember dear old Dad sawing logs on the La-Z-Boy after dinner? He wasn't just dodging the dishes. He was responding to one of the body's most inflexible commands: "First you eat, then you sleep."

"When you put food in your stomach at night, you should be able to sleep better," says David Levitsky, Ph.D., a professor of nutrition and psychology at Cornell University in Ithaca, New York. "Eating draws blood into the gastrointestinal tract and away from the brain. And if you draw blood away from the brain, you're going to get sleepy."

This doesn't mean that stuffing yourself at bedtime will send you off to dreamland, he adds. In fact, eating too much too late in the evening can leave you feeling bloated and gassy, which is more likely to keep you awake than help you sleep. But having a light snack just before bedtime will help give your body the message that it's time to nod off.

TALKING TURKEY

Have you ever wondered why you always nod off in front of the television after a Christmas or Thanksgiving feast? It's not because of the company. Traditional holiday foods such as turkey and chicken are very high in an amino acid called tryptophan, which has been shown to affect the part of the brain that governs sleep, says Dr. Levitsky. Dairy foods are also high in tryptophan, he adds.

The body converts tryptophan into serotonin, which is then converted into melatonin. Both serotonin and melatonin make you feel relaxed and sleepy. Tryptophan may be so effective, in fact, that for a long time doctors recommended tryptophan supplements to help people sleep. Even though the pills were eventually banned (due to a tainted batch imported from Japan), doctors believe that the amino acid found in foods is safe and effective as a sleep aid.

For tryptophan to be most effective, however, it's important to get it in combination with starches, according to Judith Wurtman, Ph.D., a nutrition research scientist at the Massachusetts Institute of Technology in Cambridge and author of *The Serotonin Solution*. When you eat starches—a bagel, for example—the body releases insulin, which pushes all the amino acids except tryptophan into muscle cells. This leaves tryptophan alone in the bloodstream, so it's first in line to get into the brain.

Obviously, you don't want to stuff yourself with turkey before climbing into bed at night. But having a glass of milk or a piece of cheese at bedtime will boost your levels of tryptophan, which will make getting to sleep a little bit easier.

A Natural Sleep Aid

Until recently, scientists thought that melatonin was only produced in the body. As it turns out, however, this sleepy-time hormone is also found in a variety of foods, such as oats, sweet corn, rice, ginger, bananas, and barley, says Russell Reiter, Ph.D., professor of neuroendocrinology at the University of Texas Health Science Center in San Antonio and author of *Melatonin: Your Body's Natural Wonder Drug*.

Doctors often recommend that people who have trouble sleeping take melatonin supplements. The research is preliminary, so it's not clear what amount of foods containing melatonin you'd have to eat to get the same benefits. When the Sandman is running late, however, having a banana or a bowl of oatmeal will slightly boost your melatonin levels and help prepare your body for sleep.

Sound Body, Sound Sleep

Even though scientists have identified a few key substances that help improve sleep, there's simply no substitute for having an overall healthful diet, says James G. Penland, Ph.D., research psychologist at the U.S. Department of Agriculture Human Nutrition Research Center in Grand Forks, North Dakota. "A deficiency of minerals or vitamins may affect your sleep," says Dr. Penland. "So the better your diet, the better your sleep is likely to be."

Studies have shown, for example, that when people don't get enough iron or copper in their diets, it can take longer to fall asleep, and the sleep they do get may be less than refreshing.

The easiest way to get more of these minerals in your diet is to put shellfish on the menu. Just 20 small steamed clams, for example, will provide just over 25 milligrams of iron, 139 percent of the Daily Value (DV), and 0.62 milligram of copper, 31 percent of the DV. Lentils, nuts, and whole-grain foods are also good sources of iron and copper.

Magnesium is another mineral that's essential for good sleep. "It's been shown that having low magnesium levels will stimulate brain-activation neurotransmitters, which leads to overstimulation of the brain," says Dr. Penland. Not getting enough magnesium is especially common in the elderly, he adds, since they may be taking medications that block its absorption. "That's a double whammy that puts them at high risk for sleep problems," he says.

Good sources of magnesium include dried beans such as pinto and navy beans and green leafy vegetables such as spinach and Swiss chard. You can also get magnesium from soybeans, pumpkin seeds, wheat germ, and almonds.

Finally, getting plenty of B vitamins in your diet may help take the edge off insomnia. The body uses B vitamins to regulate many amino acids, including tryptophan. Niacin is particularly important because it appears to make tryptophan work even more efficiently. Lean meat is an excellent source of all the B vitamins, including niacin. Canned tuna is another good source, with 3 ounces providing 11 milligrams of niacin, 55 percent of the DV.

The Sleep Robbers

You already know that coffee can keep you up at night, but did you know that chocolate can also send your brain into overdrive? A serving of chocolate doesn't have as much caffeine as a cup of coffee or a cola, but it can have the same effect on your sleep, says Michael Bonnet, Ph.D., a sleep specialist and director of the Veterans Affairs Medical Center in Dayton, Ohio.

It's not just late-night caffeine that leaves you staring at the ceiling, Dr. Bonnet adds. Since it takes 6 to 8 hours for the body to eliminate caffeine from your system, even the coffee you had at lunch—or the chocolate bar you had in the afternoon—can keep you up at night.

Alcohol is one of the most common disturbers of sleep, Dr. Bonnet says. Even though a glass of wine or a drink at bedtime can make you drowsy, these small amounts of alcohol can make the sleep you do get less restful. When you're having trouble getting to sleep at night, it's a good idea to skip the nightcap and maybe have a little milk instead.

IRRITABLE BOWEL SYNDROME
KEEPING YOUR INSIDES CALM

Doctors still aren't sure what causes irritable bowel syndrome (IBS), a miserable intestinal problem that often causes cramps, gas, diarrhea, and constipation. What they do know is that by eating a healthy diet—getting more of some foods and less of others—you can control IBS instead of having it control you.

Perhaps the trickiest part of managing IBS is knowing which foods are most likely to trigger attacks. Since this varies from person to person, it takes time to learn which foods are safe and which aren't. "A lot of it is trial and error," says David E. Beck, M.D., chairman of the department of colon and rectal surgery at the Ochsner Clinic in New Orleans.

Even though everyone with IBS reacts to different foods differently, there are a few common denominators. Dairy foods, for example, are often a problem. Although children can usually enjoy milk and cheese to their hearts' content, up to 70 percent of adults worldwide produce insufficient amounts of the enzyme (lactase) needed to digest the sugar (lactose) found in dairy foods. For people with IBS, having dairy foods can be especially uncomfortable, Dr. Beck says.

You don't necessarily have to give up milk and cheese entirely, he adds. But you'll certainly want to try cutting back to see if your symptoms improve. Over time, you'll get a good idea of how much of a dairy food you can enjoy without having problems.

Eating beans often causes problems for people with IBS. Again, you don't have to rule them out entirely, Dr. Beck says. You may find that some kinds of beans bother you more than others, and some may not bother you at all.

Another food that's hard to digest is the sugar (fructose) found in sodas and apple and pear juices, says Samuel Meyers, M.D., clinical professor of medicine at Mount Sinai School of Medicine in New York City. In addition, sweeteners like sorbitol, which are found in diet candy and chewing gum, can also be a problem. For many people with IBS, cutting back on juices and candies may be all it takes to ease the discomfort, he says.

A common cause of IBS flare-ups is fat. This is because the bowel normally contracts following a high-fat meal. For people with IBS, these normal contractions can be extremely painful, Dr. Meyers explains. Getting no more (and preferably less) than 30 percent of your total calories from fat will go a long way toward calming an irritable bowel, he says.

While you're cutting back on fat, it's also a good idea to get more fiber. Fiber helps relieve IBS in several ways. It makes stools larger, so the intestine doesn't have to squeeze as much to move them along, Dr. Beck says. In addition, the larger stools help sweep potential irritants from the bowel before they cause cramping, gas, or other symptoms. At the same time, getting more dietary fiber will help relieve both diarrhea and constipation, which often occur in people with IBS, Dr. Beck says.

The Daily Value for fiber is 25 grams. Simply eating more whole grains, fruits, and vegetables will significantly boost your fiber intake. "If all Americans ate low-fat, high-fiber diets, irritable bowels would be very uncommon," Dr. Meyers says.

It's also a good idea to drink less coffee. For many people, drink-

NATURAL RELIEF

Just as the right foods can help calm an irritable bowel, there are also a number of herbs that will help keep the problem under control, says Daniel B. Mowrey, Ph.D., director of the American Phytotherapy Research Laboratory in Salt Lake City. Here's what he recommends.

Licorice root. This sweet-tasting herb, which you can use to make tea, is a natural anti-inflammatory that can help relieve irritation in the bowel, Dr. Mowrey says.

Peppermint. In one study, people with IBS who took peppermint capsules were able to eliminate all or most of their symptoms, Dr. Mowrey says. Peppermint tea is also effective, he adds.

Psyllium. The main ingredient in a number of over-the-counter laxatives, psyllium seeds, which are very high in fiber, have been shown to help relieve the pain of IBS as well as the diarrhea and constipation that may accompany it.

ing coffee (regular or decaf) makes the bowel more sensitive, Dr. Beck says. He recommends limiting yourself to a cup or two each day.

Finally, it's helpful to eat smaller meals. The more food you put into your body at one time, the harder the intestines have to work, and that can cause problems for people with IBS. Having several small meals is usually easier for the body to handle than having two or three big meals, says Douglas A. Drossman, M.D., professor of medicine and psychiatry at the University of North Carolina at Chapel Hill School of Medicine.

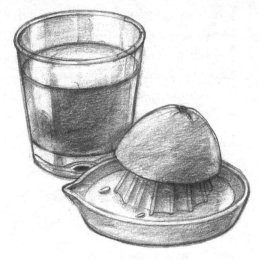

JUICING
POUR A GLASS OF HEALTH

HEALING POWER
CAN HELP:
Prevent cancer
and heart disease

Boost immunity

Like disco and leisure suits, juicing became a craze in the 1970s, only to fizzle shortly thereafter. Now, as research regarding the health benefits of eating plenty of fresh fruits and vegetables mounts, people are rediscovering juicing.

For some, whipping fresh fruits and vegetables through a juicer and extracting glassfuls of vitamin-packed pulpy nectar ensures that they'll get the recommended five to seven servings of these foods every day. Others turn to juicing as a way to get more carotenoids and flavonoids, healing compounds that experts believe can fight major diseases like cancer and heart disease. Still others see juicing as a way to cleanse the body of toxins, boost immunity, and help treat a variety of diseases, from anemia and constipation to arthritis.

MORE THAN A MULTIVITAMIN

For millions of Americans, a handful of vitamin and mineral pills is as much a part of their morning fare as a bowl of cereal and a tall glass of orange juice. And while this isn't a bad way to supplement your diet, there may be a better one.

"Juices are a multivitamin/mineral supplement for people who don't want to take pills and capsules," says Eve Campanelli, Ph.D., a holistic health-care practitioner in Beverly Hills, California. "And your body absorbs the nutrients from juices far, far better than it does from a pill."

Indeed, your body absorbs nutrients from juices better than it does from the foods themselves, says Steven Bailey, a naturopathic doctor in private practice in Portland, Oregon. Although plants are full of vitamins, minerals, and other healing compounds, these substances are bound to fibrous tissue and contained within cellulose walls. When you grind up vegetables or fruits to make juice, you break down the cellulose, releasing these compounds and making them available for absorption, says Dr. Bailey.

"Unless you chew very, very well—and few people do—you won't get all the nutrients from food that you can get from juice. Juice is one of the most powerful whole foods that you can put in your body," says Dr. Bailey. "It takes very little energy to digest it, so you maintain almost all of the energy and nutrients that it gives."

Plus, it takes a mountain of vegetables to get the same amount of nutrients found in one glass of juice. "To get all the vitamins you get from just 6 ounces of carrot juice, you'd need to eat eight carrots," says Dr. Campanelli. "Not too many people are going to eat eight carrots. But they'll drink a little glass of carrot juice."

A 6-ounce glass of carrot juice contains large amounts of beta-carotene, which, when it's converted to vitamin A in the body, delivers 948 percent of the Daily Value (DV). This same glass of juice also has 16 milligrams of vitamin C, 27 percent of the DV; 0.4 milligram of vitamin B_6, 20 percent of the DV; 537 milligrams of potassium, 15 percent of the DV; and 0.2 milligram of thiamin, 11 percent of the DV.

Despite their nutritional payload, juices should be used to supplement fresh fruits, vegetables, and grains in your diet, not replace them, says Dr. Campanelli. As good as juices are, they doesn't contribute much toward the 20 to 35 grams of fiber that adults need each day. For example, while eight carrots provide 17 grams of fiber, a 6-ounce glass of juice has a measly 2 grams. Diets high in fiber have been linked with lower incidence of certain cancers, digestive problems, and high cholesterol.

BEYOND VITAMINS AND MINERALS

Fresh juices supply more than the necessary vitamins and minerals. They also contain a variety of phytonutrients, compounds in plants that may help prevent serious health threats like cancer and heart disease.

Perhaps the best-known of the phytonutrients is beta-carotene, a plant pigment that puts the orange glow in sweet potatoes, carrots, and cantaloupe. Studies have shown that people who eat diets high in fruits and vegetables, particularly those containing large amounts of beta-carotene, have much lower

DELICIOUS COMBINATIONS

There's virtually no limit to the tastes and textures that you can create by mixing a variety of fruits and vegetables in your juicer. Here are a few simple combinations you may want to try.

- Carrots and celery, which are often combined, are considered universal mixers, which means that they combine well with any other vegetable. Try juicing three carrots for every stalk of celery.
- Combining the juice from a couple of tomatoes with juice from a few slices of sweet green peppers makes a refreshing, sodium-free alternative to salt-laden store-bought tomato juice.
- For a surprisingly refreshing drink, combine one large peeled cucumber and a small onion. Using different varieties of onions, from sweet reds to hot whites, will create a range of interesting flavors.

cancer risks than those who do not.

Beta-carotene isn't the only phytonutrient found in fruits and vegetables. There are hundreds of compounds, like lutein, lycopene, and alpha-carotene, that have shown disease-fighting mettle as well. Drinking the juices of carotenoid-rich foods, particularly carrots, tomatoes, and dark green vegetables, gives your body a full arsenal of these compounds, says Dr. Bailey.

Fruit and vegetable juices also contain compounds called flavonoids, which show strong antioxidant powers. That is, they help prevent disease by sweeping up harmful, cell-damaging oxygen molecules called free radicals that naturally accumulate in your body.

Antioxidants help prevent low-density lipoprotein cholesterol, the dangerous form of cholesterol, from oxidizing. This is the process that makes cholesterol stick to artery walls and contributes to heart disease. Studies show that people who eat flavonoid-rich foods such as apples and onions have lower risks of heart attack than those who do not.

"Drinking a large variety of vegetable and fruit juices is a wonderful way to get therapeutic amounts of all of these healing compounds," says Dr. Campanelli.

For maximum healing benefits, Dr. Bailey recommends drinking about a pint to a quart of mixed vegetable juices each day.

GET THE TOXINS OUT

Pollution, pesticides, preservatives, artificial colorings—these are a mere smattering of the toxic elements that your body takes in every day. Your body, of

In the Kitchen

There's more to juicing than merely dropping the pick of the day into the blender. To get the freshest flavors while preserving the most nutrients, here's what experts advise.

Scrub it. Be sure to wash all produce thoroughly and cut away bruised or damaged portions.

Remove the skin. While not all fruits and vegetables require peeling, many do, for a variety of reasons. The skins of oranges and grapefruits, for example, contain chemicals that can be toxic if consumed in large quantities. Waxed produce should be peeled before juicing, as should tropical fruits, which often are grown in countries where the use of pesticides isn't well-regulated.

Remove the pits and seeds. Apple seeds, which contain trace amounts of cyanide, should be removed before juicing. Seeds in melons, lemons, and limes and pits from peaches, plums, and other stone fruits should also be removed. Grape seeds are safe, however, and can be placed in the juicer along with the fruit.

Use the whole vegetable. Most vegetables can be juiced in their entirety—leaves, stems, and all. Two exceptions are rhubarb and carrots; rhubarb leaves and carrot tops both contain toxic compounds.

Chunk it. The openings of most juicers are quite small, so you should cut your produce into manageable pieces. Also, small chunks put less strain on the motor, which will help your juicer last longer.

Blend your bananas. When juicing fruits or vegetables that contain little water, like bananas and avocados, it's helpful to juice other items first, then add the drier produce to produce a thick, smooth drink.

Drink it quickly. Just as juices give up their nutritional benefits soon after they are made, their flavor is also fleeting. Some juices, such as cabbage, become rancid in a few hours. So it's a good idea to make only as much as you plan to drink right away.

Or freeze it. Carrot, apple, and orange juices are quite hardy and will keep for three to four weeks when frozen in a sealed plastic container.

course, being a good housekeeper, tries to eliminate these toxins through cleansing organs like the liver. But just as you empty vacuum cleaner bags to help the sweeper work properly, you should occasionally flush the toxins from your body, says Dr. Campanelli.

Although this theory is largely discounted by the mainstream medical community, natural-health doctors recommend "cleaning house" periodically with a juice fast. This means abstaining from solid food for a couple of days and getting your nourishment from fresh fruit and vegetable juices.

"When you spend a couple of days getting most of your nutrition from juices, not only do you get a higher portion of vitamins, minerals, and natural enzymes but your body doesn't have to work very hard at digestion, so you have more nutritionally rich blood with more time to clean up, heal overworked cells, and help the body regenerate," says Dr. Bailey.

You could also see an enhancement of your immune system, says Dr. Bailey. As a result of juice fasting, "symptoms of chronic conditions like arthritis, sinusitis, and allergies generally decrease dramatically," he says. While natural-health doctors agree that juice fasting isn't a cure for these conditions, it may help provide temporary relief.

Although juice fasts are generally safe, there are certain conditions, such as Type I (non-insulin-dependent) diabetes, that can be aggravated by them. Don't do any fasting without first consulting your doctor, warns Dr. Bailey.

Getting the Most

Sip it quickly. Once the fruit or vegetable goes through the juicer, natural enzymes in the food begin to break down the nutrients. Juice loses nutritional value quickly, says Dr. Bailey. For optimal benefits, drink juices within 30 minutes of making them, he advises.

Canned juices, of course, will keep almost forever if unopened. The trade-off is that they lack many of the nutrients found in fresh juices. The most wholesome juice, Dr. Bailey says, is always made at home.

Focus on vegetables. While a tall glass of fruit juice can be a sweet summer treat, it's better to concentrate on vegetable juices. "Fruit juices are too high in sugar and too acidic to drink in large quantities," says Dr. Bailey. "Vegetable juices are better nutritionally, and they have a higher alkaline (meaning not acidic) content."

Enjoy a variety. For maximum healing benefits, drink juices from a variety of vegetables, says Dr. Bailey. "The more variety you can work into your diet, the better. This is easy with juices, because you can combine several vegetables into one drink."

KIDNEY STONES
RELIEF FROM THE KITCHEN

There's pain. There's agonizing pain. And then there are kidney stones.

Actually, calling them kidney barbs would be more fitting since these stones, which consist mainly of mineral salts, are sometimes studded with sharp spikes. While it's possible to pass small stones without knowing you had them, larger stones, which can range from about the size of the tip of a pen to that of a pencil eraser, cause excruciating pain as they move from the kidney through the ureter, the long tube through which urine flows. Passing a large stone has been compared to the pain of childbirth. Some women say it's worse.

There are several types of kidney stones, with the most common being those formed from calcium. Experts aren't entirely sure what causes kidney stones to form. But one thing is certain. Diet can play a key role, says Lisa Ruml, M.D., assistant professor of medicine at the University of Texas Southwestern Medical Center in Dallas. What you eat affects the kinds and amounts of minerals that accumulate in your urine—minerals that, in some people, lead to the formation of stones.

Perhaps the most important point is this: If you've passed one stone, the odds are good that you'll pass another. So pay attention when your doctor tells you what kind of stones you have, since this will affect the changes you make in your diet.

The stones that respond best to dietary changes are uric acid and calcium stones. The dietary changes recommended in the next few pages are given primarily with these types of stones in mind.

STONE-CRUSHING POTASSIUM

Once you've experienced the pain of a kidney stone, you don't want a repeat performance. So consider making a handful of dried apricots or a baked potato a regular part of your anti-stone diet. Along with a variety of fruits and vegetables, these foods are somewhat alkaline, which helps neutralize stone-forming acids in the body.

Here's how it works. Alkaline foods increase the level of a mineral called citrate in the urine, and citrate, Dr. Ruml explains, helps block the formation of stones.

To raise your levels of citrate, Dr. Ruml says, you need to get more fruits and vegetables into your diet. "Many of the foods that are high in citrates, like citrus fruits and vegetables, are also good sources of potassium," she says.

Another way to increase your levels of stone-dissolving citrates is to drink more orange juice. In a study at the University of Texas Southwestern Medical Center in Dallas, men with histories of kidney stones were given either three glasses of orange juice a day or potassium-citrate supplements. The researchers found that the juice was almost as effective as the supplements. "We recommend drinking at least a liter (a little more than 32 ounces) a day if you have stones, because of its content of potassium and citrate," says Dr. Ruml.

Help from Magnesium

Your body is full of minerals that are constantly being adjusted for balance. Eating foods that are rich in magnesium, Dr. Ruml says, can help prevent stones by lowering the amount of another mineral, called oxalate. Oxalate can be a problem because it's one of the main components of kidney stones.

Fish, rice, avocados, and broccoli all are rich in magnesium. A 3-ounce fillet of baked or broiled halibut, for example, has 91 milligrams of magnesium, 23 percent of the Daily Value (DV). A half-cup of cooked long-grain brown rice has 42 milligrams and a floret of cooked broccoli has 43 milligrams, 11 percent of the DV.

Here's another easy way to get more magnesium. Drink some fortified, low-fat milk. If your doctor has recommended that you restrict dairy foods, however, don't drink more than 8 ounces a day, says Dr. Ruml.

Of course, it's also helpful to get less oxalate in your diet, Dr. Ruml says. If you're prone to kidney stones, it's a good idea to limit yourself to one serving a week of oxalate-rich foods such as black tea, chocolate, peanuts and other nuts, spinach, and strawberries.

Fiber for the Stone-Prone

If you want to leave no stone unturned, getting more fiber in your diet can be a smart strategy. In a study at the Stone Clinic at Halifax Infirmary Hospital in Nova Scotia, 21 people were put on a low-stone (low-protein, low-calcium, and low-oxalate) diet. After 90 days, they followed the same diet but also were given 10 grams (a little more than ⅓ ounce) of dietary fiber in the form of high-fiber biscuits. While the original diet helped reduce the amount of calcium in the urine, the extra fiber reduced it even more.

Doctors still aren't sure how effective fiber is at treating or preventing kidney stones, Dr. Ruml adds. "It's probably safe to say that the higher your fiber intake, the more likely you are to bind calcium and oxalate in the intestine, which will lower the urinary levels of these minerals," she says.

One more point about fiber: While reducing the amount of calcium in the urine may be beneficial for people with stones, it's not so good for those trying to prevent osteoporosis, the bone-thinning disease caused by low levels of calcium. "Some people with kidney stones may be prone to osteoporosis," Dr. Ruml says. The bottom line for the stone-prone: Check with your doctor before substantially increasing your fiber intake.

The Calcium Controversy

While people with kidney stones are sometimes told to reduce their intakes of high-calcium foods, the jury is still out on whether consuming large amounts of calcium increases the risk of developing stones. New research suggests that the reverse may be true. A Harvard study of nearly 46,000 men found that those who ate the most calcium were actually the least likely to form stones. In another Harvard study, women who consumed at least 1,100 milligrams of dietary calcium a day had one-third the risk of developing kidney stones compared with those who consumed less than 500 milligrams a day.

While vegetables such as broccoli and turnip greens have some calcium, the easiest way to get adequate amounts is by drinking milk and eating other dairy foods. A glass of protein-fortified skim milk, for example, has 351 milligrams of calcium. A cup of low-fat yogurt has 414 milligrams, and 1½ ounces of mozzarella cheese made from skim milk has 270 milligrams.

LACTOSE INTOLERANCE
DAIRY ALTERNATIVES

As we get older, milk gets harder to enjoy because we gradually start producing less of the enzyme (lactase) needed to digest the sugar (lactose) found in milk and other dairy foods. This means that undigested lactose collects in the intestine, often causing gas, cramps, and diarrhea. Doctors call this problem lactose intolerance.

Lactose intolerance usually isn't serious for the simple reason that it's easy to cut back on milk, cheese, and other dairy foods, says Talal M. Nsouli, M.D., clinical associate professor of allergy and immunology at Georgetown University School of Medicine and director of the Watergate Allergy and Asthma Center, both in Washington, D.C. On the other hand, giving up dairy foods means that you risk losing out on their greatest nutritional benefit—calcium, which you can't do without.

But there are ways to get the benefits of dairy foods without the problems. Supermarkets sell reduced-lactose milk, for example, which has about 70 percent of the lactose removed. You can also buy reduced-lactose cheeses.

Yogurt is another great food for people with lactose intolerance. Although live-culture yogurt does contain lactose, it also has beneficial bacteria that help break it down into lactic acid, which is easier to digest. Low-fat yogurt is also full of calcium, with 414 milligrams per serving.

In addition, lactose is easier for the body to digest when you have it in combination with other foods. "Many people won't have a problem when they drink milk or have cheese with a meal," says Sheah Rarback, R.D., a spokesperson for the American Dietetic Association in Miami.

Even if you've had trouble digesting dairy foods in the past, it's a good idea to periodically test the waters, she adds. Some people build up a tolerance to lactose over time and can increase the amount of dairy foods they can eat.

Another way to reduce problems from dairy foods is to take a lactase supplement. Available in drugstores and supermarkets, these supplements can be stirred into milk or taken as a pill or caplet along with dairy foods.

If you find it's simply too uncomfortable to have dairy foods, you'll want to find other ways to get more calcium in your diet. Rarback recommends shopping for calcium-fortified foods such as juices and cereals. "A glass of calcium-fortified orange juice is the calcium equivalent of a glass of milk."

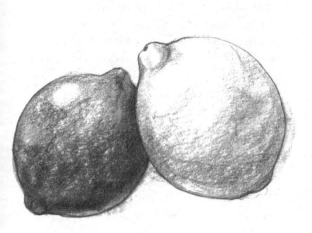

LEMONS AND LIMES
PUCKER POWER

HEALING POWER
CAN HELP:
Heal cuts and bruises

Prevent cancer and
heart disease

You may love the tartness of lemons and limes, but it's a good bet that you've never taken a big bite from the whole fruit. Back in the nineteenth century, however, people literally craved them, not for the tart blast but for the remarkable health benefits these colorful fruits conferred.

British sailors, for example, who typically spent months at sea without fresh fruits or vegetables, would quaff lime juice to prevent scurvy, a terrible disease caused by vitamin C deficiency. (It was because of the British Navy's dependence on limes that they became known as limeys.) And in California during the Gold Rush, when fresh fruits were equally scarce, miners paid top dollar for lemons.

A SEA OF C

Of all the nutrients we're most familiar with, vitamin C is perhaps the most impressive. During cold season it's always in hot demand, since it lowers levels of histamine, a naturally occurring chemical that can cause red eyes and runny noses. Vitamin C is also a powerful antioxidant, meaning that it helps disarm powerful oxygen molecules in the body that contribute to cancer and heart disease. The body also uses vitamin C to manufacture collagen, the stuff that glues

In the Kitchen

If you've ever used a grater to remove citrus zest, you've probably also experienced the pain of grated knuckles.

An easier way to remove citrus zest is to use a zester. This inexpensive kitchen gadget looks a bit like a bottle opener. The business end contains a strip of stainless steel lined with sharp-edged holes. As you pull the zester across the peel, it removes a thin, curly strip of zest that piles up nicely—without a single zinged knuckle.

cells together and is needed to help heal cuts and wounds.

The pulp and juice from lemons and limes are rich sources of vitamin C. A large lemon, for example, contains about 45 milligrams of vitamin C, 75 percent of the Daily Value (DV). Limes are also good, with a small lime containing about 20 milligrams, 33 percent of the DV.

Quest for the Zest

There's more to lemons and limes than just vitamin C. These citrus fruits also contain additional compounds such as limonin and limonene, which appear to help block some of the cellular changes that can lead to cancer.

Limonene, which is found mainly in the colorful skin, or zest, of the fruit, has been shown to increase the activity of proteins that help eliminate estradiol, a naturally occurring hormone that has been linked with breast cancer. Limonene has also been shown to increase the level of enzymes in the liver that can remove cancer-causing chemicals.

Food Alert
Citrus Sunburn

People who handle large amounts of citrus fruits may find themselves at risk for a curious condition that could be called lime (not Lyme) disease.

Lemons and limes contain furocoumarins, compounds that sensitize the skin and make it susceptible to sunburn. In one case, described in the *New England Journal of Medicine*, a man's left hand blistered and swelled after he squeezed about 60 limes to make margaritas. The researchers called this painful condition margarita photodermatitis.

Anytime you're squeezing or zesting large numbers of lemons and limes, be sure to wash your hands thoroughly to remove the oils, and also apply a strong sunscreen before going outdoors.

In Europe, food companies add citrus zest to baking flour to provide added health benefits, says Antonio Montanari, Ph.D., research scientist with the Florida Department of Citrus Research Center in Lake Alfred. "Here in America, we throw away what may be the best part of the fruit," he says.

Getting the Most

Zest up your flavors. Whether you're making a lemon meringue pie or simply adding flavor to store-bought lemon yogurt, be sure to add plenty of zest. The healing compound limonene makes up about 65 percent of oils in the peel, says Michael Gould, Ph.D., professor of human oncology at the University of Wisconsin Medical School in Madison.

Use it dried. While fresh citrus peel contains the most healing compounds, dried lemon peel isn't bad, says Dr. Montanari. You'll find dried lemon peel in the spice rack at the supermarket.

LEMON DESSERT SAUCE

½ **cup sugar**

1 **tablespoon cornstarch**

1 **tablespoon grated lemon rind**

⅓ **cup fresh lemon juice**

½ **cup fat-free egg substitute**

2 **teaspoons unsalted butter**

PER 3 TABLESPOONS

calories	**95**
total fat	**1.3 g.**
saturated fat	**0.8 g.**
cholesterol	**3.5 mg.**
sodium	**4 mg.**
dietary fiber	**0.2 g.**

In a small saucepan, mix the sugar, cornstarch, and lemon rind. Whisk in the lemon juice until smooth. Cook over low heat for 5 to 6 minutes, whisking frequently, until the sauce is hot and slightly thickened.

Place the egg substitute in a small bowl. Add 2 tablespoons of the sauce and whisk to mix and warm the egg substitute. Add to the saucepan. Cook over low heat, whisking, for 2 to 3 minutes, or until the sauce thickens. Remove from the heat and stir in the butter. Set aside to cool.

Makes about 1 cup

Cook's Note: Serve the sauce over fruit, nonfat frozen yogurt, gingerbread, angel food cake, or other cakes.

Low-Fat Diet

Keeping Your Machine Clean

Healing Power

Can help:
Reduce the risk
of heart disease

Prevent cancer

Promote weight loss

Preserve good vision

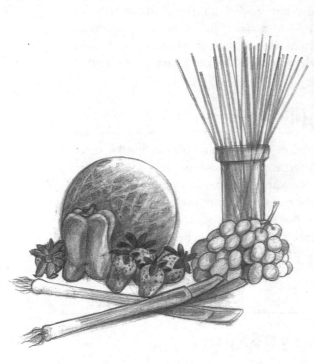

During the past decade, the evidence has become overwhelming that few things are better for your health than reducing the amount of fat in your diet. Fatty foods can dramatically increase your risk of heart disease, diabetes, high blood pressure, certain types of cancer, and many other conditions. Plus, eating too much fat has made us all, well, fatter. Thirty years ago, about 25 percent of Americans were overweight. Today, that percentage is about 33 percent, and it seems to be rising.

And it's not only adults who are carrying the extra pounds. A large percentage of children are also overweight, and studies show that the incidence of Type II (non-insulin dependent) diabetes, a condition that is often associated with overweight, among children is 10 times greater today than it was a decade ago.

To put ourselves and our children on a healthier track, researchers say, we need to switch to low-fat diets. This means not only eating lower fat foods but also getting more fruits, vegetables, legumes, and other healthful foods.

A Weighty Issue

The key to losing weight is cutting the number of calories in our diets. And the easiest way to cut calories is to eat less fat, says Judy Dodd, R.D., of Pittsburgh, a nutrition education consultant and former president of the American

Dietetic Association. Gram for gram, fat packs more energy, which is measured in calories, than any other nutrient. One gram of fat delivers 9 calories, more than twice as many as the same amount of protein or carbohydrate. Plus, your body likes fat. It's much more likely to store calories from fat than calories from other sources.

In one study, Danish researchers found that those who trimmed the amount of fat in their diets from 39 to 28 percent of total calories and increased their intake of carbohydrates were able to lose an average of 9 pounds in just 12 weeks. What's more, people who stuck to lower-fat diets were able to keep the weight off long after the study ended.

Cutting fat from your diet does more than make you healthier. Research suggests that a low-fat diet can increase your general sense of well-being as well. In a study of more than 550 women, researchers at the Fred Hutchinson Cancer Research Center in Seattle found that when the women cut their daily fat intake in half—from 40 percent to 20 percent of total calories—they felt more vigorous, less anxious, and less depressed than they had while eating their former diets.

Health for the Heart

Even if you're one of those lucky folks who can eat whatever you want and never gain an ounce, fat in the diet has to go somewhere, and all too often, that "somewhere" is inside your arteries.

There's a direct link between the amount of fat in your diet and your risk for heart disease, Dodd says. This is particularly true of saturated fat, the dangerous, artery-clogging fat found mainly in meats, full-fat dairy products, and snack foods. Research has shown that eating a low-fat diet is perhaps the best way to lower this risk. In one study, researchers put people on a very low fat diet, with only 5 percent of total calories coming from fat. After 11 days, their cholesterol levels had dropped an average of 11 percent and their blood pressures went down an average of 6 percent. This 11 percent decrease in cholesterol may have reduced their chances of dying from heart attacks by almost 33 percent.

You don't have to go on an extremely low fat diet to get the benefits. Even reducing the amount of fat in your diet just a little bit can lead to a reduction in cholesterol levels, Dodd says.

A Defense against Cancer

There is a compelling reason to make the switch to a low-fat diet. "Several studies indicate that a low-fat diet offers great protection against many diseases, including cancer," says Leena Hilakivi-Clarke, Ph.D., assistant professor of psychiatry at Lombardi Cancer Center at Georgetown University Medical Center in Washington, D.C.

In a study at the University of Benin in Nigeria, researchers found that

MAKING THE CUT

You can't open a magazine or tune in to late-night television without being bombarded with information about the latest new diets—weight loss guaranteed! But in fact, there's nothing complicated about embarking on a low-fat diet. Eating less red meat, for example, will automatically lower your intake of saturated fat. So will swapping full-fat yogurt for the low-fat kind and eating more fruits, vegetables, legumes, and whole grains. In addition, there are quite a few "sneaky" ways to get the drop on fat. Here are a few you may want to try.

Try some new cheeses. Even though cheese is usually one of the first foods to be labeled off-limits when you're switching to a low-fat diet, some cheeses are naturally lower in fat than others. Feta, camembert, and part-skim mozzarella, for example, have less than 10 grams of fat in a 1½-ounce serving. While not exactly fat-free, they are better choices than cheddar, for example, which has almost 14 grams of fat per serving.

Do the napkin test. Those big, fluffy muffins at the supermarket bakery sure look healthful, but they often contain enormous amounts of fat. Before you bring home a bag of monster muffins, put them to the test. Buy one muffin and place it on a paper napkin. If it leaves a telltale oil mark, you can bet it contains more than 3 grams of fat, and you'll want to find a lower-fat variety.

Make the good better. Pizza is one American favorite that doesn't entirely deserve its junk-food reputation. In fact, a steaming slice can be a smart choice, as long as it's not swimming in its own oil slick. To make pizza a little bit healthier, spread a napkin on top of each slice and gently blot up the excess oil.

Be wary of no-fat foods. Supermarkets seem to be bursting with fat-free versions of

when laboratory animals were fed high-fat diets, they began producing enzymes that led to cancerous changes in their colons in just three weeks.

What works in the laboratory is also effective in real life. In a study of 450 women, researchers in the department of epidemiology and public health at Yale University School of Medicine found that cutting just 10 grams of saturated fat a day—the equivalent of switching from two glasses of whole milk to the same amount of skim—could reduce the risk of ovarian cancer by 20 percent.

In another study, researchers from the University of Iowa in Iowa City compared the diets of women with cancer to the diets of women who did not have the disease. They found that women who ate the most red meat were about 50 percent more likely to get cancer than women who ate the least. This is significant, since red meat is one of the major contributors of saturated fats.

just about everything these days. But even though reduced-fat mayonnaise, salad dressings, and cheese can be great tools to help you stay within your daily fat budget, "fat-free" isn't the same thing as "calorie-free." Moderation is still important, says Judy Dodd, R.D., of Pittsburgh, a nutrition education consultant and former president of the American Dietetic Association.

Enjoy some old favorites. There's simply no reason to give up desserts just because you're following a low-fat diet. In fact, many traditional favorites like gingersnaps, vanilla wafers, and graham crackers are also very low in fat.

Go lean on meat. Even though a richly marbled Porterhouse steak can blow a hefty percentage of your fat budget (a 3-ounce serving has 9 grams of fat), many cuts of meat are low in fat. Meats labeled "loin" or "round," for example, can have as little as 3 grams of fat per serving.

Make the dairy switch. Milk is a good source of protein and an excellent source of calcium. Unfortunately, it can also be a great source of fat. To get the benefits of milk without all the fat, you simply have to give up the full-fat kind, which has 8 grams of fat in an 8-ounce serving.

One-percent low-fat milk is good choice, with 3 grams of fat per serving. Better yet, drink more skim, which has virtually no fat yet contains just as much (or even more) calcium as whole milk.

Enjoy ice cream alternatives. Just a few years ago, the tastes of low-fat and fat-free frozen desserts certainly didn't compare very favorably to traditional ice cream. But today, manufacturers have gotten very good at making lean frozen desserts that have the same rich taste and creamy texture as their high-fat kin.

A low-fat diet is protective not only because of what it doesn't contain but also because of what it does. When you cut back on fat, you generally eat more fruits, vegetables, whole grains, and legumes, all of which have been shown to keep us healthier, says JoAnn Manson, M.D., associate professor of medicine at Harvard Medical School.

Good for the Eyes

Finally, there's some evidence that eating a low-fat diet may protect you against conditions such as macular degeneration, the leading cause of vision loss in older adults.

In a survey of more then 2,000 people, researchers from the University of

Wisconsin in Madison found that those who reported getting the most saturated fat were 80 percent more likely to get macular degeneration than those getting the least.

Getting Started

Even when you're trying to reduce the amount of fat in your diet, it isn't always easy to know where to begin. For starters, you need to figure out how much fat you're actually getting each day. Ideally, you should be getting between 25 and 30 percent of your total calories from fat, Dodd says.

Suppose, for example, that you normally get 2,000 calories a day. When you're following a low-fat diet, no more than 600 of those calories should come from fat. This adds up to about 67 grams of fat a day.

Reading food labels is perhaps the easiest way to keep track of your daily fat intake, Dodd says. When you're shopping for cheese, for example, you might notice that a 1-ounce serving of cheddar has a little more than 9 grams of fat. Since that may represent a large percentage of your daily fat budget, you may decide to choose a lower-fat cheese, instead. When you're eating out or buying foods that don't have labels, you can find out how much fat you're getting by picking up a nutrition reference guide at the bookstore or supermarket. These guides list the amount of fat in most common foods, including foods that are served in restaurants.

The most important fat to watch is saturated fat, which is found in animal foods like meats, butter, cheese, and eggs. Not only is saturated fat bad for your health, but the same foods that are high in saturated fat also tend to be high in cholesterol. So when you cut one, you automatically cut the other. The American Heart Association recommends that we get no more (and preferably less) than 10 percent of our total calories from saturated fat.

Although margarine and vegetable shortening have been touted as healthy alternatives to saturated fat, they're not always good choices. Studies indicate that hydrogenated fats—the kinds used in making margarine and shortening—can clog the arteries just as much as saturated fats.

Even though it's generally a good idea to reduce the amount of all fats in your diet, some fats, such as monounsaturated and polyunsaturated fats, aren't so bad. These fats, which are abundant in vegetable and seed oils such as olive, sesame, and safflower oils and in nuts and seeds, have been shown to actually lower cholesterol and may help prevent it from sticking to artery walls. Of course, these fats contain just as many calories as other, less healthful fats, so you don't want to eat a lot of them, Dodd adds.

There's one other kind of fat that plays an essential role in a healthful, low-fat diet. The fat found in fish, called omega-3 fatty acids, has been shown to reduce clotting and inflammation in the arteries, which can significantly lower the risk of heart disease and stroke. You don't have to eat a lot of fish to get the benefits. When you're following a low-fat diet, having two fish meals a week will go a long way toward keeping your arteries in the swim, Dodd says.

POACHED COD WITH MIXED VEGETABLES

4   cod fillets (6 ounces each)
1   fennel bulb
2   carrots, cut into matchstick pieces
1   small zucchini, cut into matchstick pieces
2   shallots or 1 small onion, thinly sliced
1   cup apple juice
¼   teaspoon salt
2   cups water
    Ground black pepper

PER SERVING
calories	**202**
total fat	**1.5 g.**
saturated fat	**0.3 g.**
cholesterol	**80 mg.**
sodium	**269 mg.**
dietary fiber	**3.8 g.**

Rinse the cod with cold water and pat dry with paper towels.

Trim the fennel, reserving the narrow top stems and some of the feathery leaves. Cut the bulb in half lengthwise. Cut out and discard the core. Cut into matchstick-size strips.

Coat a large skillet with no-stick spray. Warm over medium-high heat. Add the fennel, carrots, zucchini, and shallots or onions. Cook, tossing, for about 1 minute. Stir in ¼ cup of the apple juice and ⅛ teaspoon of the salt. Cook for 2 to 3 minutes, or until the vegetables are crisp-tender. Season to taste with the pepper. Transfer the vegetables to a platter and cover to keep warm.

In the same skillet, combine the water, the reserved fennel stems and leaves, and the remaining ¾ cup apple juice. Bring to a simmer over medium heat. Reduce the heat to low and add the cod. Cook, turning once, for 4 to 5 minutes, or until the cod is opaque in the center. Test for doneness by inserting the tip of a sharp knife in 1 fillet.

Remove the cod with a slotted spatula. Set over the reserved vegetables. Sprinkle with the remaining ⅛ teaspoon salt. Season to taste with pepper.

Makes 4 servings

Cook's Note: Fresh fennel is labeled "anise" in many supermarkets. Swordfish, halibut, or whitefish would also work well in this recipe.

CHOCOLATE MINT PUDDING CAKE

1 **cup unbleached all-purpose flour**

¾ **cup granulated sugar**

1 **teaspoon baking soda**

¾ **teaspoon baking powder**

¼ **teaspoon salt**

½ **cup cocoa powder**

½ **cup skim buttermilk**

½ **cup unsweetened applesauce**

1 **teaspoon vanilla**

½ **teaspoon peppermint extract**

¾ **cup packed light brown sugar**

1 **cup + 2 tablespoons boiling water**

PER SERVING
calories	**208**
total fat	**1 g.**
saturated fat	**0.5 g.**
cholesterol	**1 mg.**
sodium	**293 mg.**
dietary fiber	**5 g.**

Preheat the oven to 350°F. Coat a 12" × 8" baking dish with no-stick spray. Set aside.

In a large bowl, combine the flour, granulated sugar, baking soda, baking powder, salt, and ¼ cup of the cocoa. Whisk to mix.

Add the buttermilk, applesauce, vanilla, and peppermint extract. Stir just until the dry ingredients are well-incorporated. Do not overbeat; the batter will look like brownie batter and will look a bit lumpy because of the applesauce. Pour into the prepared pan.

In a small bowl, combine the brown sugar and the remaining ¼ cup cocoa. Mix well. Sprinkle over the batter. Pour on the water; do not stir.

Transfer carefully to the oven. Bake for 25 to 30 minutes, or until the top is set and the cake moves away from the sides of the pan. Cool on a wire rack for 20 to 30 minutes.

To serve, scoop the cake out of the pan with a pancake turner, turning each piece upside down on a plate so the pudding is on top.

Makes 8 servings

Cook's Note: This cake tastes best warm. If the cake has cooled, place individual pieces on a microwaveable plate and microwave on high power for 30 seconds, or until warm.

Lupus
Eating to Fight Inflammation

It's a mysterious disease—a case of the body's protective forces turning traitor. Lupus erythematosus, or lupus for short, occurs when the immune system, which usually protects the body, instead turns against it, attacking and damaging healthy tissues.

For reasons that aren't entirely clear, lupus, which is a form of arthritis, strikes eight times as many women as men, probably due to the effects of female hormones on the immune system. There are two types of the disease. Discoid lupus, the less serious form, affects the skin. Systemic lupus, which is more serious, can affect the whole body, including the heart, lungs, kidneys, joints, and nervous system.

There is no cure for lupus, but there's increasing evidence that how you eat—choosing certain foods and avoiding others—can give you an edge in battling it.

Healing Yourself with Food

While you may associate linseed oil with the smell of a paint factory, the grain from which it's extracted has been shown to significantly help people whose kidneys have been damaged by lupus.

Linseed, which is also known as flaxseed, has an abundance of two compounds that may help improve kidney function. One is alpha-linolenic acid, an omega-3 fatty acid (the same type of beneficial fats found in fish). Alpha-linolenic acid stops both inflammation and clogging of the arteries, both of which play some role in damaging the tiny and very fragile blood vessels supplying blood to the kidneys.

Flaxseed is also high in lignans, compounds that can help prevent clots from forming in the bloodstream. Such clots can damage and clog the tiny blood vessels of the kidneys.

In one study, researchers at the University of Western Ontario in Canada gave flaxseed to nine people whose kidneys were damaged by lupus. They found that the people who were given ¼ cup of raw ground flaxseed a day, which they stirred into juice or sprinkled on breakfast cereal, had better kidney function.

More research needs to be done, but preliminary evidence also suggests that

THE SPROUT CONNECTION

For years, stories have circulated that eating alfalfa sprouts (or taking alfalfa supplements) can make lupus symptoms worse, or even bring on the disease. Paradoxically, folklore has it that alfalfa is good for arthritis, and since lupus is a form of arthritis, that would mean that alfalfa should be good for lupus. Which is true?

According to Victor Herbert, M.D., professor of medicine at Mount Sinai School of Medicine and Bronx Veterans Affairs Medical Center, both in New York City, and co-editor of *Total Nutrition*, alfalfa does appear to affect the immune system in a detrimental way in people with systemic lupus.

The best advice? If you have lupus, you may want to keep a food diary during flare-ups to help you keep track of what you were eating when symptoms appeared. Then you will know which foods (including alfalfa) appear to cause problems.

flaxseed may help improve the immune system, thus helping to control lupus flare-ups. In addition, the lignans in flaxseed appear to have antibacterial and antifungal capabilities. This is significant because people with lupus are more prone to infections than people without the disease.

"It takes just a little flaxseed to confer the benefits," says Lilian Thompson, Ph.D., professor of nutritional sciences at the University of Toronto. For most people, ¼ cup a day is about right, she says.

You can buy flaxseed in health food stores. In order to get the benefits of the lignans, however, the flaxseed must be ground before you eat it. You can buy ground flaxseed that's been vacuum-packed to preserve freshness, says Stephen Cunnane, Ph.D., professor of nutritional sciences at the University of Toronto. Or you can buy whole flaxseed and grind it at home. You can use ground flaxseed to replace some of the wheat flour in muffins or breads, or try sprinkling it on cereal or into stews and soups.

CUTTING THE FAT

We all know how important it is to eat less fat, particularly the saturated fat found in meats and many dairy products. It's particularly important for people with lupus. "Lupus patients get more artery-clogging heart disease than people in the general population, and they also get it at younger ages," says Michelle Petri, M.D., director of the Lupus Center at Johns Hopkins University School of Medicine in Baltimore. Reducing fat in the diet is one of the best ways to reduce this risk.

Another reason to cut back on fat has to do with immunity; since people on high-fat diets appear to have more immunity-related problems. As you might expect, eating too much red meat, which is usually high in saturated fat, can be a problem. A Japanese study of more than 150 women, for example, showed that those who ate meat frequently were nearly 3½ times more likely to develop lupus.

It's not only meat or saturated fat that's a problem. Laboratory studies showed that when mice with lupus were given smaller-than-usual amounts of polyunsaturated fats, such as those in vegetable oils like safflower and corn oil, their symptoms were reduced.

In short, if you have lupus, it's important to cut back on all types of fat in your diet. Here are some ways to get started.

Cut back on meat. Since meat is often one of the main sources of fat in the diet, cutting back automatically reduces the total amount of fat you consume. It's a good idea to limit yourself to 2- to 3-ounce servings of baked, broiled, or grilled meat.

Put vegetables on the menu. Eating more vegetarian meals, which typically include fresh vegetables, grains, and legumes, is another way to keep fat levels down. At the very least, try to substitute vegetarian meals for meat meals at least twice a week.

Open the spice cabinet. Rather than automatically adding butter or margarine to your food, look for other, healthier seasonings. By using spices, fresh herbs, and a splash of lemon or flavored vinegar, you'll get all the good tastes with a lot less fat.

Choose oils wisely. Since lupus may be aggravated by polyunsaturated fats, it's a good idea to switch to oils that are higher in monounsaturated fats, such as olive and canola oils.

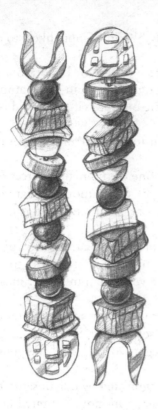

MEAT
A MINE
OF MINERALS

HEALING POWER

CAN HELP:
Prevent iron-deficiency
anemia

Boost the immune system

Prevent pernicious
anemia

Americans are back in the saddle
again. After a decade of searching for greener pastures, we've decided that the
grass was actually pretty tasty back at the ranch. So we're stampeding back, steaks
in hand, ready to hit the backyard barbecue.

Does this latest swing back to red meat mean that we're headed straight
for imminent health disaster? Not at all. In moderation, lean meats—not just
beef but also pork, venison, and other meats with less than 25 to 30 percent of
calories from fat—can provide significant health benefits, from preventing vitamin and mineral deficiencies and boosting immunity to building stronger
blood.

"People read these reports that red meat causes cancer and heart disease,
so they think that they have to stop eating meat," says Susan Kleiner, R.D.,
Ph.D., owner of High Performance Nutrition in Mercer Island, Washington.
"What they don't realize is that the people in these studies are eating 10 ounces
of red meat a day."

"Moderation is the key," urges Dr. Kleiner. "When it comes to red meat,
you should have no more than 3 to 5 ounces a day. That's about the size of a
deck of cards. For a lot of people, that looks like a garnish. But if you use just
enough meat to accent a meal, you'll be able to get all the benefits without the
potential detriments."

Ironing Out Anemia

Iron deficiency is the most common nutritional deficiency in the United States. Maybe that's why fatigue, the main symptom of iron deficiency anemia, is the number one reason that people drag themselves to see their doctors.

Meat is an important source of iron, a mineral that's essential for boosting the oxygen-carrying capability of blood. Once you've depleted your iron stores, your red blood cells get smaller. This makes it difficult for your lungs to send enough oxygen to the rest of your body. Without enough oxygen, you start feeling worn out.

"Women especially don't get enough iron," says Dr. Kleiner. "Mostly because, unlike men, they deny themselves foods that are rich in this mineral, like red meats." This is especially troubling, she says, because women generally need more iron than men to replace what is lost each month during their menstrual cycles.

In addition, women who exercise are at higher risk for anemia, says Dr. Kleiner. That's because the body uses more iron during exercise to meet the increased demand for oxygen. If you don't have enough iron to begin with, it's easy to run out while you're working up a sweat.

In one study, researchers had 47 inactive women step up the pace in a 12-week moderate-intensity aerobic exercise program. After just 4 weeks, all of them had significant dips in their iron stores. If you're active, it's particularly important to keep an eye on your iron intake.

What's so special about meat when you can also get iron from nonmeat sources like fortified breakfast cereals, tofu, and beans? Or, for that matter, when you can take an iron supplement?

For one thing, meats are unusually rich in iron. A 3-ounce serving of top round, for example, contains 3 milligrams of iron, 20 percent of the Recommended Dietary Allowance (RDA) for women and 30 percent of the RDA for men. A 3-ounce serving of pork tenderloin has 1 milligram of iron, 7 percent of the RDA for women and 10 percent for men.

Even though some plant foods are rich in iron—a baked potato, for example, contains 3 milligrams—it comes in a form that's harder for your body to absorb than the iron found in meats.

Meats contain a type of iron called heme iron, which is up to 15 percent more absorbable than nonheme iron, the kind found in plant foods. Plus, when you eat heme iron from meats, it helps your body absorb nonheme iron, so you get the maximum iron absorption from all your food, says Dr. Kleiner.

Zinc Immunity

Your immune system's duty is to keep your body from falling down on the job. Zinc's duty is to keep your immune system from doing the same. Not getting

In the Kitchen

Lean meats like flank steak and pork loin have all but supplanted their high-fat predecessors in healthy kitchens. To be truly good, however, they do require special handling.

"Because they're so low in fats, lean meats can end up very dry and tough, unless you prepare them properly," explains Michael Hughes, president of Broken Arrow Ranch, a game distributor in Ingram, Texas.

To ensure that your meat meals are moist and flavorful, try the following cooking tips.

- Start with a marinade. Marinating lean meats in the refrigerator several hours prior to preparation will infuse them with flavor and add extra liquid to help keep them moist during cooking.
- Simmer it. Forget roasting, broiling, and other dry cooking methods when preparing lean beef; the meat simply does not contain enough fat to be self-basting. You're more likely to be successful when you braise, simmer, or poach your lean meats.

enough of this important mineral means that your immune system will have a harder time fending off infections, colds, and other health invaders.

As with iron, you can get zinc from foods besides meats, such as whole grains and wheat germ. But again, your body has a harder time retrieving zinc from plant sources, whereas the zinc in meats is readily absorbed, explains Dr. Kleiner.

By including a little meat in your diet, it's easy to meet the Daily Value (DV) of 15 milligrams of zinc. Three ounces of top round steak, for instance, provides 5 milligrams, or about a third of the DV for this essential mineral.

The Best of the Bs

For most of us, getting enough vitamin B_{12} (the Daily Value is 6 micrograms) isn't a problem. If you eat meats, fish, eggs, poultry, or dairy products on a regular basis, you're almost certainly getting enough.

But if you don't eat these foods, and many strict vegetarians don't, you could be headed for trouble. Low levels of vitamin B_{12} can result in a rare and sometimes fatal blood disorder, called pernicious anemia, that causes fatigue, memory loss, and other neurological problems. And worse, you may not even know that there's a problem until it's already well-advanced.

"Pernicious anemia comes on very slowly and can take up to seven years to develop," says Dr. Kleiner. "And because one of the symptoms of the illness is deteriorating mental function, lots of people aren't even aware that there's anything wrong with them. It can take a long time to straighten this problem out, and the damage can be irreversible, especially in children."

Including small amounts of meats or other animal foods in your diet on a regular basis makes it easy to get enough vitamin B_{12}, says Dr. Kleiner. If you're a strict vegetarian who doesn't get vitamin B_{12} from animal foods, it's essential that you take a daily supplement or eat soy foods such as tempeh and miso, which are high in this nutrient. In addition, many cereals, pastas, and other packaged foods have been fortified with vitamin B_{12}, she points out.

Most meats are full of other B vitamins as well. They generally provide 10 to 20 percent of the DV for B-complex vitamins: riboflavin (essential for tissue repair), vitamin B_6 (needed for immunity), niacin (vital for skin, nerves, and digestion), and thiamin (which helps the body convert blood sugar into energy).

SAFER GRILLING

Grilled foods taste great, but for a long time researchers have worried about their safety. The problem is that grilling causes certain compounds in meats to change into compounds called heterocyclic amines, which may increase the risk for cancer.

What's a grill-chef to do? The answer, some researchers say, can be summarized in one word: marinade. In one study, researchers found that when medallions of chicken breast were marinated (or even dipped) in a mixture of olive oil, brown sugar, mustard, and other spices before being grilled, they contained 90 percent less of the dangerous compounds than nonmarinated meat that was cooked the same way.

Getting the Most

Buy free-range. For the best healing meats, some experts advise, look for "free-range" meats. These are meats that come from livestock that is allowed to roam free instead of being restricted in close quarters. Because the animals aren't crammed together, the ranchers generally use fewer antibiotics and skip the growth hormones, explains Dr. Kleiner.

"Although I recommend organic, chemical-free meat, if the higher price is going to keep you from eating it, don't worry about the chemicals, and get the nutrients," recommends Dr. Kleiner. "In the long run, that's more important."

Add some variety. Although much of the research on the health benefits of meats has been done in studies with lean beef, experts are quick to note that you shouldn't limit yourself to eating beef alone. Other meats such as pork and lamb can also play a role in a healthful diet. "In the same way that you should eat a wide variety of grains and vegetables, you should also eat a variety of meats to ensure that you get all the nutrients they have to offer," advises Dr. Kleiner.

You might also want to take a walk on the wild side and go with game. Many people believe that game meats such as venison are tastier than more pedestrian meats such as beef. In addition, game is generally much leaner—deriving less than 18 percent of its calories from fat—while delivering the same powerhouse of B vitamins and minerals. A lean cut of beef, such as tip round steak, has 34 percent calories from fat.

HORSERADISH–SPIKED PORK AND APPLES

12 **ounces pork tenderloin, trimmed of fat**

2 **medium apples**

2 **tablespoons unbleached all-purpose flour**

1 **cup apple cider**

1 **tablespoon extra-hot horseradish**

PER SERVING

calories	**218**
total fat	**6.3 g.**
saturated fat	**2.2 g.**
cholesterol	**52 mg.**
sodium	**38 mg.**
dietary fiber	**1.6 g.**

Cut the pork crosswise into ¼" slices. Core the apples and cut into thin slices.

Coat a large no-stick skillet with no-stick cooking spray and place over medium-high heat. Add the pork and cook for 2 minutes, or until lightly golden on the bottom. Turn and cook for 2 to 3 minutes, or until lightly golden and cooked through. Test for doneness by inserting the tip of a sharp knife in a piece of the pork. Remove the pork to a clean plate and set aside.

Reduce the heat to medium. Add the apples and cook, stirring occasionally, for 3 to 4 minutes, or until they begin to turn light golden. Sprinkle with the flour and continue cooking, tossing to coat evenly with the flour.

Stir in the cider. Cook, stirring, for 3 to 4 minutes, or until the sauce thickens. Stir in the horseradish. Spoon the apples and sauce over the pork.

Makes 4 servings

Lamb Shanks in Tomato-Orange Sauce

4   **lamb shanks (12 ounces each)**

1   **can (16 ounces) crushed tomatoes**

1   **tablespoon minced garlic**

1   **orange**

2   **tablespoons finely chopped fresh mint**

¼   **teaspoon salt**

Per serving

calories	**270**
total fat	**12.2 g.**
saturated fat	**5.1 g.**
cholesterol	**96 mg.**
sodium	**482 mg.**
dietary fiber	**2.4 g.**

Coat a Dutch oven with no-stick spray and place over medium heat. Add the lamb and cook, turning as needed, for 10 minutes, or until lightly browned on all sides. Add the tomatoes, 1 cup water, and garlic.

Grate the rind from the orange and add it to the pan. Squeeze the juice and add it to the pan. Bring to a simmer.

Cover, reduce the heat to low, and cook for 2 to 3 hours, or until the meat is tender and falling off the bone.

Stir in the mint and salt. Simmer for 1 to 2 minutes to allow the flavors to blend.

Makes 4 servings

Cook's Note: Serve the lamb over hot cooked pasta, rice, couscous, or potatoes.

Beef and Spinach Stir-Fry

1   **pound beef eye of round, trimmed of fat**

1   **tablespoon cornstarch**

2   **teaspoons canola oil**

2   **teaspoons grated fresh ginger**

1   **small onion, thinly sliced**

1   **bag (6 ounces) spinach, washed and trimmed**

⅓   **cup defatted beef broth**

2   **tablespoons ketchup**
    Ground black pepper

Per serving

calories	**207**
total fat	**7.6 g.**
saturated fat	**2.1 g.**
cholesterol	**61 mg.**
sodium	**263 mg.**
dietary fiber	**1.6 g.**

Cut the beef across the grain into very thin slices. Place in a medium bowl. Add the cornstarch and toss to combine.

Heat the oil in a wok or large skillet over medium-high heat until it is nearly smoking. Add the beef and ginger. Stir-fry for 2 minutes, or until the beef is no longer pink on the surface. Transfer to a plate.

Add the onions to the pan and stir-fry for 1 to 2 minutes, or until softened. Add the spinach and stir-fry for 30 seconds, or until just wilted.

In a small bowl, combine the broth and ketchup. Add to the pan. Add the beef. Stir-fry for 2 to 3 minutes, or until the sauce is heated through and coats the beef and vegetables. Season to taste with pepper.

Makes 4 servings

Cook's Note: Serve over rice or noodles.

THE BEST CUTS

While meats can play a valuable role in a healthful diet, it's important to shop only for those items that are suitably low in fat—preferably with no more than 25 to 30 percent of calories coming from fat. In the following tables, we've listed a few meats (and a variety of cuts) that you may want to try. Only prominent nutrients—those providing more than 10 percent of the Daily Value (DV)—are mentioned. All nutritional information is based on 3-ounce servings.

Beef

Eye Round

Calories	143
Fat	4 grams
Calories from fat	26 percent
Vitamin B_{12}	2 micrograms (33 percent of DV)
Zinc	4 milligrams (27 percent of DV)
Iron	2 milligrams (20 percent of RDA for men and 13 percent for women)
Niacin	3 milligrams (15 percent of DV)
Vitamin B_6	0.3 milligram (15 percent of DV)

Top Round

Calories	153
Fat	4 grams
Calories from fat	25 percent
Riboflavin	0.2 milligram (33 percent of DV)
Potassium	376 milligrams (33 percent of DV)
Iron	3 milligrams (30 percent of RDA for men and 20 percent for women)
Niacin	5 milligrams (25 percent of DV)
Vitamin B_6	0.5 milligram (25 percent of DV)

Vitamin B_{12}	2 micrograms (12 percent of DV)
Zinc	5 milligrams (11 percent of DV)

Pork Tenderloin

Calories	141
Fat	4 grams
Calories from fat	26 percent
Thiamin	0.8 milligram (53 percent of DV)
Vitamin B_6	0.4 milligram (20 percent of DV)
Niacin	4 milligrams (20 percent of DV)
Zinc	3 milligrams (20 percent of DV)
Riboflavin	0.3 milligram (18 percent of DV)
Potassium	457 milligrams (13 percent of DV)
Iron	1 milligram (10 percent of RDA for men and 7 percent for women)

Lamb Foreshank

Calories	159
Fat	5 grams
Calories from fat	29 percent
Niacin	14 milligrams (70 percent of DV)
Zinc	7 milligrams (47 percent of DV)

Vitamin B_{12} 2 micrograms
                        (33 percent of DV)

Deer
Calories   134
Fat   3 grams
Calories from fat   18 percent
Iron   4 milligrams
                        (40 percent of RDA
                        for men and 27
                        percent for women)
Niacin   6 milligrams
                        (30 percent of DV)
Riboflavin   0.5 milligram
                        (29 percent of DV)
Thiamin   0.2 milligram
                        (13 percent of DV)
Zinc   2 milligrams
                        (13 percent of DV)

Elk
Calories   124
Fat   2 grams
Calories from fat   12 percent
Iron   3 milligrams
                        (31 percent of RDA
                        for men and 21
                        percent for women)
Zinc   3 milligrams
                        (20 percent of DV)

Veal Leg
Calories   128
Fat   3 grams
Calories from fat   20 percent
Niacin   9 milligrams
                        (45 percent of DV)
Zinc   3 milligrams
                        (20 percent of DV)
Riboflavin   0.3 milligram
                        (18 percent of DV)

Vitamin B_{12} 1 microgram
                        (17 percent of DV)
Vitamin B_6 0.3 milligram
                        (15 percent of DV)

Moose
Calories   114
Fat   1 gram
Calories from fat   6 percent
Iron   4 milligrams
                        (40 percent of RDA
                        for men and 27
                        percent for women)
Niacin   5 milligrams
                        (25 percent of DV)
Zinc   3 milligrams
                        (20 percent of DV)
Riboflavin   0.3 milligram
                        (18 percent of DV)

Bison/Buffalo
Calories   122
Fat   2 grams
Calories from fat   15 percent
Iron   3 milligrams
                        (30 percent of RDA
                        for men and 20
                        percent for women)
Zinc   2 milligrams
                        (13 percent of DV)

Emu
Calories   103
Fat   3 grams
Calories from fat   23 percent
Iron   4 milligrams
                        (40 percent of RDA
                        for men and 27
                        percent for women)

Mediterranean Diet

A Model for Good Health

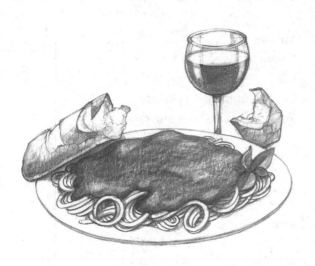

Healing Power

Can help:
Reduce the risk of heart disease and cancer

Lower cholesterol

During the early 1960s, when the rate of heart disease in the United States was skyrocketing, people in Greece had some of the lowest heart disease rates in the world.

Here's the curious part. They were enjoying this robust good health even though their diet racked up nearly 40 percent of its calories from fat, plus they generally washed down their meals with a glass or two of wine.

Scientists wanted to know more. So they searched the shores of the Mediterranean Sea and discovered that it wasn't only in Greece that people were living longer and healthier but also in neighboring nations like France, Italy, and Spain. Clearly, these folks were onto something.

But what?

"For one thing, the traditional Mediterranean diet includes a lot of vegetables and legumes, along with fruits, fresh whole-grain breads, dates, and nuts," says Christopher Gardner, Ph.D., research fellow at Stanford University Center for Research in Disease Prevention in Palo Alto, California. "Meats like lamb and chicken are consumed infrequently and in small portions, and the main source of fat in the diet is monounsaturated fat from olives and olive oil rather than the saturated fat from animal foods. In addition, physical activity is a significant part of the daily routine," he adds.

THE HEART OF THE MATTER

Just how healthful is traditional Mediterranean fare? In one study, French researchers looked at 600 men who had recently had a heart attack. They put half of the men on a traditional Mediterranean diet and half on a low-fat, low-cholesterol diet that people with heart disease are typically told to follow. Those following the traditional Mediterranean diet had a 70 percent lower rate of recurrent heart problems than those following the prudent low-fat diet.

Other studies had similar results. When researchers examined the diets and disease rates of people in seven different countries, for example, they found that while heart disease accounts for 46 percent of deaths of middle-aged men in America, only 4 percent of men in Crete, an island in the Mediterranean, had similar problems. In fact, the death rate from all causes in Crete during this 15-year study was lower than that of the other countries.

THE FAT FACTOR

There are many reasons that the Mediterranean diet is good for the heart, but perhaps most important is where it gets its fat.

Even though people in Mediterranean countries eat as much fat as we do (or more), they eat relatively little meat. This means that they consume only minuscule amounts of artery-clogging saturated fat. "The biggest bang for the buck comes from limiting saturated fat and replacing it with monounsaturated fat, like olive oil," says Dr. Gardner. Olive oil is not only a monounsaturated fat, it also contains antioxidant compounds that help prevent chemical changes in the body that can cause the dangerous low-density lipoprotein (LDL) cholesterol to stick to artery walls.

The second most-common source of fats in the Mediterranean diet is nuts and seeds. Nuts contain alpha-linolenic acid, which the body coverts to the same kind of heart-healthy fats found in fish (which people in the Mediterranean also eat). Studies show that people who get the most of these fatty acids are the ones least likely to have heart disease.

"This doesn't mean people should run out and start adding tons of olive oil and nuts to their diets," warns John A. McDougall, M.D., medical director of the McDougall Program at St. Helena Hospital in Napa Valley, California, and author of *The McDougall Program for a Healthy Heart*. It's not only diet that makes people in Mediterranean countries so healthy. They also tend to walk a lot, do hard physical labor, and generally stay active. So even though they take in a lot of calories from fat, they're usually able to keep their weight under control.

"Americans who got all that fat from olive oil would just get fat, which itself is a major heart disease risk," Dr. McDougall says. But some olive oil is good, particularly when you use it to replace the less healthy saturated fats in your diet.

THE MEDITERRANEAN PLAN

Unless you've been living on popcorn and Twinkies for the last 10 years, you're already familiar with the U.S. Department of Agriculture (USDA) Food Guide Pyramid, which recommends that everyone eat approximately 15 to 26 servings of fruits, vegetables, beans, grains, and proteins every day. In this country, the pyramid is considered the optimal eating plan.

However, the USDA's isn't the only pyramid going. There's also a Mediterranean Pyramid, based on the traditional diet of southern Europe. Unlike our pyramid, which includes meats as a way of getting enough proteins every day, the Mediterranean Pyramid depends instead on legumes, fish, and nuts to supply the necessary proteins. Red meat is reserved for a few times a month.

The Mediterranean Pyramid also calls for large amounts of olive oil and daily doses of cheese and yogurt, all washed down with a healthy splash of red wine. Regular physical activity is also an essential part of the plan.

To the right is the traditional Mediterranean Pyramid. You should choose most of your foods from the base of the pyramid and save those at the top for special occasions.

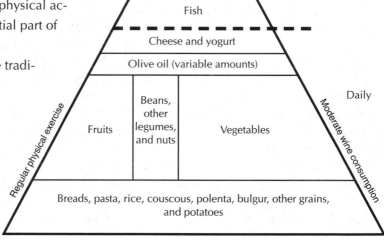

Adapted from "The Traditional Healthy Mediterranean Diet Pyramid"
Copyright © 1994 by Oldways Preservation & Exchange Trust

FIVE-A-DAY PROTECTION

The folks at the American Heart Association would be delighted if they could get us to eat the five servings (or more) of fruits and vegetables that the Mediterraneans eat every day. Studies have shown that people who eat the most fruits and vegetables have fewer problems with heart disease. Presumably this is due to the antioxidant vitamins and other healing compounds in these foods.

In addition, fruits, vegetables, and beans, which are another Mediterranean staple, are among the best sources of folate, a vitamin that may work hard in the fight against heart disease, says Dr. Gardner.

Folate helps decrease levels of an amino acid called homocysteine. There is a link between too much homocysteine and heart disease. Research has shown that healthy people who have high levels of homocysteine are about 14 times more likely to have heart disease than those with low or moderate levels.

In addition, the Mediterranean diet is extremely high in fiber. High-fiber foods not only help keep your weight down by filling you up without a lot of fat and calories, they also help block the absorption of certain fats and cholesterol. This means that some of these harmful substances are flushed away before making it into the bloodstream.

So powerful are the effects of fiber that a study of nearly 44,000 men ages 40 to 75 found that men who added just 10 grams of fiber a day to their diet decreased their risk of heart disease by almost 30 percent.

LIGHT ON THE CHEESE

In the Mediterranean diet, cheese is part of most meals. How can people who eat so much cheese, which is often high in saturated fat, be so healthy?

There are several explanations. The cheeses popular in the Mediterranean are not the high-fat cheeses we eat here, like American, Swiss, or cheddar. Rather, they are cheeses that are naturally lower in fat, such as feta and Parmesan.

"The people on the Mediterranean also use these cheeses in small amounts," says Christopher Gardner, Ph.D., research fellow at the Stanford University Center for Research in Disease Prevention in Palo Alto, California. "They don't eat ounces and ounces of them every day. Nor should we."

While cheese can be an important source of calcium, limit your servings to about an ounce a day—approximately the size of three dominoes—or less. Also, look for reduced-fat cheese or cheese that is naturally low in fat.

A DRINK FOR HEALTH

It's not only olive oil and fruits and vegetables that make the Mediterranean diet so good for the heart. Another factor appears to be the wine, especially red wine, that people in these countries drink with almost every meal.

Wine contains compounds called phenols that help prevent LDL cholesterol from sticking to artery walls. It also keeps platelets in blood from sticking together and causing clots. "In moderation, wine can be a nice addition to a healthy diet," says Robert M. Russell, M.D., of the Jean Mayer USDA Human Nutrition Research Center on Aging at Tufts University in Boston.

Beyond the Heart

Although the Mediterranean diet is most renowned for its role in keeping the heart healthy, it also appears to reduce the risks of other health threats, among them cancers of the breast and colon.

Studies show that compared to women elsewhere in the world, women in some Mediterranean countries have half the risk (or less) of getting breast cancer. This could be due to their low intake of saturated fat and high intake of mono-unsaturated fats, fruits, and vegetables.

Indeed, Italian researchers have found that people in the Mediterranean region who follow the traditional diet—that is, those who eat lots of fruits and vegetables and not much fat and protein—are less likely to get cancer than those who eat more modern, less healthful diets.

"The message here is simple," says Dr. Gardner. "For optimal health, choose a plant-based diet, which is naturally high in vitamins, minerals, fiber, and antioxidants and low in fat, cholesterol, and sodium."

MEDITERRANEAN-STYLE PENNE

8 **ounces penne**

½ **cup dry-packed sun-dried tomatoes, cut into 3 or 4 strips each**

2 **tablespoons olive oil**

2 **cloves garlic, minced**

1 **can (15 ounces) cannellini or Great Northern beans, rinsed and drained**

2 **tablespoons minced fresh sage**

¼ **teaspoon salt**

Ground black pepper

PER SERVING

calories	**394**
total fat	**11.8 g.**
saturated fat	**1.5 g.**
cholesterol	**0 mg.**
sodium	**413 mg.**
dietary fiber	**7.6 g.**

In a large pot of boiling water, cook the pasta according to the package directions. About 1 minute before the pasta is scheduled to be done, add the tomatoes to the pot.

Scoop out ¼ cup of the cooking water and set aside. Drain the pasta and tomatoes. Place in a large bowl. Add the reserved cooking water and toss to mix.

In a medium saucepan over medium heat, warm the oil. Add the garlic and cook for 30 seconds, or until fragrant. Remove from the heat. Stir in the beans, sage, and salt. Cook for 1 minute, stirring, or until the beans are warm. Season with the pepper.

Pour over the pasta and toss gently to mix.

Makes 4 servings

Vegetable Pitas with Creamy Mint Sauce

Mint Sauce

- ½ cup nonfat plain yogurt
- 1 tablespoon minced fresh mint
- 1 clove garlic, minced

Pita Sandwiches

- 2 medium eggplants (1 pound each)
- 4 teaspoons olive oil
- ⅛ teaspoon salt
- 4 rounds pita bread (6" diameter)
- 2 large tomatoes, each cut into 8 slices

PER SANDWICH	
calories	**301**
total fat	**6 g.**
saturated fat	**0.9 g.**
cholesterol	**1 mg.**
sodium	**428 mg.**
dietary fiber	**7.5 g.**

To make the sauce: In a small bowl, mix the yogurt, mint, and garlic.

To make the sandwiches: Preheat the broiler. Coat a broiler pan with no-stick spray.

Cut the eggplants lengthwise into ⅛"-thick slices. Discard the outer slices that are mostly skin. Place the eggplant slices, slightly overlapping, on the broiler pan. Brush lightly with the oil. Sprinkle with the salt.

Broil 6" from the heat for 5 to 6 minutes, or until the pieces begin to lightly brown. Turn the slices and coat lightly with no-stick spray. Broil for 3 to 4 minutes, or until the slices are almost soft. Transfer to a plate. Set aside for 1 to 2 minutes, so the steam will finish softening the slices.

Cut the pitas in half and open the halves. Fill each pocket with several slices of eggplant and 2 tomato slices. Spoon 1 tablespoon of the sauce into each pocket.

Makes 4 servings

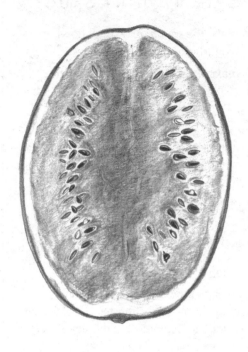

MELONS
HEALTH FROM THE VINE

HEALING POWER
CAN HELP:
Prevent birth defects

Reduce the risk of cancer and heart disease

Keep blood pressure low

Summer picnics don't really come alive until the barbecue is cold and the potato salad has been put away. That's when it's time to pick up a knife and cut into the tough green rind of an ice-cold watermelon, revealing the sweet red flesh within.

There's always something exciting about cutting open a watermelon, crenshaw, or honeydew. For one thing, they come encased in protective rinds, so what's inside always comes as a surprise. And even before you cut, most melons whet your appetite by releasing a rich, penetrating scent, which is why they're sometimes called the "perfumy fruits."

Here's another reason melons are so marvelous. Researchers have found that they contain a number of substances that are very good for your health. Both watermelons and muskmelons—which include honeydews, crenshaws, and a few other melons—provide folate, a B vitamin that has been shown to lower the risks of birth defects and heart disease. Melons also contain potassium, which is essential for keeping blood pressure at healthy levels. And because melons are low in calories and fat, they're the perfect food for waist-watchers.

Cantaloupes are especially healthful, and they contain certain nutrients that other melons don't, which is why they're discussed in a separate chapter (see page 110).

Melons for Moms – And More

In what has been called one of the most critical discoveries of the twentieth century, researchers found that if all women of childbearing age consumed at least 400 micrograms of folate a day, the incidence of brain and spinal cord birth defects (called neural tube defects) could be cut in half or even more. For a long time, doctors weren't sure what folate did. They suspected that it played a role in preventing birth defects, but there wasn't strong evidence one way or the other.

Then a study of almost 4,000 mothers revealed that those who got enough folate were 60 percent less likely to have children with brain and spinal cord defects than women who got smaller amounts.

Folate, a B vitamin, is an essential ingredient when cells are dividing rapidly. It serves as the shuttle bus that carries fragments of proteins. When folate levels are low, these fragments, lacking transportation, may be left behind. As a result, the newly forming cells may have defects that can lead to birth defects. (Later in life, the same problem can lead to cellular changes that could lead to cancer.)

So before you start shopping for pickles, put a few melons in your cart because they're very good sources of folate. A cup of honeydew, for example, contains 11 micrograms of folate, 3 percent of the Daily Value (DV). Casaba melons are even better, with the same cup providing 29 micrograms of folate, 7 percent of the DV.

If 7 percent doesn't sound like a lot, remember that a cup of melon is the equivalent of about five good bites. Most people eat two or more cups of melon at a time, making it a very good folate find.

Incidentally, it's not only moms-to-be who should be making the most of

Melons without Motion

There's a good chance that whoever invented the wheel was a watermelon fan. As you've probably noticed, a watermelon's smooth, cylindrical shape gives it a tendency to roll—usually off a table or the seat of your car—creating instant melon puree.

There's another problem with the shape of watermelons. Since they can't be stacked, they take a lot of room to store, which is expensive for melon growers. In Japan, where space is at a premium, growers have hit upon an ingenious solution: the square watermelon.

When melons are young and still on the vine, Japanese growers sometimes place them in boxes. As the melons grow to fit the space, they develop flat bottoms and sides, making them perfect for stacking. Square watermelons aren't yet available in this country, but just for fun, if you have a backyard garden, you may want to try growing your own.

IN THE KITCHEN

Unlike most fruits and vegetables, which are easy to check for ripeness, melons hide their succulence—or their toughness—behind a protective rind. To get the best taste every time, here are a few tips you may want to try.

Check the bottom. A watermelon that's pale-yellow or beige on the bottom was allowed to ripen on the vine and will probably be at the peak of freshness. If the color is uniform, however, it may have been picked early and won't deliver its full flavor.

Take a sniff. Most melons (with the exception of watermelon) release a rich, fragrant odor when they're fully ripe. If you can't smell it in the store, don't take it home.

Check the stem. When muskmelons are allowed to ripen in the field, the fruit slips off the vine, leaving the stem behind. So if you see a muskmelon with the stem attached, you'll know that it was picked early and isn't fully ripe. It's okay, though, if watermelons still have their stems.

Give it a slap. Although thumping is the time-honored method for testing a watermelon's ripeness, a slap works better. If the melon sounds hollow rather than solid, it's ready to go.

melons. The same nutrient that protects against birth defects is also good for the heart.

The body uses folate to control levels of a chemical in the blood called homocysteine. "Although small amounts of homocysteine are normal, too much of it somehow contributes to the artery-clogging process that leads to heart disease," says Killian Robinson, M.D., a cardiologist at the Cleveland Clinic Foundation in Ohio. "We know that low levels of folate are related to too-high homocysteine levels."

Finally, folate has been shown to reduce the risk of polyps, precancerous growths in the colon that sometimes progress to full-blown cancer. Researchers at Harvard Medical School found that people getting the most folate were 33 percent less likely to develop polyps in the colon than those getting the least.

THE FIBER FIX

One thing that your digestive tract needs is a steady supply of dietary fiber. Fiber is so important, in fact, that people who don't get enough have higher risks for cancer as well as for a variety of digestive problems, says John H. Weisburger, Ph.D., senior member of the American Health Foundation in Valhalla, New York.

The type of fiber that is found in melons, called soluble fiber, is tremendously important for helping to keep the colon healthy, Dr. Weisburger explains. Because soluble fiber absorbs water as it move through the digestive tract, it causes stools to get heavier and larger. As a result, they move more quickly through the intestine, reducing the amount of time that harmful substances in the stool are in contact with the colon wall.

"Getting more fiber can reduce the number of polyps in the gastrointestinal tract and also the risk of colon cancer," says Dr. Weisburger. All melons contain some fiber, although honeydews beat out watermelon by quite a bit. Half a honeydew has nearly 3 grams of fiber, 12 percent of the DV.

MORE MELONS, LESS PRESSURE

If you have high blood pressure, you're probably already getting less salt and more minerals in your diet. It's a good idea to get more melons as well. All melons, especially honeydews and crenshaws, are good sources of potassium, which is perhaps the most important mineral for keeping blood pressure down.

The potassium in melons acts as a natural diuretic, removing excess fluids from the body. This is important because when fluid levels are high, blood pressure can rise, says Michael T. Murray, a naturopathic doctor in Bellevue, Washington, and author of *Natural Alternatives to Over-the-Counter and Prescription Drugs*. Plus, potassium keeps the artery walls relaxed.

Relaxed arterial walls do not contract as strongly as more "taut" or rigid walls. This means that the blood pressure created with each heartbeat is not as great. The result, of course, is lower blood pressure—which can reduce the risk of stroke, heart disease, and other serious conditions.

People with high blood pressure are often advised to get at least the DV of 3,500 milligrams of potassium a day. Melons make it easy. Half a honeydew, for example, has about 1,355 milligrams of potassium, over a third of the DV. Watermelons also contain potassium, but only about half as much as honeydews or crenshaws.

Getting the Most

Make it a honey. Even though watermelon is a decent source of nutrients, it contains so much water that they're very diluted. Ounce for ounce, honeydews have over twice the potassium and almost three times more folate.

Buy them whole. Supermarkets often sell watermelons, honeydews, and other melons cut into halves or slices. This can save space in your refrigerator, but it won't save much in the way of nutrients. When the flesh of melons is exposed to light, the nutrients start to break down. So it's a good idea to buy melons whole. And once you've cut them, keep them covered in the refrigerator to prevent the vitamins from breaking down.

Keep them cold. Folate is readily destroyed by heat, so it's important to store melons, whole or cut, in a cool, dark place.

HONEYDEW AND BLUEBERRY SALAD

1 **honeydew melon**

1 **cup fresh blueberries**

2 **strips lemon rind (1″ × ¹⁄₂″ each)**

¹⁄₄ **cup berry vinegar (see note)**

2 **teaspoons sugar**

PER SERVING

calories	**71**
total fat	**0.2 g.**
saturated fat	**0 g.**
cholesterol	**0 mg.**
sodium	**18 mg.**
dietary fiber	**1.5 g.**

Cut the honeydew in half, scoop out the seeds, and remove the flesh from the rind; discard the rind. Cut the flesh into ³⁄₄″ cubes. Place in a large glass bowl. Add the blueberries and lemon rind.

In a small bowl, combine the vinegar and sugar. Whisk until the sugar is dissolved. Pour over the fruit and toss gently. Cover and refrigerate for 1 to 2 hours.

Toss gently to mix. Remove and discard the lemon rind. To serve, remove the honeydew and blueberries with a slotted spoon.

Makes 8 servings

Cook's Note: Raspberry vinegar is available in some large supermarkets. Blueberry vinegar, sold in some specialty shops, is especially good in this salad. The juice left from marinating the salad can be served with the salad or drained and refrigerated for a refreshing drink.

MEMORY PROBLEMS
EATING FOR RECALL

Like a Dick Tracy decoder ring, sometimes the answers to life's most perplexing memory problems are found inside a cereal box. Just ask William Regelson, M.D., professor of medicine at the Virginia Commonwealth University, Medical College of Virginia School of Medicine in Richmond.

"What we sometimes assume is the onset of 'senility' may be caused by marginal nutritional deficiencies," says Dr. Regelson. "When people say that they're losing their mental functions, one of the first things I tell them is that they should eat Total cereal. It has varying amounts of all the vitamins and minerals they need. You'd be surprised how many people are fine once they meet their nutritional needs."

Many researchers are discovering the same thing. When people are low in certain nutrients, their mental performance dips. Even not getting enough water can cause the mind to get fuzzy, says Susan A. Nitzke, R.D., Ph.D., associate professor in the nutritional sciences department at the University of Wisconsin in Madison. "The thirst mechanism slows down as we age, so we're not always aware right away that we need water," she says. "One of the symptoms of severe dehydration is mental confusion."

In addition, the body begins absorbing some nutrients a little less efficiently over time. So even though your need for calories doesn't change, you may need additional nutrients to keep your mind sharp, says Dr. Regelson.

Not all memory problems are caused by diet. But when nothing else is amiss, it may be what you're eating—or not eating—that's slowing you down.

B IS FOR BRAINS

The B vitamins are perhaps the most essential nutrients for helping to keep your mind sharp. Your body uses B vitamins to turn food into mental energy and to manufacture and repair your brain tissue. "Deficiencies in thiamin, niacin, and vitamins B_6 and B_{12} can all cause mental dysfunction," says Vernon Mark, M.D., author of *Reversing Memory Loss*. "In fact, pellagra, a niacin deficiency, used to be a leading cause for admissions into state mental hospitals," he explains.

Avoiding the Brain Drain

Killing brain cells is not the best way to get a high score in the memory department. Yet that's exactly what many of us do to our gray matter every day, says Vernon Mark, M.D., author of *Reversing Memory Loss.*

"Alcohol is a brain poison," says Dr. Mark. "Even if you're doing everything else right, drinking too much alcohol can cause a significant decrease in memory function." In fact, even small amounts of alcohol can damage cells in the part of the brain responsible for memory.

Many doctors recommend abstaining from alcohol entirely to keep your mind at its sharpest. At the very least, it's a good idea to limit yourself to one or two drinks—meaning 12 ounces of beer, 5 ounces of wine, or 1 1/2 ounces of liquor—a day.

Research has shown, in fact, that when children are given 5 milligrams of thiamin instead of the Daily Value (DV) of 1.5 milligrams, they achieve substantially higher scores when given tests of mental functioning, Dr. Mark adds.

Today, many breads, cereals, and pastas are enriched with thiamin and niacin, so most people get enough of these nutrients. Niacin deficiencies have become extremely rare, especially in this country. But in older folks or in people who frequently drink alcohol, levels of thiamin can dip low enough to cause memory problems, says Dr. Mark.

The easiest way to make sure you get enough brain-boosting B vitamins is to eat foods containing enriched grains. One cup of enriched spaghetti, for example, has 0.3 milligram of thiamin, 20 percent of the DV, and 2 milligrams of niacin, 10 percent of the DV. Meat is also a good source of these nutrients. Three ounces of pork tenderloin, for example, provide 0.8 milligram of thiamin, 53 percent of the DV. For niacin, 3 ounces of chicken breast deliver 12 milligrams, 60 percent of the DV.

It's not as easy to get additional amounts of vitamins B_6 and B_{12}, because it's harder for the body to absorb them as we get older. "After the age of 55, it's pretty common to be low in these vitamins, because the lining of the stomach is changing," says Dr. Regelson.

As you get older, it's a good idea to get more than the DV of both of these nutrients. Vitamin B_6 is abundant in baked potatoes, bananas, chickpeas, and turkey. One baked potato provides 0.4 milligram of vitamin B_6, 20 percent of the DV, and one banana provides 0.7 milligram, 35 percent of the DV. For vitamin B_{12}, meat and shellfish are good choices. Three ounces of lean ground beef will provide 2 micrograms of vitamin B_{12}, about a third of the DV. Clams are an incredible source, with 20 steamed clams providing 89 micrograms, 1,483 percent of the DV.

Maintaining the Flow

One way to alleviate memory problems is to get more blood to the brain, says Dr. Regelson. When adequate blood flow isn't maintained, the brain and memory begin performing poorly.

The lack of blood to the brain is often caused by the same thing that leads to heart disease: a buildup of cholesterol and fat in the arteries. "This condition is not only preventable through diet," says Dr. Regelson, "it's at least partially reversible."

A primary cause of cardiovascular disease—clogged arteries in the heart and the brain—is too much fat, especially saturated fat, in the diet, says Dr. Nitzke. "Keep your intake of saturated fat low by cooking with small amounts of liquid oils instead of butter or margarine and minimizing your intake of fatty foods such as mayonnaise, rich desserts, and fatty meats," she says.

Just as important, she adds, is getting more fruits and vegetables. Fruits and vegetables are packed with antioxidants—compounds that block the effects of harmful oxygen molecules called free radicals. This is important because when free radicals damage the harmful low-density lipoprotein cholesterol, it becomes stickier and is more likely to stick to artery walls.

The combination of reducing fat in your diet and eating more fruits and vegetables will help keep your arteries clear. In fact, it may even help restore blood flow through arteries that have already begun to close up, says Dr. Regelson.

The Coffee Conundrum

Millions of Americans jump-start their brains each morning with steaming cups of coffee, and for good reason. The caffeine in coffee has been shown to improve mental functioning, including memory.

In one study, researchers from the Netherlands used a chemical to block short-term memory in 16 healthy people. They found that giving these folks 250 milligrams of caffeine—about the amount in three cups of coffee—quickly restored their powers of recall.

Getting too much coffee, of course, can be more of a bane than a boon, if only because the java buzz wears off within 6 to 8 hours. For some people, at least, the after-coffee slump can result in mental fogginess.

"Everyone has different reactions to caffeine," says Suzette Evans, Ph.D., assistant professor at Columbia University College of Physicians and Surgeons and the New York State Psychiatric Institute, both in New York City. For people who rarely drink coffee, having a cup or two can definitely improve performance and memory, she says. But if you drink coffee throughout the day, you quickly build up tolerance and won't get the same benefits. In fact, too much caffeine can make you jittery and reduce your concentration.

MENOPAUSAL PROBLEMS
FOODS FOR MIDLIFE—AND BEYOND

For many women, menopause—or the change, as it is sometimes called—is a time of great exuberance. Unfettered by monthly periods, concerns about pregnancy, or the anxiety of starting a career, it's natural to feel a sudden sense of freedom—as though the rest of your life is truly your own.

"There is no more creative force in the world than the menopausal woman with zest," said anthropologist Margaret Mead, who did some of her most exciting work when she was well past her fifties.

Still, the body does undergo a number of physical changes during menopause that can take the zest from the best. Hot flashes, mood swings, and insomnia are just a few of the symptoms many women experience around this time. For years, women (and their doctors) assumed that the discomfort of menopause was an inevitable part of the process. As it turns out, however, many of the problems of menopause can be controlled or even eliminated simply by eating the right foods, says Isaac Schiff, M.D., chief of obstetrics and gynecology at Massachusetts General Hospital in Boston and author of *Menopause*.

HORMONAL SHIFTS

As a woman approaches menopause, her ovaries begin producing less of the female hormones estrogen and progesterone. At some point, they begin producing so little of these hormones that menstrual periods stop, and the physical problems, such as hot flashes and mood swings, begin.

Even more serious are some of the long-term changes in the body caused by low hormone levels. Estrogen, for example, regulates a woman's cholesterol levels. When estrogen dips, cholesterol rises, which is why women have higher risks of heart disease after they have passed menopause.

Estrogen also plays a role in keeping a woman's bones full of calcium. When estrogen levels drop, the bones lose calcium at a very fast rate. Unless women take care to get extra calcium in their diets, their bones may become thin and weak, a condition called osteoporosis.

PROTECTING THE HEART

Since many of the problems of menopause are caused by low levels of estrogen, it makes sense that replacing some of the estrogen will make women healthier. Scientists have found that a number of foods—most notably soy foods such as tofu and tempeh—contain large amounts of phytoestrogens, plant compounds that act very much like the natural hormone.

This is particularly important for protecting the heart, since a woman's risk for heart disease rises after menopause. Research has shown, however, that eating more soy foods can help bring down cholesterol levels and the risk for heart disease. In a study at the University of Kentucky in Lexington, people eating just under 2 ounces of tofu a day were able to reduce total cholesterol by over 9 percent and harmful low-density lipoprotein cholesterol by nearly 13 percent.

Of course, when you're eating more soy foods, you're automatically eating less saturated fat, and this can also help keep cholesterol levels down. "Women approaching menopause and those who are already menopausal should concentrate on having the heart-healthiest diet," adds Wulf H. Utian, M.D., Ph.D., director of the department of obstetrics and gynecology at University MacDonald Womens Hospital and chair of the department of reproductive biology at Case Western Reserve University, both in Cleveland. "It's one of the most important issues they face because of menopause."

TURN DOWN THE HEAT

Hot flashes are perhaps the best-known sign of menopause. They can come out of nowhere and leave women feeling flushed and uncomfortable. Here, too, the phytoestrogens in soy can help.

Consider this. In Asian countries, where women eat a lot of soy foods, only about 16 percent have a problem with menopausal discomfort. In fact, there isn't even a word in Japanese for "hot flash." In this country, however, where soy foods are used much less often, 75 percent of menopausal women complain of hot flashes or other uncomfortable symptoms.

It's not only soybeans that can help relieve hot flashes. Black beans (which you can cook up into great-tasting soups or sprinkle into salads) contain about the same amount of phytoestrogens as soybeans. Ground flaxseed, which can be baked into bread and muffins, is also a good source.

What's more, you don't have to eat a lot of phytoestrogen-rich foods to get the benefits. Getting just 2 ounces of tofu or tempeh (a cake made from soybeans) a day can help prevent hot flashes from coming back. Or you could have a bowl of miso soup, which is flavored with a salty condiment made from soybeans and salt.

Take Charge of Your Bones

One of the most critical issues facing women is keeping their bones strong after menopause. "Getting enough calcium before, during, and after menopause is one of the most important things a woman can do to prevent possibly disastrous bone fractures," says Dr. Utian

Here, too, soy foods can make a difference, since there's some evidence that the phytoestrogens in soy play an active role in helping bones hang on to their calcium. A laboratory study found, for example, that animals given small amounts of genistein (a phytoestrogen found in soy) were able to maintain healthy, calcium-filled bones even when they were no longer producing estrogen.

Holding on to calcium is important because many women don't get anywhere near enough of this important mineral. On average, women ages 20 to 50 get about 600 milligrams a day, and women past menopause get only about 500 milligrams a day.

Scientists at the National Institutes of Health recommend that women in their childbearing years get at least 1,000 milligrams of calcium a day. Women past menopause should aim for 1,500 milligrams a day.

Most women can get plenty of calcium in their diets. For example, 1 cup of skim milk contains 302 milligrams of calcium, 30 percent of the DV. An 8-ounce serving of yogurt has 415 milligrams, 41 percent of the DV, and 3 ounces of salmon has 181 milligrams, 18 percent of the DV.

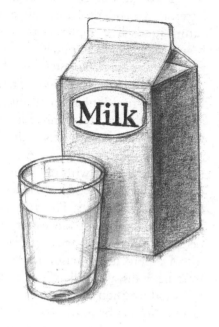

MILK
A GLASSFUL OF GOODNESS

HEALING POWER

CAN HELP:
Keep bones strong
and prevent osteoporosis

Lower blood pressure
and cholesterol

Reduce the risk of stroke

Even people who love milk often feel guilty about indulging. Despite its old-time reputation as being the perfect food, milk is extremely high in fat. A cup of whole milk is 49 percent fat. Reduced-fat (2 percent) milk isn't much better. It contains 34 percent fat. Worse, most of this fat is saturated, the kind that clogs your arteries. Not exactly what you'd call "perfect."

Before you wipe away your milk mustache forever, though, consider the lighter side: low-fat and skim milk. A cup of low-fat (1 percent) milk gets only 23 percent of its calories from fat. Skim milk (also called nonfat or fat-free) is the ultimate, with virtually no fat. Both skim and low-fat milk are two of the cheapest, easiest ways to help fulfill your daily requirements for a variety of important nutrients. Best of all, skim milk isn't the thin, gray, watery stuff it used to be. Several manufacturers, wise to the fact that consumers want the flavor of fat without the fat itself, now offer richer, creamier skims. Chances are, you won't be able to tell the difference.

"Once you get the fat out, milk is a highly nutritious food," says Curtis Mettlin, Ph.D., chief of epidemiologic research at Roswell Park Cancer Institute in Buffalo, New York. The many nutrients that milk contains can go a long way toward preventing high blood pressure, stroke, osteoporosis, and maybe even cancer—all for 85 calories, less than 5 grams of cholesterol, and less than 1 gram of fat per glassful of skim milk.

Richness
without the Fat

With a name like "buttermilk," you would expect this thick, creamy, and delectably tart drink to be very high in fat. But despite the name, buttermilk is lower in fat than regular milk, making it a healthful alternative to milk, cream, and mayonnaise in everything from salad dressings to baked goods.

A cup of buttermilk made from skim milk has about 2 grams of fat. Buttermilk made with reduced-fat (2 percent) milk contains 5 grams of fat. By contrast, 1 cup of regular milk has approximately 8 grams of fat. Making this one simple change—replacing some of the milk in your diet with buttermilk—can cut substantial amounts of fat from your diet. Just be sure to check the label before putting buttermilk in your shopping cart, since some brands are quite a bit lower in fat than others. You can buy buttermilk in skim, low-fat (1 percent), and reduced-fat versions.

Buttermilk is good in yet another way. As with low-fat and skim milk, it's among the best calcium sources you can find. A cup of buttermilk made from skim milk has more than 285 milligrams of calcium, about 29 percent of the Daily Value.

Skim Past Heart Disease

If you're concerned about cholesterol, you're probably already eating foods like apples, oats, and beans. Milk, as it turns out, is another food that can send cholesterol south.

Researchers at Kansas State University in Manhattan, Kansas, and Pennsylvania State University in University Park had 64 people drink a quart of skim milk a day. After a month, the people with the highest cholesterol levels saw their cholesterol drop almost 10 points. That's almost a 7-percent reduction. Since every 1-percent drop in cholesterol translates into a 2-percent reduction in death from heart disease, milk helped these folks reduce their risks of heart attacks or strokes by nearly 14 percent.

"Studies have shown that milk contains substances that reduce the liver's production of cholesterol," says Arun Kilara, Ph.D., professor of food science at Penn State and one of the researchers on the study.

Here's another great thing about milk. Its abundance of calcium may help reduce blood pressure as well as cholesterol. In the University Park study, drinking milk was able to lower systolic blood pressure (the top number), on average, from 131 to 126 after eight weeks, while diastolic pressure (the bottom number) dropped from 82 to 78.

Researchers aren't sure how much milk you should drink when trying to lower cholesterol or blood pressure. However, a good place to start would be with four glasses a day—the amount used in the study. If you think that's a lot, try drinking an 8-ounce glass of skim milk with each meal, then have one as a snack.

THE BEST BONE-BUILDER

Milk is best known for its ability to help strengthen bones. There's good reason for this. Milk is an excellent source of calcium, with 1 cup skim containing more than 300 milligrams, almost a third of the Daily Value (DV). That's why drinking milk is often recommended as a great strategy for preventing osteoporosis, the bone-thinning disease that affects more than 28 million people in the United States, most of them women.

In a study of 581 women past menopause, researchers at the University of California, San Diego, found that those who drank the most milk in their teens and early twenties had stronger bones than those who drank less.

The DV for calcium is 1,000 milligrams. But the amount that you need depends on your age, sex, and other factors. While men between the ages of 25 and 65 and women between the ages of 25 and 50 need 1,000 milligrams of calcium a day, men and women over 65 need 1,500 milligrams. Women who are postmenopausal and taking estrogen need 1,000 milligrams. Pregnant women or those who are breastfeeding need 1,200 to 1,500 milligrams a day.

A STRIKE AGAINST STROKE

Milk not only does the body good, research suggests it's also good for the brain. In one study, men who drank 16 ounces or more of milk a day had 50 percent lower risks of thromboembolic stroke (which occurs when a clot blocks blood flow to the brain) than those who did not drink milk.

It's not certain why milk showed such impressive results. Calcium didn't appear to have anything to do with it since people who took calcium supplements without accompanying dairy foods didn't show the same benefits, says study leader Robert Abbott, Ph.D., professor of biostatistics at the University of Virginia School of Medicine in Charlottesville. "But milk contains all kinds of nutrients besides calcium, and it did appear to be protective," he says. The benefits weren't due only to the milk, he adds. "The milk-drinkers tended to be leaner, more physically active, and to eat healthier foods than the men who didn't drink milk."

HELP FOR CANCER

Fruits and vegetables have gotten the most glory as cancer-fighting foods, and rightly so. Still, drinking skim or low-fat milk may also play a protective role.

Researchers at Roswell Park Cancer Institute, led by Dr. Mettlin, asked more than 4,600 people with and without cancer how many glasses of whole milk, skim milk, or reduced-fat milk they drank a day. They found that those who drank skim or reduced-fat milk had lower risks of developing several types of cancers, including cancers of the stomach and rectum, then those who drank whole milk. "These reduced risks were most likely due to their consuming less dietary fat from milk as well as from other foods," says Dr. Mettlin.

Another study, sponsored by the American Cancer Society, found that women who drank either skim or reduced-fat milk were three times less likely to develop ovarian cancer than women who drank more than a glass of whole milk a day.

Since a high intake of dietary fat is linked to cancer, it's not surprising that people who drank whole milk had the highest risks of cancer. What was surprising was that in both studies, people who didn't drink milk had higher risks of cancer than those who drank skim or reduced-fat milk. So there may be something in milk that helps protect against this disease, says Dr. Mettlin.

Liquid Nutrition

We've been talking about milk's role in preventing disease. Yet even for healthy, day-to-day living, milk is a truly nutritious food. Apart from its high calcium content, 1 cup of milk also contains 100 international units of vitamin D, 25 percent of the DV. Just as your bones need calcium to stay strong, they also need vitamin D, which helps the calcium be absorbed.

In addition, 1 cup of skim milk supplies about 400 milligrams of potassium, approximately 12 percent of the DV. Potassium is a key mineral for protecting against high blood pressure, stroke, and heart trouble. Milk also contains 0.4 milligram of riboflavin, more than 23 percent of the DV.

Getting the Most

Buy it in cartons. While those translucent plastic jugs are a convenient way to carry milk home from the store, they also admit light, which destroys riboflavin and vitamin A. In fact, milk stored for one day in a translucent plastic jug loses 90 percent of its vitamin A and 14 percent of its riboflavin. Further, the action of light can give milk an off-taste that many people find unpleasant. So you may want to buy the cartons instead.

Give your taste buds time to adjust. While some people take to skim milk right away, others loathe the taste, at least at first. To make skim milk part of your diet without shocking your taste buds, make the switch slowly. Try mixing a carton of whole milk with a carton of reduced-fat milk and drink that for a few weeks. Slowly reduce the amount of whole milk you add to the mix until you're drinking straight reduced-fat milk. When you're used to that, add skim milk to the reduced-fat. Eventually you'll be drinking—and enjoying—pure skim.

Add some thickening. One of the things people dislike about skim milk is its rather thin consistency. To make it thicker and creamier, try adding 2 to 4 tablespoons of nonfat milk powder to each cup of skim.

Try a new brand. If you're not happy with the milk you've been drinking, try one of the creamier versions. For example, Borden makes a product called Lite Line that's fat-free but tastes like reduced-fat. Lite-Line is available in Texas and other selected regions. Or look for fat-free milk that's fortified with nonfat milk solids. It's labeled "protein fortified."

Work it into your diet. Even if milk isn't your favorite beverage, there are other ways to get it into your diet. Using skim milk instead of water when preparing oatmeal, for example, will boost your breakfast's calcium content from 20 to 320 milligrams.

CREAMY POTATO SOUP

½	**cup water**
2	**cloves garlic, halved**
3½	**cups skim milk**
4	**medium boiling potatoes, peeled and cut into 1" chunks**
¼	**teaspoon salt**
3	**tablespoons chopped fresh parsley**
¼	**teaspoon ground black pepper**
⅛	**teaspoon ground nutmeg**
2	**teaspoons unsalted butter**

PER SERVING

calories	**212**
total fat	**2.5 g.**
saturated fat	**1.5 g.**
cholesterol	**9 mg.**
sodium	**253 mg.**
dietary fiber	**1.9 g.**

In a Dutch oven, combine the water, garlic, and 3 cups of the milk. Cook over medium heat until the mixture almost starts to simmer.

Reduce the heat to low. Add the potatoes and salt. Cover and cook, stirring occasionally, for about 30 minutes, or until the potatoes are tender. Stir in the parsley, pepper, nutmeg, and the remaining ½ cup milk.

Remove from the heat and let cool for 5 minutes. Puree in a blender or food processor, working in batches if necessary. Return the puree to the Dutch oven. Reheat briefly. Stir in the butter.

Makes 4 servings

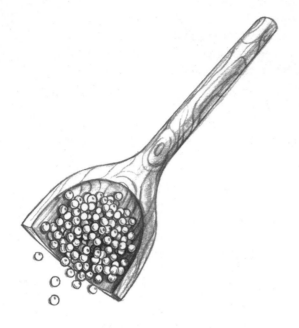

MILLET
A Grain for Women's Health

Healing Power

Can help:
Ease premenstrual
discomfort

Speed wound healing

In many parts of the world, millet, a nutritious, mild-tasting grain that looks like a tiny yellow bead, has been a staple for about 6,000 years. In Ethiopia, for example, it's cooked into a porridge. And in India, millet is used to make bread.

In this country, though, millet is eaten more by birds than people. When you pour out a tray of bird feed, you'll see pale little pellets filling the spaces between sunflower seeds. Those pellets are grains of millet.

We would do well to take a hint from our feathered friends, since millet is a very nutritious grain. It contains magnesium, an essential mineral that may help ease premenstrual discomfort. In addition, millet is higher in protein than most other grains, which is good news for those who eat little or no meat. And like all grains, millet contains dietary fiber, although much of the fiber is lost during processing. Still, a half-cup of cooked millet contains more fiber than an equal amount of cooked brown rice.

Help for Monthly Discomfort

Magnesium takes part in controlling more body functions than just about any other nutrient. It regulates the heartbeat, helps nerves function, and keeps bones strong. In addition, it may even play a role in easing women's premenstrual discomfort.

Research has shown that women with premenstrual syndrome (PMS) often have low levels of magnesium. "A marginal magnesium deficiency could make certain women more susceptible to PMS," says Donald L. Rosenstein, M.D., chief of the psychiatry consultation service at the National Institutes of Health.

A half-cup of cooked millet contains nearly 53 milligrams of magnesium, about which is 13 percent of the Daily Value (DV) for the mineral. Eating more millet, along with other magnesium-rich foods like tofu, avocados, spinach, bananas, and peanut butter, could help ease the irritability, sadness, and other emotional ups-and-downs that some women experience every month, says Dr. Rosenstein.

Essential for Repairs

The body uses protein for building and repairing muscles, connective fibers, and other tissues. Getting more protein in your diet is particularly important when you've cut yourself, been burned, or had surgery, says Michele Gottschlich, R.D., Ph.D., director of nutrition services for the Shriners Burns Institute in Cincinnati. "Without plenty of protein in the diet, wound healing can be delayed," she explains.

A half-cup of millet contains nearly 4 grams of protein, more than 8 percent of the DV. Compare that to a similar amount of brown rice, which supplies only 2.5 grams of protein.

While meat is also a potent source of protein, it also can be high in cholesterol-raising saturated fats, adds Lynne Brown, Ph.D., associate professor of food science at Pennsylvania State University in University Park. One cup of cooked millet provides about as much protein as an ounce of beef, making it a low-fat, cholesterol-free alternative.

In the Kitchen

Unlike brown rice, millet doesn't take forever to go from pot to plate. And it's very easy to make.

In a saucepan, mix 1 cup of whole millet with $2\frac{1}{2}$ to 3 cups of water, bring to a simmer and cook, covered, until the grains are tender, usually about 30 minutes. Although millet is usually cooked plain, here are some ways that you can customize the taste and texture.

- Cooking millet in apple juice instead of water will add a bit of sweetness to the dish.
- If you want millet to have a fluffy texture—more like rice than cereal—let it cook undisturbed for about 20 minutes.
- For a creamier texture, stir millet frequently while it cooks, which causes the grains to absorb more water.

Getting the Most

Shop for the whole grain. While cracked millet cooks more quickly than whole millet, it loses some of its nutrients during processing. So to get the most value, it's a good idea to shop for the whole grain.

Fit in some flour. Using millet flour in place of wheat or corn flour is an easy way to pack more of this healthful grain into your diet. However, since millet lacks gluten, the protein in wheat flour that allows yeast breads to rise, it's best used for quick breads and other recipes that don't call for yeast.

Store it carefully. Millet can go rancid rather quickly, giving up both its good taste and some of its essential nutrients. To keep millet fresh, be sure to store it in an airtight container in a cool, dry place.

MILLET-CRANBERRY MUFFINS

1	orange
1/2	cup honey
1	egg
3	tablespoons canola oil
1 1/2	cups unbleached all-purpose flour
1/2	cup whole-wheat flour
1	tablespoon baking powder
1/8	teaspoon salt
1	cup dried cranberries
3/4	cup millet

PER MUFFIN

calories	**293**
total fat	**5.2 g.**
saturated fat	**0.6 g.**
cholesterol	**18 mg.**
sodium	**152 mg.**
dietary fiber	**3 g.**

Preheat the oven to 400°F. Coat a 12-cup muffin tin with no-stick spray or line the cups with paper liners.

Grate 1 tablespoon of rind from the orange and place in a large bowl. Squeeze 1/3 cup of juice from the orange and add to the bowl.

Add the honey, egg, and oil. Whisk until blended.

In a medium bowl, combine the all-purpose flour, whole-wheat flour, baking powder, and salt. Mix and add to the honey mixture. Mix just until blended. Do not overbeat. The batter will be thick.

Stir in the cranberries and millet.

Spoon the batter into the prepared muffin tin, filling the cups about 3/4 full. Bake for 20 minutes, or until golden. Test for doneness by inserting a toothpick in the center of 1 muffin. Allow to cool slightly on a wire rack. Serve slightly warm.

Makes 12

Motion Sickness
Keeping Your Stomach Calm

Food is the last thing you want to think about when your stomach is turning upside down. But if you're among the 90 percent of Americans who occasionally suffer from motion sickness, you may want to make food the first thing on your list, even before you get on the boat or climb into the car. Research has shown that what you put—or don't put into your stomach can have a big impact on how you feel.

Some foods stimulate your body to produce more gas and acids, which can make motion sickness even worse. Other foods, by contrast, help keep your stomach calm, either by blocking the effects of natural toxins or by preventing "nausea signals" from even reaching your brain.

One of the best ways to prevent motion sickness is to have a little ginger. Ginger acts as a sponge, absorbing a lot of the acid that your stomach pumps out as a natural reaction to motion. In addition, it helps block nausea signals that sometimes travel from the stomach to the brain, says Daniel B. Mowrey, Ph.D., director of the American Phytotherapy Research Laboratory in Salt Lake City. Dr. Mowrey has studied the calming effects of ginger on thousands of motion sickness sufferers. What's more, he has firsthand knowledge of how well it works. He gives it to his own kids. "When we get in the car to take a trip, if they forgot their ginger root, they're out of it," Dr. Mowrey says. "When they have it, they're just fine."

For minor motion sickness, having ginger ale, ginger snaps, or ginger tea before and during the trip can help settle your stomach, Dr. Mowrey says. For those who need more relief, he recommends taking two 940-milligram capsules of ginger root (or an equivalent amount of smaller capsules) about 20 minutes before leaving and again every half-hour during the trip. If you tend to get really ill, Dr. Mowrey recommends increasing the amount to six capsules before leaving and six to eight capsules every half-hour during the trip. "You know you've taken enough of it to do the job when you get an aftertaste," Dr. Mowrey adds. "If you don't get that aftertaste, you can take more."

Since stomach acid can play a role in causing motion sickness, it's a good idea to eat something before traveling. Foods that are high in carbohydrates, like breads and crackers, are particularly good because they soak up large amounts of stomach acid, says William Ruderman, M.D., a gastroenterologist in private

Desperate Measures

People have been getting seasick for as long as there have been boats. The rolling waves make many people feel so sick that they'll try—or eat—anything to make the churning go away.

In *Heave Ho! My Little Green Book of Seasickness*, Charles Mazel, Ph.D., an ocean engineer and marine biologist at the Massachusetts Institute of Technology in Cambridge, has chronicled some of the more unusual strategies that people have used through the ages to cope with this miserable condition.

- Cook a fish found in the belly of another fish, season it with pepper, and eat it as you go on board.
- Poke your finger in a loaf of bread and fill the hole with Worcestershire and hot-pepper sauces. Enjoy.
- Try rice covered with horseradish sauce, herrings, and sardines.
- Eat cold stewed tomatoes with saltines.
- Take a handful of salted peanuts with breakfast each morning.
- Take a handful of wheat, pound it, pour a little water on it, and press out the juice. Take a spoonful of the juice every 10 minutes.
- Find a stone in the stomach of a cod, place it in a glass of water, and drink.

practice in Orlando, Florida. In a study of 57 pilots, researchers at the University of North Dakota in Grand Forks found that those who ate carbohydrate-rich foods such as breads and cereals before their flights tended to experience less motion sickness than those pilots who ate foods high in protein, sodium, or calories.

Not surprisingly, eating beans, chili peppers, and other gas-producing foods before flying can cause a lot of discomfort, says Dr. Ruderman. "Foods that produce a lot of gas actually distend your intestinal tract, and they can only add to your misery," he says.

It's not only what you eat that can ease motion sickness but also what you drink. It's a good idea to drink plenty of water before and during your trip, says Dr. Ruderman. It's particularly important to drink more fluids when you're flying, because the air in airplane cabins is extremely dry.

However, don't use coffee, soda, or alcohol as substitutes for water, he adds. Both caffeine and alcohol are diuretics, which means that they take away more fluids than they replace.

MUSCLE CRAMPS
A MATTER OF MINERALS

Whether you're on a treadmill, writing a letter, or even lying in bed at night, your muscles are constantly contracting and relaxing. As a result, they need a lot of nourishment. When they don't get it, they'll sometimes contract into tight, painful spasms known as muscle cramps. Cramps are a muscle's way of telling you it's tired, hungry, and in need of rest.

Muscle cramps are painful, but they play a protective role, says Leslie Bonci, R.D., a dietitian at the University of Pittsburgh Medical Center and a spokeswoman for the American Dietetic Association. Essentially, they force the muscle to remain inactive until it has time to recover, usually within a few minutes.

While you can't prevent muscle cramps entirely, choosing the right foods will make them less likely to return. Here's how it works.

HELP FROM ELECTROLYTES

Muscles don't move without orders from the brain. Before you can stand up, blink an eye, or turn the pages of this book, the brain sends electrical messages to the appropriate muscles, telling them when (and how much) to contract or relax. Minerals such as calcium, potassium, sodium, and magnesium, which are known as electrolytes, play a role in helping the messages get through, says Joel Press, M.D., medical director of the Center for Spine, Sports, and Occupational Rehabilitation at the Rehabilitation Institute of Chicago.

If you haven't been getting enough of these minerals or have sweated them out during vigorous exercise, a muscle may not get the message to relax. This can cause it to contract in a painful cramp.

Of all the electrolytes, magnesium is one of the most important, because it helps other electrolytes do their jobs, says Robert McLean, M.D., clinical assistant professor of medicine at Yale University School of Medicine. When you don't eat enough magnesium-rich foods, minerals such as calcium and potassium can't get into muscle-fiber cells. So even if you have an abundance of other electrolytes, without magnesium they may be locked out and ineffective. "People who are depleted of magnesium tend to have greater irritability of the muscles and nerves," says Dr. McLean. "This irritability may cause muscle cramping."

Many foods contain large amounts of magnesium, says Dr. McLean. For example, a serving of tofu has 128 milligrams of magnesium, 32 percent of the Daily Value (DV). A serving of spinach has about 44 milligrams, 11 percent of the DV, and a serving of mackerel has 82 milligrams, 20 percent of the DV.

You also need plenty of calcium, which helps regulate the muscles' ability to contract. Dairy foods are the best sources. A cup of skim milk, for example, has nearly 302 milligrams of calcium, 30 percent of the DV, while a serving of low-fat yogurt has 77 milligrams, 7 percent of the DV.

Getting enough potassium in your diet may also be helpful for preventing cramps, says Dr. Press. Bananas are a good source of potassium, with one banana supplying 451 milligrams, 13 percent of the DV. Potatoes are also a good source, with a half-cup containing 114 milligrams, 3 percent of the DV.

For most people, the problem isn't getting enough sodium, it's getting too much, since this mineral is found in large amounts in many foods, particularly processed foods. And for those who are sensitive, sodium can lead to fluid retention and high blood pressure. So even if you have been getting cramps, leave the sodium alone—you're almost certainly getting enough.

When it comes to fluids, however, it's almost impossible to get too much. Whenever you perspire, you lose fluids from the muscle cells, which can result in cramping, Bonci says. Sipping water frequently throughout the day will help keep electrolyte levels in balance. When you're planning on being active, it's a good idea to drink at least 16 ounces of water or juice to prime your body with the necessary minerals. You should also drink 8 ounces of water every 15 to 20 minutes during exercise, she adds.

Water provides many of the electrolytes that your body normally needs, but during vigorous exercise the muscles may need extra supplies. Sports drinks such as Gatorade, which contain carbohydrates as well as electrolytes, can help keep muscles from cramping. "They get the electrolytes into the bloodstream and then into the muscle very quickly," Bonci says. "This is especially important for exercise sessions lasting an hour or more."

Muscles need more than electrolytes and water to function well. They also need glycogen, a sugar that comes from carbohydrates. When muscle tissues run low on glycogen, they're more likely to tire and cramp, says Paul Saltman, Ph.D., professor of biology at the University of California, San Diego. Getting plenty of carbohydrates in your diet will help keep muscles working well. Good sources include potatoes, rice, bananas, and bread.

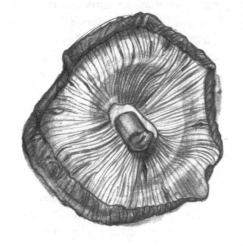

Mushrooms
The Healing Fungus

Healing Power
Can help:
Inhibit tumor growth

Boost the immune system

Lower cholesterol levels

Mushrooms are so popular in Asian countries that they're sold by streetcart vendors, just as we sell corn dogs and Italian ice. But while Americans have been slow to embrace these meaty morsels, they're becoming increasingly commonplace, both in the kitchen and in research laboratories.

Scientists are discovering what natural healers have known for ages. Mushrooms not only are important sources of nutrients but also stimulate the immune system. Researchers say that they possibly can help fight cancer and high cholesterol, and perhaps even AIDS.

Unfortunately, the common white button mushroom, our favorite from the fungus family, has no known medicinal value. It does, however, supply good amounts of some key nutrients, like the B vitamins.

A Cap on Cancer

Long esteemed in Japan for their reputed tumor-shrinking abilities, shiitake mushrooms have been attracting global attention because of the cancer-fighting compound that they contain.

These large, meaty black mushrooms contain a polysaccharide, or complex sugar, called lentinan. Polysaccharides are large molecules that are similar in

IN THE KITCHEN

Although you can buy fresh shiitake mushrooms at specialty markets, you're more likely to find them in their dehydrated form. Here's how to use them.

Soften them up. To reconstitute dried mushrooms, place them in a saucepan, cover with water, and bring them to a rolling boil. Reduce heat and simmer for 20 minutes. Then drain, slice, and add them to your recipe.

You may want to reserve the mushroom water, which adds a rich taste to soups and sauces.

Cut them fine. Reconstituted mushrooms don't look as pretty as their freshly picked brethren. Also, they have a slightly pungent flavor that in large amounts may be objectionable. Chefs usually chop them up, using them sparingly for stir-fries, casseroles, soups, and grain dishes.

structure to bacteria, explains Robert Murphy, R.N., a naturopathic doctor in private practice in Torrington, Connecticut. When you eat shiitake mushrooms, your immune system starts amassing an army of infection-fighting cells. "In essence, they fool the immune system into kicking into action," he says. Researchers have found that when they feed lentinan in the form of dried mushroom powder to laboratory animals with tumors, they can inhibit tumor growth by 67 percent.

Researchers are also looking at the maitake mushroom, also known as hen of the woods or the dancing mushroom. Like shiitakes, maitake mushrooms have a centuries-old reputation for being helpful in treating people with cancer. Only recently are they getting the attention that they deserve in Western nations.

The active polysaccharide in maitake mushrooms, called beta-glucan or D-fraction, has been highly effective in shrinking tumors in lab-oratory animals—maybe even more effective than lentinan, say experts.

"You definitely get some of these polysaccharides that activate the immune system when you eat a healthy serving—about a half-cup—of these mush-rooms," says Dr. Murphy. "I tell people that they can go to the market and buy shiitake and maitake mushrooms and include them in their diets." Both types are usually found in Asian food stores and some supermarkets.

IMMUNITY BOOSTING AND AIDS

Because the shiitake and maitake mushrooms have proven so effective in bolstering the immune system, some scientists have tested their mettle, with some success, against HIV, the virus that causes AIDS.

In laboratory studies, an extract of the maitake mushroom's beta-glucan was able to prevent HIV from killing T cells, the immune system's crucial white blood cells. "Eating these mushrooms on a regular basis seems to be a very good way to keep your immune system up and running," says Dr. Murphy.

Cutting Cholesterol

If your cholesterol levels are hovering near the danger zone—200 and above—you might want to consider making mushrooms a regular side dish on your table.

During the 1970s and 1980s, human and animal studies in Japan showed that one of the compounds in shiitake mushrooms, eritadenine, could effectively lower cholesterol levels. More recently, researchers from Slovakia have found that by feeding mice 5 percent of their diets in dried mushrooms, particularly oyster mushrooms, they could reduce blood cholesterol by 45 percent, even when the mice were given high-cholesterol foods.

Researchers still can't say how many mushrooms people have to eat to get the same effect. But experts agree that adding a couple of these large, meaty morsels to your plate each day certainly can't hurt, and it may help play a role in bringing your cholesterol levels down.

A Boost of Bs

Mushrooms offer two important B vitamins, niacin and riboflavin, that are not often found in vegetables. For once, the common white button mushroom may be a key player. While dried shiitake mushrooms have a higher nutrient concentration, they also have a strong flavor; most people won't use them in large quantities. But white mushrooms, with their mild taste, can be eaten with virtually every meal.

Niacin is important because it helps your body form the enzymes needed to convert sugars into energy, to use fats, and to keep your tissues healthy. White button mushrooms are a good source, containing 4 milligrams of niacin, 20 percent of the Daily Value (DV).

Like niacin, riboflavin is a "helper nutrient." It's needed to convert other nutrients, like niacin, vitamin B_6, and folate, into usable forms. If you're low on

Raw sliced mushrooms are a salad bar favorite. But you don't want to make a habit of eating too many uncooked mushrooms, warn experts.

Raw mushrooms contain hydrazines, toxic chemicals that studies show can produce tumors in laboratory animals. Though nobody really knows how many raw mushrooms people have to eat to get a similar effect, experts recommend eating your mushrooms cooked because hydrazines are eliminated during heating.

riboflavin, you could also be low on these other nutrients. A half-cup of boiled white mushrooms contains 0.2 milligram of riboflavin, 12 percent of the DV.

Getting the Most

Cook 'em up. For both taste and nutrition, mushrooms are better cooked than raw. This is because they are mostly water. When you cook them, you remove the water and concentrate the nutrients as well as the flavor.

Eat the exotic. To get optimal healing power from mushrooms, stick to Asian varieties, particularly shiitake and maitake, say experts. Other mushrooms that may provide therapeutic benefits are enoki, oyster, pine, and straw varieties.

GLAZED SHIITAKE MUSHROOMS

1 **pound shiitake mushrooms**

1 **teaspoon canola oil**

⅓ **cup defatted reduced-sodium chicken broth**

1 **teaspoon cornstarch**

2 **teaspoons reduced-sodium soy sauce**

1 **tablespoon dry sherry**

PER SERVING

calories	**89**
total fat	**1.6 g.**
saturated fat	**0.2 g.**
cholesterol	**0 mg.**
sodium	**99 mg.**
dietary fiber	**2.7 g.**

Rinse the mushrooms and pat dry with paper towels. Trim and discard the stems. Cut each cap into 3 or 4 slices.

In a large no-stick skillet over medium heat, warm the oil. Add the mushrooms and 2 tablespoons of the broth. Cook, stirring often, for 5 to 6 minutes, or until the mushrooms are hot and start to give off liquid.

In a small bowl, dissolve the cornstarch in the remaining broth. Stir in the soy sauce and sherry. Add to the skillet. Cook, stirring constantly, for 2 minutes, or until the sauce is clear and the mushrooms are glazed.

Makes 4 servings

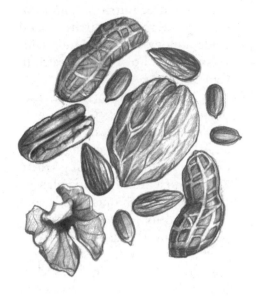

NUTS
A Shell Game You Can Win

Healing Power

Can help:
Lower cholesterol

Protect against heart disease

Prevent cancer

The ancient Persians believed that eating five almonds before drinking alcoholic beverages would prevent intoxication, or at least the hangover that might follow. They also believed that almonds would ward off witches and stimulate milk production in nursing mothers.

As nutty as this seems today, it's not surprising that ancient civilizations took their nuts seriously. Not only are nuts a compact source of energy, they also are easily stored through cold winters and hot summers, making them available throughout the year. What's more, nuts contain a number of compounds that may help prevent heart disease and cancer.

The Fat Factor

Before we talk about the health benefits of nuts, it's important to discuss one of their potential drawbacks. While nuts are high in nutrients, they're also high in fat. One-third cup of nuts typically contains anywhere from 240 to 300 calories and 20 to 25 grams of fat.

Not all types of nuts are loaded with fat, but most are. The coconut, for example, contains a lot of fat, and most of it is the dangerous saturated kind. "On the other end of the spectrum is the chestnut, which is extremely low in

In the Kitchen

Blending your own peanut butter is a lot of fun. Not only does it taste good but also, depending on the amount of oil you add, it has a bit less fat than the store-bought kind. Plus, it's very easy to make. Here's how.

- Buy roasted peanuts, the kind that come in a vacuum-sealed can or jar. You can also use roasted peanuts in the shell, but shelling them requires more work.
- For each cup of peanuts, add 1 1/2 to 2 tablespoons of canola or another light-flavored oil. Some people will add 1/2 teaspoon of salt per cup of peanuts, but this is optional.
- Put the peanuts and oil in a blender and puree until you get the texture you want—extra-chunky, chunky, or creamy.
- Transfer the peanut butter to a jar and store in the refrigerator. It will stay fresh for three to four months. However, the oils in "natural" peanut butter will separate, so be sure to stir it well before using.

fat and almost all of it is unsaturated," points out Joan Sabaté, M.D., Dr. P.H., chairman of the department of nutrition and associate professor of nutrition and epidemiology at Loma Linda University School of Public Health in California.

"It's very unfortunate that people shun nuts just because they're high in calories," Dr. Sabaté adds. "The trick to eating nuts is not overdoing it—fitting them wisely into a healthy eating plan."

Even though nuts mainly contain a healthy form of fat, it's important not to eat too many of them. Or if you do, be sure to get less of other, less healthy fats, such as butter, hydrogenated margarines, and nutrient-empty snack foods such as chips and cookies, Dr. Sabaté says.

Good for the Heart

One great thing about nuts is that they contain a number of compounds that help keep the arteries open and blood flowing smoothly.

It was quite by accident that researchers at Loma Linda University discovered that eating nuts seems to protect against heart disease. They asked 26,000 members of the Seventh-Day Adventist Church, an extremely health-conscious bunch, to indicate the frequency with which they ate 65 food items.

As it turns out, the Adventists are very fond of nuts. Twenty-four percent ate nuts at least five times a week. In the population at large, by contrast, only 5 percent of people eat them that often. As the researchers discovered, this difference in nut consumption made a colossal difference in heart disease risk. Eating nuts just one to four times a week reduced the risk of dying from artery-clogging heart disease by 25 percent. People who ate them five or more times per week slashed their risks in half.

Researchers aren't sure which nuts made the most difference. Among the most popular choices were peanuts, almonds, and walnuts. (Even though peanuts are technically a legume, they're nutritionally similar to nuts and, in fact, are sometimes referred to as groundnuts.)

What is it about nuts, which are practically dripping with oil, that amazingly defats arteries? "With a few exceptions, most nuts are high in monounsaturated and polyunsaturated fats," says Dr. Sabaté. "When these types of fats replace saturated fats in the diet, they can help lower total cholesterol as well as the unhealthy low-density lipoprotein (LDL) cholesterol." At the same time, nuts don't affect levels of the heart-healthy high-density lipoprotein (HDL) cholesterol.

Another thing that makes nuts healthy for the heart is an amino acid called arginine. Some arginine may be converted in the body to nitric oxide, a compound that helps expand the blood vessels. In fact, it acts much like the drug nitroglycerin, which is used to rapidly dilate arteries to permit more blood to reach the heart. Nitric oxide also appears to help keep the platelets in blood from clumping, which can further reduce heart disease risk.

"Nuts are also high in vitamin E, which may keep LDL cholesterol from oxidizing," says Dr. Sabaté. This is the process that makes cholesterol more likely to stick to artery walls and block blood flow. Nuts have more vitamin E than any other food, with the exception of oils. Almonds and walnuts are particularly good choices. One-third cup of either nut contains about 12 international units, or 40 percent of the Daily Value (DV).

Nuts also contain generous amounts of heart-healthy copper and magnesium. Magnesium appears to regulate cholesterol and blood pressure as well as heart rhythms, while copper may play a role in lowering cholesterol.

PREVENTING CANCER

Just as nuts contain compounds that may help prevent heart disease, they also contain compounds that may help stop cancer.

Walnuts, for example, contain a compound called ellagic acid that appears to battle cancer on several fronts. "Ellagic acid is a good antioxidant, disabling harmful oxygen molecules, called free radicals, that are known to instigate the cancer process," says Gary D. Stoner, Ph.D., director of the cancer chemoprevention program at the Ohio State University Comprehensive Cancer Center in Columbus. Ellagic acid also helps detoxify potential cancer-causing substances, while at the same time helping to prevent cancer cells from dividing.

In one study, laboratory animals given ellagic acid as well as a cancer-causing substance were 33 percent less likely to develop esophageal cancer than animals given only carcinogens. In another study, laboratory animals were 70 percent less likely to develop liver tumors when they were given purified ellagic acid.

A Nutritional Payload

All nuts are richly endowed with protein, and most contain a generous supply of vitamins and minerals as well as dietary fiber.

While the plain old peanut doesn't hit the charts for healing potential, it's the highest in protein of any nut, with ⅓ cup containing more than 11 grams, 22 percent of the DV. That's more protein than you'll get from the same amount of beef or fish. Better yet, the protein in peanuts is a complete protein, meaning that it contains all the essential amino acids we can't do without. Brazil nuts, cashews, walnuts, and almonds also are good sources of protein, each containing at least 6 grams in ⅓ cup, 12 percent of the DV.

In addition, all nuts are a good source of fiber, with ⅓ cup typically containing 1 to 2 grams—about the amount in a similar amount of Cheerios. Among the most fiber-rich nuts are pistachios (nearly 5 grams per ⅓ cup, almost 20 percent of the DV), and almonds (just over 6 grams, about 24 percent of the DV).

SPICED ALMOND CEREAL SNACK MIX

1	egg white
1½	teaspoons Cajun seasoning blend
1	teaspoon Worcestershire sauce
½	teaspoon garlic powder
1	teaspoon water
2	cups whole-wheat cereal squares
1½	cups whole almonds

PER ⅓ CUP

calories	163
total fat	11.4 g.
saturated fat	1.1 g.
cholesterol	0 mg.
sodium	146 mg.
dietary fiber	2.9 g.

Preheat the oven to 300°F. Coat a jelly-roll pan with no-stick spray.

In a large bowl, combine the egg white, Cajun seasoning, Worcestershire sauce, garlic powder, and water. Whisk to thoroughly mix. Add the cereal and almonds. Toss well to coat.

Spread out evenly in the prepared pan. Bake for 30 minutes, or until golden and crisp. Allow to cool. Store in an airtight tin or jar.

Makes about 3⅓ cups

WALNUT AND RED-PEPPER TOPPING

2/3 cup chopped walnuts

2/3 cup chopped roasted sweet red peppers

2 cloves garlic, minced

2 tablespoons minced fresh parsley

1/8 teaspoon salt

1/8 teaspoon crushed red-pepper flakes

PER 1/3 CUP

calories	**149**
total fat	**12.7 g.**
saturated fat	**1.2 g.**
cholesterol	**0 mg.**
sodium	**240 mg.**
dietary fiber	**1.4 g.**

Place the walnuts in a large no-stick skillet over medium heat. Cook, shaking the pan frequently, for 1 to 2 minutes, or until toasted and fragrant.

Stir in the roasted peppers, garlic, parsley, salt, and red-pepper flakes. Cook, stirring frequently, for 3 minutes, or until heated through. If the mixture starts to stick to the pan, add a little water.

Makes 1 1/3 cups

Cook's Notes: Store in a covered container in the refrigerator for up to 1 week. Reheat before tossing with cooked pasta.

If using jarred roasted sweet red peppers, drain and rinse. Pat dry with paper towels before adding to the skillet.

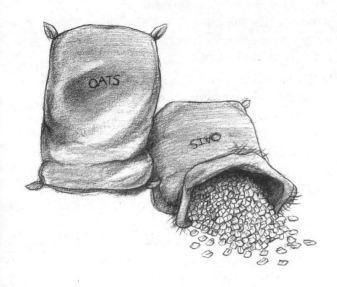

Oats
Mopping Up Cholesterol

Healing Power

Can help:
Lower cholesterol
and blood sugar

Improve insulin
sensitivity

Control appetite

Reduce the risk of heart
disease and cancer

If it weren't for horses, we probably wouldn't even know about oats, to say nothing of the great health benefits they provide. When horses were introduced in various parts of the world, oats went along as their feed. Not surprisingly, however, humans were a bit reluctant to take a taste. Samuel Johnson's 1755 *Dictionary of the English Language* defined oats as "a grain which in England is generally given to horses, but which in Scotland supports the people." It seems that the Scots were ahead of their time.

Oats are a very healthy grain. For one thing, unlike wheat, barley, and other grains, processed oats retain the bran and germ layers, which is where most of the nutrients reside. In addition, oats contain a variety of compounds that have been shown to reduce heart disease, fight cancer, lower blood sugar, improve insulin sensitivity, and help with dieting.

Help for High Cholesterol

For years, we've been hearing that oatmeal and oat bran can help lower cholesterol, a critical move in reducing the risk of heart disease. Studies show that getting more oats in the diet not only lowers total cholesterol but, more encouragingly, lowers the bad low-density lipoprotein (LDL) cholesterol while leaving the beneficial high-density lipoprotein cholesterol alone.

Oats contain a type of soluble fiber called beta-glucan, which traps dietary cholesterol within a sticky gel in the intestine. Since this gel isn't absorbed by the body, it passes through the intestine, taking unwanted cholesterol with it.

Soluble fiber isn't the only thing doing the trapping. Oats also contain compounds called saponins, which in preliminary animal studies appear to bind to cholesterol and usher it out of the body. Saponins also glom onto bile acids. This is good because high levels of bile acids can cause cholesterol levels to rise.

"We used to think that saponins had only negative effects on the body," says Joanne L. Slavin, Ph.D., professor of nutrition at the University of Minnesota in St. Paul. "In fact, we call them antinutrients because they inhibit the absorption of various nutritional substances. But their positive health benefits are clearly stronger than their negative attributes."

It doesn't take a loaf of oats to lower cholesterol. Having about ¾ cup of dry oatmeal (which cooks up to about 1½ cups) or just under ½ cup of dry oat bran (which cooks up to about 1 cup) a day can help lower total cholesterol 5 percent.

A STABLE OF PROTECTION

Like all plant foods, oats contain a variety of compounds that provide different kinds of protection. Three of these compounds—tocotrienols (related to vitamin E), ferulic acid, and caffeic acid—are antioxidants. That is, they help control cell-damaging particles called free radicals, which, when left unchecked, can contribute to heart disease, cancer, and certain eye diseases.

Tocotrienols, which are richly abundant in oats, pack at least two punches against heart disease. They're very effective at stopping oxidation, the process

In the Kitchen

Oats are among the easiest foods to cook. Just add 1 part oatmeal to 2 parts water, cover, simmer, and serve. Here are a few ways to change both the texture and the taste of oats to suit your personal preference.

Cream them with milk. Cooking oats in milk instead of water yields a much creamier porridge, which some people prefer to the firmer, water-cooked variety.

Make them coarser. If you prefer your oats with a firm, slightly coarse texture, chefs advise adding the oats to water that's already boiling rather than mixing them with cold water and then raising the heat.

Change the taste. To add extra flavor to oats, you can eliminate the water or milk altogether and cook them in apple, pear, or peach juice.

Since the sugars in juices can readily scorch and give the cereal a slightly burnt taste, be sure to use a heavy-bottomed pan or use a double boiler over a slow, steady heat and watch the time carefully.

that causes LDL cholesterol to turn rancid and stick to artery walls. Indeed, tocotrienols are 50 percent more powerful than vitamin E, says David J. A. Jenkins, M.D., Sc.D., Ph.D., professor of nutritional sciences and medicine at the University of Toronto. In addition, tocotrienols act on the liver, which might turn down the body's own production of cholesterol.

Battling Cancer

Some of the same compounds in oats that protect against heart disease may also help prevent cancer, says A. Venket Rao, Ph.D., professor of nutrition at the University of Toronto.

We've already discussed how the saponins in oats bind to bile acids. This is important because, while bile acids are necessary for the absorption and digestion of fat, they also cause problems. In the large intestine, they get converted by bacteria into a form called secondary bile acids. Secondary bile acids can damage intestinal cells, possibly setting in motion the events that lead to cancer. "By binding up bile acids and reducing the amount that can be transformed into a toxic version, saponins may help lower cancer risk," says Dr. Rao.

In addition, saponins appear to strengthen the immune system, making the body better able to detect and deactivate foreign invaders such as bacteria, viruses, and cancer cells. "In animal experiments, the addition of saponins to the diet increased the number of natural killer cells, which translates into a stronger immune surveillance system," says Dr. Rao.

Other compounds in oats protect against cancer in much the same way that they help prevent heart disease—by neutralizing cell-damaging free radicals before they cause harm.

Finally, oats contain generous amounts of a compound called phytic acid, says Dr. Slavin. "Although we haven't identified the exact mechanism, there's some evidence that phytic acid binds up certain reactive minerals, which may be important in preventing colon cancer."

KEEPING BLOOD SUGAR STEADY

Another benefit of oats is that they appear to help keep the body's blood sugar levels in balance. This is important for the estimated 21 million Americans with impaired glucose tolerance, a condition that is similar to diabetes and that increases the risks of heart disease and strokes.

In people with this condition, blood sugar levels are higher than they should be, but not so high that the people are actually diabetic. Yet even slightly elevated blood sugar levels may be cause for concern because they cause the body to pump out larger amounts of insulin to bring them down.

The soluble fiber in oats lays down a protective gummy layer in the intestine. This slows the rate at which carbohydrates are absorbed by the body, which in turn helps keep blood sugar levels stable. In addition, soluble fiber appears to reduce the output of hormones in the digestive tract, which indirectly lowers the body's production of insulin.

Here's an additional benefit of the soluble fiber in oats. Because it soaks up lots of water, it creates a feeling of fullness. This means that when you eat oats, you feel satisfied longer and so are more likely to eat less, which is good news for anyone who's trying to lose weight.

HELP FOR HIV

Although the evidence is still preliminary, the saponins in oats may be effective in disabling HIV, the virus that causes AIDS.

It's long been a puzzling fact that while some people infected with HIV develop AIDS relatively quickly, others don't become sick for years. Scientists are working to discover what makes HIV stronger, or more virulent, in some people.

It could be that various compounds found in food, including the saponins in oats, may play a role in squelching HIV. "Although this research is in its very early stages, it certainly is something to pursue," says Dr. Rao.

Getting the Most

Eat for convenience. Unlike many foods, in which the processed versions are often the least nutritious, oats retain their goodness in different forms. So when time is an issue, go ahead and enjoy quick oats. They provide just as many vitamins and minerals as the traditional, slower-cooking kind. Keep in mind, however, that quick oats do contain more sodium than their slower-cooking kin.

For protein, take your pick. Both rolled oats and oat bran are good sources of protein. One cup of cooked oat bran contains 7 grams, 14 percent of the Daily Value (DV), while a serving of rolled oats has 6 grams, 12 percent of the DV.

Cut calories with bran. When you're trying to eat lean, oat bran is often a better choice than oatmeal. A 1-cup serving of cooked oat bran contains 87 calories, whereas the same amount of oatmeal has 145.

OATMEAL-APRICOT COOKIES

⅔ **cup dried apricots, coarsely chopped**

⅓ **cup boiling water**

1 **cup packed light-brown sugar**

¼ **cup unsalted butter, at room temperature**

¼ **cup fat-free egg substitute**

1½ **teaspoons vanilla**

½ **cup unbleached all-purpose flour**

1 **teaspoon ground cinnamon**

1 **teaspoon baking soda**

¼ **teaspoon salt**

2½ **cups quick-cooking rolled oats**

PER COOKIE

calories	**78**
total fat	**2.1 g.**
saturated fat	**1.1 g.**
cholesterol	**4 mg.**
sodium	**70 mg.**
dietary fiber	**1 g.**

Preheat the oven to 350°F. Coat 2 baking sheets with no-stick spray.

Combine the apricots and water in a food processor. Process until well-blended (some small chunks may remain).

Transfer to a large bowl. Add the brown sugar and butter. Beat with an electric mixer until well-blended. Add the egg substitute and vanilla. Beat to mix.

Add the flour, cinnamon, baking soda, and salt. Beat just until well-mixed. Sprinkle with the oats. Stir with a large spoon to mix.

Drop by tablespoonfuls onto the prepared baking sheets. Bake 1 sheet at a time for 10 to 12 minutes, or until the cookies are golden. Transfer the cookies to a wire rack to cool. Store in a cookie jar or other covered container that's not airtight.

Makes 28 cookies

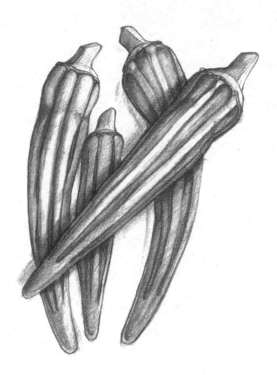

OKRA
A FOOD FOR HEALTHY CELLS

HEALING POWER
CAN HELP:
Prevent cancer

Ease cold symptoms

Reduce the risk
of heart disease

Prevent constipation

Even in the deep South, where gumbo is eaten all the time, okra isn't everyone's favorite vegetable. It can be tough. It can be slimy. It has an unusual, tart taste. No wonder it's usually hidden inside a bowl of this thick, aromatic broth.

But okra's status as a secondary player may be about to change. A study from Emory University in Atlanta found that it contains a powerful compound that shows promise for fighting cancer and heart disease. In addition, okra contains a variety of healthful nutrients like vitamin C, calcium, and potassium.

"It does have a little bit of everything," says Belinda Smith, R.D., research dietitian at the Veterans Administration Medical Center at the University of Kentucky College of Medicine in Lexington. "And it's very low in calories."

PROMISING PROTECTION

A key ingredient in gumbo, okra contains a compound that researchers say shows promise for tackling cancer. The compound, called glutathione, attacks cancer in two ways. It's an antioxidant, which means that it hampers the effects of free radicals, unstable oxygen molecules that can damage healthy cells and cause them to become cancerous. In addition, glutathione prevents other cancer-causing chemicals called carcinogens from damaging DNA, the chemical blueprint that tells cells how to function. It does this by ushering chemicals away from cells, into the urine, and eventually out of the body.

In a study of more than 1,800 people, researchers at Emory University discovered that those who had the highest intake of glutathione, which is found not only in okra but also in watermelons, avocados, and grapefruit, were 50 percent less likely to develop oral and throat cancers than those with low levels of the compound.

Okra isn't the highest source of glutathione, but it isn't the lowest, either. A study at the University of Louisville in Kentucky that measured glutathione levels in food found that okra scored in the medium range, according to Calvin A. Lang, Sc.D., professor of biochemistry at the University of Louisville School of Medicine.

Researchers aren't sure how much glutathione people need to stay healthy, but they know one thing. It's better to have more than less. "If you keep your glutathione at a high level, you lower your risk of getting a serious illness," Dr. Lang says.

A Mixed Pod of Nutrients

Just like the gumbo in which it's often cooked, okra contains a hodgepodge of ingredients. Topping the list is vitamin C. A half-cup of cooked okra contains more than 13 milligrams, 22 percent of the Daily Value (DV). A powerful antioxidant, vitamin C has been shown to help fight cancer, prevent heart disease, and even help calm the common cold.

Okra provides a good amount of magnesium as well. A half-cup of cooked okra has about 46 milligrams, 11 percent of the DV. This mineral may help you avoid heart disease, fight chronic fatigue syndrome, lower blood pressure, ward off diabetes, and slow bone loss.

In addition, okra is a good source of fiber, Smith says. Whether frozen or cooked, a half-cup serving of okra has about 2 grams of fiber, 8 pecent of the DV. That's about the same amount as a half-cup of raw carrots or apples.

The two kinds of fiber in okra help in different ways. The soluble fiber lowers cholesterol and helps control symptoms of diabetes. In addition, it can help with weight control because it forms bulk in the stomach, making you feel full. Insoluble fiber (what used to be called roughage) has been shown to help prevent colon cancer and digestive disorders such as constipation.

Getting the Most

Put water to work. Okra is traditionally served fried, which adds a tremendous amount of fat to the diet. A better way to prepare it is by steaming, Smith says. Cooking with moist heat requires no added fat. Plus, it has the added advantage of preserving more of the nutrients than other cooking methods.

Savor the slime. When cooked, okra releases a thick, slimy fluid that's a rich source of nutrients. Rather than discarding the juice, you can use it as a natural thickening ingredient for gumbos, stews, and soups.

CREOLE-STYLE OKRA

1 **pound fresh okra**

1½ **cups chopped onions**

1 **can (16 ounces) reduced-sodium tomatoes (with juice)**

½ **teaspoon dried basil**

½ **teaspoon hot-pepper sauce**

½ **teaspoon packed light-brown sugar**

¼ **teaspoon dried thyme**

⅛ **teaspoon salt**

PER SERVING

calories	**81**
total fat	**0.6 g.**
saturated fat	**0.1 g.**
cholesterol	**0 mg.**
sodium	**92 mg.**
dietary fiber	**5.7 g.**

Trim the okra and cut into ½" slices.

Coat a large saucepan with no-stick spray. Add the onions and cook over medium heat, stirring frequently, for 7 to 8 minutes, or until lightly golden.

Meanwhile, drain the tomatoes through a fine sieve set over a medium bowl; set aside the juice. With a spoon, lightly crush the tomatoes.

Add the tomatoes to the saucepan. Stir in the basil, hot-pepper sauce, brown sugar, thyme, salt, and ¼ cup of the reserved tomato juice. Cook, stirring, for 2 minutes.

Add the okra. Cook, stirring frequently, for 10 to 15 minutes, or until the okra is tender. Add the remaining tomato juice, if needed, to keep the okra from sticking.

Makes 4 servings

Cook's Note: If fresh okra is unavailable, substitute frozen. Do not thaw before using. Add 2 to 3 minutes to the cooking time.

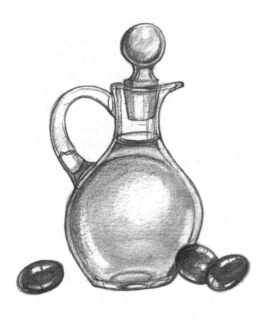

OLIVE OIL
AN ELIXIR FOR YOUR HEART

HEALING POWER
CAN HELP
Lower cholesterol

Reduce the risk
of heart disease
and breast cancer

Researchers were amazed more than 40 years ago when they first started studying Greeks living on the island of Crete. Even though the traditional Greek diet is very high in fat, people had exceptionally low rates of heart disease. "They have to be doing something right, and olive oil seems to play a critical role." says Dimitrios Trichopoulos, M.D., professor of epidemiology and cancer prevention at the Harvard School of Public Health.

We would do well to follow their example. Olive oil not only appears to lower the risk of heart disease, it may reduce the risk of breast cancer as well.

A BETTER FAT

All fats, from butter and margarine to olive oil, contain almost the same number of calories. But they behave quite differently inside the body. Saturated fats, for example, which are found mainly in meats and dairy foods, are incredibly destructive because they make it difficult for the body to rid itself of harmful low-density lipoprotein (LDL) cholesterol, the kind that blocks arteries and raises the risk of heart disease.

Olive oil, however, is a monounsaturated fat. Replacing saturated fats in the diet with olive oil lowers levels of LDL cholesterol while leaving the beneficial high-density lipoprotein cholesterol alone.

In the Kitchen

Some olive oils are quite rare and exquisitely flavored—and exquisitely priced. Others are much more affordable and, of course, the flavors reflect that. Many cooks keep two (or more) kinds of olive oil in the kitchen—a gourmet oil for drizzling on salads or pastas and a heartier oil to use for cooking.

- **Extra-virgin** is the Cadillac of olive oils. It's usually used as a flavoring oil and not for cooking. When buying extra-virgin olive oil, look at the color. The deeper the color, the more intense the olive flavor.
- **Pure (also called virgin) olive oil** is paler than extra-virgin and has a milder flavor. It's usually used for low- to medium-heat frying.
- **Light olive oil** is often used by people who want the heart-healthy benefits of monounsaturated fats but don't want the strong olive taste. It stands up to heat well, so you can use it for high-heat frying.

The olive oil–loving Greeks eat very little butter or margarine, Dr. Trichopoulos adds. What's more, their main meals usually consist of vegetables or legumes instead of meats. So even though they use a lot of olive oil, they get very little saturated fat.

One scientific project, called the Seven Countries Study, found that while 46 percent of deaths among middle-aged American men were due to heart disease, the number in Crete was a mere 4 percent—more than 10 times lower.

Chemicals for the Heart

It's not only the monounsaturated fat that makes olive oil so good for the heart. It also contains other disease-fighting compounds that can stop damage in the arteries before it starts.

Here's why. The body naturally produces harmful oxygen molecules called free radicals. These molecules damage LDL cholesterol in the bloodstream, making it more likely to stick to artery walls. But several of the compounds in olive oil, such as polyphenols, are powerful antioxidants. This means that they're able to disable free radicals before they do damage, Dr. Trichopoulos explains. As a result, getting more olive oil in your diet can help keep your arteries clear.

A Woman's Best Friend

Even though olive oil is best known for protecting the heart, evidence suggests that it may play a role in protecting the breasts as well. In a study of more than 2,300 women, researchers from the Harvard School of Public Health and the Athens School of Public Health in Greece found that women who used olive oil more than once a day had 25 percent lower risks of breast cancer compared to those who used it less often. And in fact, women in Greece are much less likely to die of breast cancer than their American counterparts.

"We're still not certain what accounts for this apparent protective effect," says Dr. Trichopoulos. Olive oil is rich in vitamin E, which has been shown to stop cellular damage that can lead to cancer. And of course, the same polyphenols that help prevent free radicals from damaging the heart may play a role in preventing cancer as well.

Getting the Most

Look for extra-virgin. All olive oils are high in monounsaturated fats, but they don't contain equal amounts of disease-fighting polyphenols. To get the most of these compounds, look for olive oil labeled "extra-virgin." This type of oil is made from the first pressing of perfectly ripe olives, which leaves the polyphenols in and the bitter acids out.

Keep it cold. Because people don't always use a lot of olive oil, it tends to go bad on the shelf, giving up both its good taste and its protective compounds. To keep olive oil fresh, store it in the refrigerator or another dark, cool place. Bringing it to room temperature will quickly restore its pourable nature.

LEMON-ROSEMARY DRESSING

1 sprig fresh rosemary
1 small clove garlic
1 strip lemon rind (1" × ½")
¾ cup olive oil
¼ cup fresh lemon juice

PER 1 TABLESPOON

calories	**90**
total fat	**10.1 g.**
saturated fat	**1.4 g.**
cholesterol	**0 mg.**
sodium	**0 mg.**
dietary fiber	**0 g.**

Place the rosemary and garlic on a cutting board. Lightly crush both with the side of a heavy knife. Place the rosemary, garlic, and lemon rind in a clean bottle with a tight-fitting cap. Pour in the oil and lemon juice. Cap the bottle and shake well. Refrigerate if not using right away. Shake before serving.

Makes 1 cup

Cook's Note: Pure olive oil will make a dressing with a mild olive flavor. For a more assertive olive flavor, you can use a mixture of half extra-virgin olive oil and half pure olive oil. The dressing can be stored in the refrigerator for up to 1 week. Drizzle on steamed vegetables, fish, or seafood. Or use as a dressing for pastas, potato salads, or other salads.

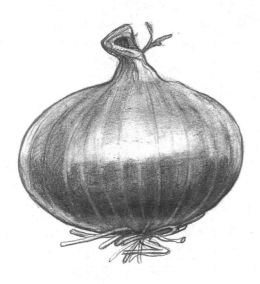

ONION FAMILY
ROOTS OF GOOD HEALTH

HEALING POWER
CAN HELP:
Raise beneficial HDL
cholesterol

Lower blood pressure

Decrease the risk
of cancer

Relieve congestion

Reduce inflammation

Scene: The Civil War, 1864. The Union soldiers are ailing with dysentery. General Ulysses S. Grant wires a directive to the War Department to save his troops.

"I will not move my army without onions!"

Three trainloads are shipped the next day. The rest, as they say, is history.

It's a stretch to say that onions won the war between the states. And scientists haven't proven that onions can stave off dysentery. But onions and other members of the allium family—such as leeks, shallots, and scallions—contain dozens of compounds that provide protection from other conditions, including cancer, high blood pressure, heart disease, high cholesterol, and asthma.

So grab an onion, a sharp knife, and a hanky and start chopping your way to better health.

ONION RINGS AND HEART STRINGS

Don't be offended the next time your honey suggests you "go Dutch" when you go out to dinner. He may be suggesting you take a cue from a group of

386

heart-healthy men who ate their fill of onion-laden delights as part of a ground-breaking study in the Netherlands.

In this much-acclaimed study, researchers found that men who ate a quarter-cup of onions a day, along with an apple and four cups of tea, had one-third the risk of dying from heart attacks compared to those who ate the least amounts of these foods.

What's so important about onions? Wrapped beneath their papery skins are dozens of compounds that help lower cholesterol, thin the blood, and prevent hardening of the arteries—all of which can go a long way toward preventing heart disease.

The first family of heart-healthy compounds in onions is the flavonoids. Flavonoids are substances in plants that have potent antioxidant powers, meaning that they help prevent disease by sweeping up harmful, cell-damaging oxygen molecules called free radicals, which naturally accumulate in your body.

One particular onion-dwelling flavonoid called quercetin has been shown to help knock out heart disease in two ways. One, it helps prevent the dangerous low-density lipoprotein form of cholesterol from oxidizing, which is the process that makes it stick to artery walls. Two, it helps prevent platelets in blood from sticking together and forming harmful clots.

A second group of protective compounds in onions are the same ones that make you cry—the sulfur compounds. Experts say that these compounds raise your levels of beneficial high-density lipoprotein cholesterol, which helps keep plaque from sticking to artery walls. At the same time, they lower levels of dangerous blood fats called triglycerides, which helps make blood thinner, keeping your blood pressure in the safety zone.

You don't need a lot of onions to keep your pump primed with protective compounds. In fact, studies show that you can reap the benefits by eating just one medium onion, raw or cooked, a day.

CANCER PROTECTION

You can hold the pickles if you like, but when you're looking for cancer protection, don't skimp on the onions. They may be a key player in cancer prevention, especially cancers of the gastrointestinal tract, say experts.

"The primary flavonoid found in onions—quercetin—actually halts the progression of tumors in the colons of animals," says Michael J. Wargovich, Ph.D., professor of medicine at the M. D. Anderson Cancer Center at the University of Texas in Houston. This means that onions do double duty in suppressing tumors, because the sulfur compounds also fight cancer, adds Dr. Wargovich.

In a large study in the Netherlands, researchers looked at the diets of nearly 121,000 men and women. The more odoriferous bulbs these onion-loving Hol-

Even though eating raw or cooked onions may help fight the airway inflammation that accompanies asthma attacks, eating certain pickled onions may have the opposite effect, warn researchers.

In a study in Spain, scientists found that some people with asthma experienced attacks after eating Spanish pickled onions (but not the Dutch variety), presumably because high levels of sulfites are added as preservatives.

If your doctor has told you that you're sensitive to sulfites, the best advice is to get your onions out of the ground. Or if you do buy pickled onions, check the label to make sure they're made without sulfites.

landers included in their daily diets, the lower their risks of stomach cancer.

Scientists suspect that onions prevent cancer not only by putting the brakes on tumor development but also by stomping out harmful bacteria that may get stomach cancer started.

A Good Kind of Onion Breath

Putting a few layers of raw onions on your turkey burger can give you industrial-strength breath, but those very same onions also may give people with asthma or other respiratory ailments clearer airways.

"There are sulfur compounds in onions that inhibit the allergic, inflammatory response like that seen in asthma," says Eric Block, Ph.D., professor of chemistry at the State University of New York at Albany.

Although more research needs to be done on onions' asthma-attacking abilities, you can see the anti-inflammatory effect for yourself. The next time you have an insect bite or other type of minor inflammation on your skin, rub a cut onion on it. This should help reduce the inflammation, says Dr. Block.

You only need to eat a few servings of onions a day to keep your breathing passages free and clear. "Unlike some foods, where it's just not conceivable that you could eat enough to produce a significant effect, you can with onions," says Dr. Block. "If you like onions, you can consume them in pretty large quantities. And there's good evidence that you should."

Combined Benefits

Whether you're eating for health or good taste, there's no reason to limit yourself to onions. Scallions, shallots, and other allium vegetables not only pack the same sulfur compounds and flavonoids as their bigger brothers, they also have a few of their own nutrients that can help fight disease and boost immunity.

Scallions, also called spring or green onions, are actually just young, underdeveloped onions. But they are higher in nutrients, particularly folate and vitamin C, than their adult counterparts.

A half-cup of chopped raw scallions provides 32 micrograms, or 8 percent of the Daily Value (DV) of folate, a nutrient that's essential for normal tissue growth and that may protect against cancer, heart disease, and birth defects. In that half-cup you'll also get more than 9 milligrams (almost 16 percent of the DV) of vitamin C, an immunity-boosting antioxidant nutrient that helps vacuum up tissue-damaging oxygen molecules in the body.

Shallots, another miniature member of the allium family, have their own benefits. Just 1 tablespoon of chopped shallots contains 600 international units of vitamin A, 12 percent of the DV. This essential nutrient helps keep immunity strong and also guards against vision problems associated with aging, like cataracts and night blindness.

IN THE KITCHEN

A lot of people would love more onions in their diets if it weren't for the tears required to chop them. Here's how to get the benefits of onions without the pain.

1. Chill the onion for 30 minutes.
2. Don't slice through the root end (the root end is opposite the stem end or top of the onion) since that will release a cloud of sulfur compounds that are concentrated in the root.
3. Using a sharp knife will allow you to cut more quickly, minimizing the time you're exposed to the onion's tear gases. It also helps to run the blade of the knife under cold water periodically while chopping.

Getting the Most

Add some color. To get the most nutrients from your daily dose of onions, eat several different kinds. Red and yellow onions and shallots have the highest flavonoid content, while white onions have the least.

Save your breath. If the fear of having horrific halitosis is keeping you from enjoying the health benefits of onions, here's a freshening tip. Eat a sprig of fresh parsley. This will help neutralize the sulfur compounds before they turn into offending breath. A breath freshener made with parsley seed oil can also help.

Keep your eyes peeled. Even if you like onions, you may not love them enough to eat a half-cup or so a day. That's why scientists are trying to develop new onion strains with high concentrations of flavonoids like quercetin. Experts aren't sure when these new onions will be on the market, but keep your eyes open for special displays at your supermarket.

Braised Red Onions

1 **teaspoon unsalted butter**
2 **large red onions, cut into quarters**
2 **tablespoons frozen pineapple juice concentrate**
1 **tablespoon white-wine vinegar**
1/8 **teaspoon salt**
   Ground black pepper

Per serving

calories	**53**
total fat	**1.1 g.**
saturated fat	**0.6 g.**
cholesterol	**3 mg.**
sodium	**69 mg.**
dietary fiber	**0.9 g.**

In a large saucepan over medium heat, melt the butter. Add the onions and cook, stirring to separate them into pieces, for 5 minutes, or until they begin to soften. Stir in the pineapple juice concentrate, vinegar, and salt.

Partially cover, reduce the heat to low, and cook for 10 to 15 minutes, or until the onions are tender. Season to taste with the pepper.

Makes 4 servings

Scallion Orange Sauce

1 **bunch scallions**
1 **teaspoon olive oil**
3/4 **cup fresh orange juice**
1 **teaspoon grated orange rind**
3/4 **teaspoon reduced-sodium soy sauce**
1 **teaspoon cornstarch**
1 **tablespoon cold water**

Per 1/2 cup

calories	**78**
total fat	**2.4 g.**
saturated fat	**0.4 g.**
cholesterol	**0 mg.**
sodium	**68 mg.**
dietary fiber	**0.8 g.**

Trim the scallions and slice finely, including the bulbs and the green tops.

In a small saucepan over medium heat, warm the oil. Add the scallions and cook for about 30 seconds, or until fragrant. Add the orange juice, orange rind, and soy sauce. Bring to a simmer. Reduce the heat to low.

In a cup, dissolve the cornstarch in the water. Add to the saucepan and cook, stirring constantly, for 1 to 2 minutes, or until the mixture thickens and turns translucent.

Makes about 1 cup

Cook's Note: Serve the sauce over grilled chicken or fish and also over noodles, rice, or other grains. You can easily double or triple the recipe.

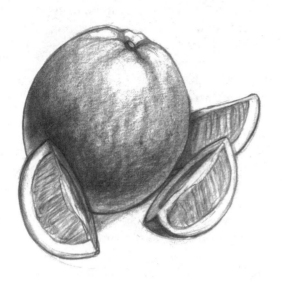

ORANGES
THE SWEET TASTE OF CITRUS

HEALING POWER

CAN HELP:
Lower the risk
of heart disease
and stroke

Stop inflammation

Fight cancer

The orange is nearly the perfect fruit. Not only is it high in vitamin C and fiber; it's also rich in natural sugars for quick energy. And because it comes ready-wrapped in its own protective skin, you can eat it anywhere, anytime.

Yet oranges are more than just a wholesome (and convenient) food. They also contain a quartet of compounds—limonin, limonene, limonin glucoside, and hesperidin—that show promise for blocking cancer. Plus, they contain compounds that may be able to stop heart disease even before it starts.

HELP FOR THE HEART

Studies have shown that the vitamins and other compounds in oranges are surprisingly effective antioxidants. That is, they're able to block free radicals, corrosive oxygen molecules in the body that can damage cells, before they do harm. This is important because free radical damage can set the stage for clogging of the arteries, a key risk factor for heart disease and stroke.

Vitamin C has long been recognized as a powerful antioxidant. Yet there appear to be other compounds in oranges that are even more powerful.

"We measured the total antioxidant capacity of oranges and found that vitamin C only accounted for maybe 15 to 20 percent of the total activity," says

One of the nicest things about oranges is their pleasant, citrusy zing. But for some people these natural acids can deliver a painful bite.

While few people have severe allergic reactions to oranges, some may have a condition called oral allergy syndrome, which causes itching and burning in the mouth or throat. This can be caused by eating oranges and other citrus fruits as well as other fresh fruits and vegetables, says Carol G. Baum, M.D., director of allergy and clinical immunology at Kaiser Permanente in White Plains, New York.

While reactions to citrus fruits are rare in adults, they occur more often in young children. "Infants may get a rash around their mouths because of the natural acid in foods like oranges," says Marianne Frieri, M.D., Ph.D., director of the allergy and immunology training program at Nassau County Medical Center–North Shore University Hospital in East Meadow and Manhasset, New York.

She adds, however, that in most cases the discomfort is only temporary. Healing quickly occurs once the offending food is taken away.

Ronald L. Prior, scientific program officer at the Jean Mayer USDA Human Nutrition Research Center on Aging at Tufts University in Boston. "The other compounds in oranges turned out to be very strong antioxidants—anywhere from three to six times as potent as vitamin C."

In one study researchers gave rats an extract from the peel and pith of oranges. The extract, which contained the compound hesperidin, significantly raised the animals' levels of healthful high-density lipoprotein cholesterol, while at the same time lowering the dangerous low-density lipoprotein cholesterol. If hesperidin works the same way in human tests, oranges could be used to help temper high cholesterol, which is one of the main risk factors for heart disease.

Hesperidin may have other benefits as well. In laboratory studies, for example, Brazilian researchers found that hesperidin was able to help stop inflammation. And since it doesn't damage the delicate stomach lining the way aspirin can, it someday could be used to help relieve swelling in people who are sensitive to other anti-inflammatory drugs such as aspirin or ibuprofen.

CANCER CONTROL

Laboratory studies have shown that the limonene found in oranges can help block lung and breast cancers, says Bill Widmer, Ph.D., research scientist with the Florida Department of Citrus Research Center in Lake Alfred.

In a study at Duke University Medical Center in Durham, North Carolina, laboratory animals given a diet consisting of 10 percent limonene showed a 70 percent reduction in cancerous tumors. Among the tumors that remained, 20 percent shrank to less than half their former size.

In another study researchers at Cornell University in Ithaca, New York, fed animals with early stages of liver cancer an extract of orange juice concentrate from which the vitamin C had been removed. The incidence and size of precancerous lesions dropped 40 percent.

"The rats were drinking the human equivalent of a gallon of orange juice a day for four months," adds Robert S. Parker, Ph.D., professor of nutritional and food sciences at Cornell. "That's an unrealistic amount for humans, but since we fed the animals only certain components of the juice, the actual protective effect of whole juice may be greater than the results suggested. Humans may be able to obtain protective effects at lower levels, particularly if they consume the juice regularly over a long period of time."

The research on limonene has been so promising that researchers in England are testing its effects on breast cancer.

"The way that limonene acts on tumor cells or lesions is really interesting and unique," says Michael Gould, Ph.D., professor of human oncology at the University of Wisconsin Medical School in Madison. Essentially, the compound gets cancer cells to self-destruct. It assists them in their own suicides.

SEIZE THE Cs

Oranges are best known for their vitamin C, and with good reason. One orange contains about 70 milligrams of vitamin C, almost 117 percent of the

Daily Value (DV). Vitamin C is critical not only for controlling harmful free radicals but also for aiding healing and boosting immunity. It's vitamin C's immune-boosting power that gives it its reputation for fighting the symptoms of a cold.

The vitamin also helps the body absorb iron from food, which is particularly important for women, who lose a little bit of iron (and blood) each month during menstruation.

In one large study, Gladys Block, Ph.D., professor of epidemiology and director of the public health nutrition program at the University of California, Berkeley, reviewed 46 smaller studies looking at the effects of vitamin C. Most of those studies found that people who got the most vitamin C had the lowest risks of cancer.

Filled with Fiber

An orange contains 3 grams of fiber, about 12 percent of the DV. Because insoluble fiber adds bulk to the stool, it can help relieve a host of intestinal problems, from constipation and hemorrhoids to diverticulosis. By speeding digestion, it can also help reduce the risk of colon cancer by moving the stool and any harmful substances it might contain through the colon more quickly.

Oranges also contain a second form of fiber, called soluble fiber. This type of fiber, which includes pectin, breaks down to form a gel-like barrier in the small intestine. Studies show that it can help lower cholesterol as well as help control changes in blood sugar, critical for those with diabetes.

If you were to eat more than seven oranges a day, you could lower your total cholesterol by about 20 percent. Of course, it's unlikely that anyone likes oranges that much. But by eating a variety of fruits and vegetables, including oranges whenever possible, you can do a lot to keep your cholesterol levels down.

Getting the Most

Stock your freezer. Drinking orange juice is one of the easiest ways to get more vitamin C in your diet. Fresh juice is delicious, but it's also a bother to make. Fortunately, frozen orange juice retains most of the nutrients. In fact, since juice manufacturers squeeze every last drop from their fruit, a lot of the potent compounds in the peel wind up in the concentrate, providing additional health benefits along with good taste.

Eat the sections. Half of an orange's pectin is contained in the albedo, the inner white spongy layer that lies right under the colorful part of the skin. So don't be too neat when you eat. Eating a little of this spongy layer with each section will provide more of this important fiber.

Orange-Onion Salad

4   **large navel oranges**

$^1/_2$ **small red onion, very thinly sliced**

$^1/_4$ **cup nonfat plain yogurt**

2   **tablespoons fresh orange juice**

$^1/_4$ **teaspoon dried tarragon**

Per serving

calories	**104**
total fat	**0.3 g.**
saturated fat	**0 g.**
cholesterol	**0 mg.**
sodium	**12 mg.**
dietary fiber	**3.8 g.**

Peel the oranges and cut each crosswise into 4 or 5 slices. Arrange decoratively on a platter, alternating with the onion slices.

In a small bowl, combine the yogurt, orange juice, and tarragon. Whisk to mix. Drizzle over the oranges and onions.

Makes 4 servings

OSTEOPOROSIS
DAIRY FOR BETTER BONES

For years now we've been trying to reduce the fat in our diets in order to control weight and reduce the risk of high cholesterol and heart disease. But in the rush to save our hearts, we may be losing our bones.

While milk, cheese, and other dairy foods can be very high in fat, they're among the best sources of calcium, the nutrient that's essential for keeping bones strong, says Daniel Baran, M.D., professor of medicine, orthopedics, and cell biology at the University of Massachusetts Medical Center in Worcester. But by forsaking these foods for fear of fat, you're at risk for developing osteoporosis, a condition in which bones become thin and brittle.

It's no mystery why osteoporosis is so prevalent in this country. The average American woman only gets 450 milligrams of calcium a day—nowhere near the 1,000 to 1,500 milligrams that's needed to ward off the disease, says Susan Broy, M.D., director of the Osteoporosis Center at the Advocate Medical Group in Chicago. Ironically, women, who need calcium even more than men do, are more likely to turn away from calcium-rich foods because they're more worried about their waistlines than their bones, Dr. Broy says.

Getting enough calcium is especially important for women approaching menopause, when estrogen levels decline. Estrogen helps bones absorb and keep calcium. When estrogen levels fall, in many cases the bones become weaker. In fact, the highest rate of bone loss occurs in the first five to seven years after menopause.

The sad thing about osteoporosis, says Dr. Broy, is that it's often preventable—if you get enough calcium. In one study, for example, researchers in the Netherlands found that women who got at least 1,000 milligrams of calcium a day—about the amount in three glasses of milk—were able to reduce their bone loss by 43 percent. Another study, this one done by researchers at Radcliffe Infirmary in Oxford, England, found that women who drank the most milk had bone densities 5 percent higher than those who did not drink milk.

Thanks to low-fat dairy foods, it has become very easy to get more calcium without having to worry about weight, adds Dr. Baran. A glass of whole milk for example, has more than 8 grams of fat, while a glass of low-fat (1 percent) milk has 3 grams—almost three times less. A glass of skim milk is even better, with barely 0.5 gram per serving.

BONING UP ON SOY

In an effort to turn back the clock, doctors often recommend that women past menopause take estrogen replacement therapy to keep their bones strong. But it may be possible to restore estrogen without taking drugs—just by eating a little more soy.

Research has shown that tofu, tempeh, and other soy foods contain compounds called isoflavones, which are very similar to (although weaker than) the estrogen women produce naturally, says Jeri W. Nieves, Ph.D., nutritional epidemiologist at Columbia University in New York City and director of the bone mineral measurement laboratory at Helen Hayes Hospital in West Haverstraw, New York. There's some evidence that getting enough isoflavones in the diet may play a powerful role in keeping bones strong.

In a study at the University of Illinois, women were given either 55 milligrams or 90 milligrams of isoflavones a day. (A half-cup of tofu contains 35 milligrams.) After six months, women getting the larger amount had an increase in bone density of 2 percent.

The research is preliminary, Dr. Nieves adds, and researchers aren't sure what quantity of isoflavones you'd need to keep your bones strong. However, 90 milligrams, the amount used in the study, is a good starting point. It's easy to get this much in your diet. A cup of soy milk, for example, has 30 milligrams, and a cup of roasted soy nuts has 60 milligrams.

Not all soy foods contain the beneficial compounds, though. Soy sauce, soybean oil, and soy hot dogs, for example, may share the name, but they won't provide the benefits.

Low-fat doesn't mean low in calcium, adds Dr. Broy. Low-fat dairy foods have just as much calcium as their full-fat counterparts. In fact, skim milk has even more calcium, because manufacturers replace some of the fat with the calcium-rich portions of whole milk. So while a glass of whole milk has about 290 milligrams of calcium, a glass of fortified skim has nearly 352.

Even if you're not a milk-drinker, you can still get plenty of calcium by adding nonfat milk powder to cereals or baked goods, like muffins and cakes, says Edith Hogan, R.D., a spokeswoman for the American Dietetic Association. A half-cup of skim milk powder contains almost 420 milligrams of calcium, and it has little effect on the texture or flavor of foods, Hogan says.

Of course, you can also add milk powder to foods that already contain milk. When Hogan makes her morning oatmeal, for example, she substitutes 1 cup of low-fat milk for the cooking water, then adds a half-cup of milk powder to the finished cereal. This one-two punch provides 720 milligrams of calcium—twice as much as many Americans get in an entire day.

Putting more cheese on the menu is an excellent way to get more calcium, Hogan says. A half-cup of ricotta cheese has 337 milligrams of calcium, more

STRENGTHEN WITH SUPPLEMENTS

In today's fast-paced, eat-on-the-run world, it's not always easy to get all the calcium your bones need. When your diet falls short, taking a calcium supplement makes good sense, says Daniel Baran, M.D., professor of medicine, orthopedics, and cell biology at the University of Massachusetts Medical Center in Worcester.

Women who are past menopause, when bone loss is greatest, need 1,500 milligrams of calcium a day. (Post-menopausal women taking estrogen need less, about 1,000 milligrams a day.) All calcium supplements, whether they're made from bone meal, oyster shells, or calcium citrate, are effective, says Dr. Baran. But the best supplements, as well as the least expensive, are those containing calcium carbonate, which is the same ingredient found in many antacids, says Dr. Baran.

than you'd get in an 8-ounce glass of low-fat milk.

It's very easy to work more cheese into your diet, she adds. Ricotta, for example, can be added to casseroles, lasagnas, enchiladas, and other dishes that call for a little cheese. Or you can simply sprinkle a little low-fat Parmesan on pastas or salads. One tablespoon provides almost 70 milligrams of calcium and very little fat.

Even though green, leafy vegetables don't contain as much calcium as dairy foods, they can still help you get the calcium you need. A half-cup serving of kale, for example, has nearly 47 milligrams of calcium, while the same amount of broccoli provides 36 milligrams. And you don't have to eat salads to get the benefit, Hogan adds. Mixing a cup of chopped kale into a soup, for example, will add a little taste, and with it an extra 94 milligrams of calcium.

While dairy foods and produce are the best natural sources of calcium, many packaged foods, such as orange juice, have been fortified with calcium, says John Bilezikian, M.D., professor of medicine in the division of endocrinology and director of the metabolic bone diseases program at Columbia University College of Physicians and Surgeons in New York City. Fortified orange juice has as much calcium as a glass of milk. So when you're at the supermarket, read the labels on packaged breads, juices, and breakfast cereals to make sure that you're getting all the calcium that you can.

BEYOND THE BASICS

While calcium is *the* mineral for strong bones, it doesn't work alone. In fact, it can't even get into your bones without help from other nutrients, especially vitamin D. "Without vitamin D, you absorb very little of the dietary calcium," Dr. Baran says.

You can get some vitamin D by eating salmon and other fatty fish, but fortified foods such as milk and breakfast cereals are often the best sources, says Dr. Baran. The DV for vitamin D is 400 international units, about the amount you'd get in four glasses of vitamin D–fortified milk.

Actually, if you spend any time outdoors, you really don't need to worry about vitamin D because your body produces it whenever sunshine strikes your skin. Even if you were to get no vitamin D in your diet, spending about 15 minutes a day in full sunlight, with only your face and hands exposed, would provide all you need, Dr. Baran says.

In addition to vitamin D, you also need a variety of minerals, like zinc, copper, and manganese, to help calcium be absorbed, says Paul Saltman, Ph.D., professor of biology at the University of California, San Diego.

Each of these minerals is very easy to get in your diet, Dr. Saltman adds. Seafood and lean meats, for example, are excellent sources of zinc, with 3 ounces of oysters providing more than 28 milligrams of zinc, about 188 percent of the DV. A 3-ounce serving of flank steak has just under 4 milligrams, approximately 26 percent of the DV.

STOP THE BONE ROBBERS

When trying to prevent osteoporosis, what you eat is generally more important than what you avoid. A number of foods and beverages can prevent calcium from being absorbed, however, so it's important to watch what you eat and to cut back on the worst offenders.

Coffee and colas, for example, contain caffeine, which can substantially reduce the amount of calcium you're able to absorb. To keep bones strong, doctors often advise having no more than two or three servings of coffee or soda a day, says Elaine Feldman, M.D., professor emeritus of medicine, physiology, and endocrinology at the Medical College of Georgia in Augusta.

When you do have coffee, it's a good idea to pour in a bit of milk, adds Jeri W. Nieves, Ph.D., nutritional epidemiologist at Columbia University in New York City and director of the bone mineral measurement laboratory at Helen Hayes Hospital in West Haverstraw, New York. Milk essentially blocks the effects of caffeine, preventing it from pulling calcium from your bones.

Getting too much salt in your diet can also be bad for bones. Not only does it decrease the amount of calcium your body is able to absorb; it also increases the amount of calcium that's excreted from the body. You don't have to give up salt entirely, Hogan adds, but a little moderation will help keep your bones healthy.

OVERWEIGHT
EATING AWAY THE POUNDS

Lose a pound a day—without dieting!"

"Burn fat—while you sleep!"

Yeah, right. When it comes to diets, most of us have swallowed enough snake oil to float a tanker. The only miracle about so-called miracle diets is that we keep trying them.

Losing weight and keeping it off doesn't take a miracle. It rests on one simple premise: "Energy in equals energy out," says Simone French, Ph.D., assistant professor of epidemiology at the University of Minnesota in Minneapolis. "If you take in more energy than you expend, you gain weight. If you take in less energy than you expend, you lose weight."

In other words, calories count. The number of calories you take in has to be less than the number of calories you burn. Exercise also counts because it helps you burn more calories.

Moreover, researchers are finding that what you eat is just as important as how much of it you eat. For example, the body doesn't process the calories in a high-fat chocolate-chip cookie the same way it does the calories in a potato or a plate of carbohydrate-loaded pasta. Further, studies show that while some foods fuel the impulse to eat, others seem to "switch off" the appetite.

So the real miracle may be that certain foods can actually help, rather than hinder, your efforts to lose weight.

THE LOW-FAT SOLUTION

Most people trying to lose weight can count calories in their sleep. But calories, while important, are just part of the weight-loss equation. To trim the fat from your middle, you have to get it off your plate.

There are several reasons why focusing on fat is such a critical part of any weight-loss plan. First, fat is incredibly calorie-dense. One gram of fat contains 9 calories, while a gram of carbohydrate or protein has only 4 calories. This is why a raw carrot contains only 31 calories, while a similar-size serving of carrot cake holds a whopping 314 calories.

Compared with protein and carbohydrates, fat has a natural tendency to stick around. In the process of storing fat, your body burns only 3 percent of the fat calories. With carbohydrates, by contrast, it burns 23 percent of the calories prior to storage.

In a study at Indiana University in Bloomington, researchers examined the diets of 78 people and found, not surprisingly, that those who were overweight consumed more fat than their leaner peers. What was surprising was that the overweight folks ate fewer calories. This suggests that the fat you eat is much more likely to become the fat you wear.

To maintain good health, most experts agree that you should limit fat intake to no more than 25 percent of calories. But to lose weight, you should cut it even more, to 20 percent.

The Fat-Free Danger

Following a low-fat diet isn't without pitfalls, however, especially when it comes to low-fat snacks. "Many people think that they can eat as many low-fat foods as they want, but these foods can contain a significant amount of calories," says Dr. French. "And if you take in a lot more calories than you need, even if they're fat-free calories, you gain weight."

That's not to say that you can't enjoy low-fat snacks. You just need to be smart about how and when you indulge. Since "fat-free" doesn't mean "calorie-free," you don't want to be gobbling low-fat or nonfat foods on a regular basis. However, you can put them to good use by eating them in small amounts between meals. By satisfying your snack tooth before lunch or dinner, you'll be less likely to overeat at mealtimes, says Joanne Curran-Celentano, R.D., Ph.D., associate professor of nutritional sciences at the University of New Hampshire in Durham.

While fat-free (or even high-fat) snacks are fine as a treat, you can't depend on them to keep your appetite satisfied and your waistline trim. Whenever possible, select snacks that are naturally low in fat, like fruits, vegetables, and whole grains, says Dr. Curran-Celentano.

The Case for Carbs

It wasn't so long ago that people who were trying to lose weight avoided bread, potatoes, and pasta because it was believed that these and other "starchy" foods went straight to the hips. Research shows, however, that people who lose weight and keep it off tend to eat more of these foods rather than less.

Foods high in complex carbohydrates, including rice, beans, starchy vegetables, and pasta, make you feel full because they have a lower "energy density"—that is, they weigh more than high-fat foods but contain fewer calories, says Barbara Rolls, Ph.D., professor of nutrition department at Pennsylvania State University in University Park. "The lower a food's energy density, the more likely it is to fill you up," she says.

To grasp the importance of energy density, consider an average 1,600-calorie day. To get that many calories from high-carbohydrate foods, you would have to eat one of the following: 17 whole-wheat pancakes, 11 baked potatoes, 8 cups of spaghetti, or 8 toasted cinnamon-raisin bagels. Now suppose that you decided to get those calories from high-fat foods. Here's what's on the menu: only three fast-food fish sandwiches with cheese and tartar sauce.

See the difference? When you're eating high-carbohydrate foods, you can keep yourself satisfied and still not go over a healthy number of calories, says Dr. French.

What's more, research suggests that people prefer following a high-carbohydrate, low-fat diet when they're trying to lose weight. In a study at the University of Minnesota in Minneapolis, women following a low-fat diet were encouraged to eat as much as they wanted of foods that were low in fat but high in complex carbohydrates, like fruits, vegetables, grains, and beans. Women in another group, by contrast, followed a low-calorie diet that nonetheless was higher in fat, with up to 30 percent of total calories coming from fat.

After six months, women in both groups had lost about the same amount of weight—9.7 pounds for the low-fat group, compared to 8.4 pounds for the calorie cutters. But women in the low-fat group associated the experience with a better quality of living and rated their diets as tastier, compared with those in the low-calorie group. In addition, women in the low-fat group consumed 17 percent fewer calories than the calorie cutters without even trying.

Dr. Curran-Celentano suggests splitting your diet into 60 percent carbohydrate, 20 percent protein, and 20 percent fat. "It's a good idea to select high-fiber foods as your carbohydrate choices," she says. "You'll get more nutrients and avoid dips in blood sugar, which can cause food cravings and hunger pangs."

High-Satisfaction Foods

If your idea of a weight-loss plan is to "eat light," you may want to consider doing just the opposite. Research suggests that controlling appetite and weight gain may be as simple as choosing "high-satisfaction" foods.

Researchers at the University of Sydney in Australia had volunteers eat 240-calorie portions of a variety of foods, including fruits, baked goods, snack foods, high-carbohydrate foods, high-protein foods, and cereal. After eating, the participants rated their feelings of hunger every 15 minutes. The goal was to see which foods kept them feeling satisfied the longest.

White bread was assigned an automatic score of 100 points, and all other foods were measured against that. Here's how the menu lined up. A potato topped the list, receiving a score of 323 and making it more than three times as satisfying as white bread. It was followed by fish (with a score of 225), oatmeal (209), oranges (202), apples (197), and whole-wheat pasta (188). Surprisingly, baked goods got the least satisfactory ratings. Even more surprising, the more fat a food contained,

SATISFACTION GUARANTEED

Controlling appetite is perhaps the key to successfully losing weight, according to a study at the University of Sydney in Australia. Researchers there have identified a number of "high-satisfaction" foods, which help keep you feeling full longer. In the accompanying table, anything with a rating of 100 or better (the score given to white bread) is considered satisfying. Foods that scored less than 100 tend not to stick around, so you'll probably wind up eating more of them—and gaining weight.

Food	Rating	Food	Rating
Potatoes	323	Crackers	127
Fish	225	Cookies	120
Oatmeal	209	White pasta	119
Oranges	202	Bananas	118
Apples	197	Cornflakes	118
Whole-wheat pasta	188	Jelly beans	118
Steak	176	French fries	116
Baked beans	168	White bread	100
Grapes	162	Ice cream	96
Grain bread	154	Potato chips	91
Popcorn	154	Yogurt	88
Bran cereal	151	Peanuts	84
Eggs	150	Candy bar	70
Cheese	146	Doughnut	68
White rice	138	Cake	65
Lentils	133	Croissant	47
Brown rice	132		

the less likely it was to rank high on the scale. A croissant, for example, received a score of 47, which meant that it was less than half as satisfying as a piece of white bread. Foods containing more protein, fiber, and water received higher scores.

To put the results of this study to work, always select satisfying foods like vegetables and fruits over their higher-fat, lower-fiber counterparts, recommends Dr. Rolls. For example, choose a baked potato over a serving of french fries. Between meals, snack on a cup or two of air-popped popcorn, which is more likely to satisfy you than the same amount of potato chips. Better yet, grab an apple or an orange. The idea is to satisfy your hunger immediately and help control your appetite for the next few hours, without loading you up with unwanted calories.

PARKINSON'S DISEASE
FOODS THAT PROTECT THE BRAIN

Every move you make, from turning the pages of this book to swallowing a sip of water, is controlled by a chemical called dopamine. Dopamine is a brain chemical that transmits signals to muscles throughout your body. But in people with Parkinson's disease, the cells that make dopamine are damaged or destroyed. As dopamine levels decline, the simplest movements become increasingly difficult to perform.

There isn't a cure for Parkinson's disease, but research suggests that what you eat can help slow, if not stop, damage to these essential cells. In fact, getting enough of a few key nutrients may help prevent damage even before it starts.

PROTECTING THE BRAIN

Scientists believe that Parkinson's disease is caused, in part, by harmful oxygen molecules called free radicals. These molecules, which are missing electrons, careen like pinballs through the body, stealing electrons wherever they can find them. In the process, they may damage dopamine-producing cells in the brain, says James David Adams Jr., Ph.D., associate professor of molecular pharmacology and toxicology at the University of Southern California School of Pharmacy in Los Angeles.

One of the best ways to stop this damage is to get more antioxidant vitamins, especially vitamins C and E, in your diet. These nutrients come between free radicals and your body's cells, offering up their own electrons and preventing further harm. Studies have shown, in fact, that people with Parkinson's disease tend to have low levels of antioxidants. "The antioxidants appear to be very protective," says Christine Tangney, Ph.D., associate professor of clinical nutrition at Rush–Presbyterian–St. Luke's Medical Center in Chicago.

It's easy to get vitamin C in your diet, but getting extra vitamin E can be a challenge because it's mainly found in oils like sunflower and peanut oils. One way to get more vitamin E is to have several servings a day of nuts or wheat germ, says Dr. Tangney. One serving of wheat germ (just under 2 tablespoons) provides almost 5 international units of vitamin E, nearly 17 percent of the Daily Value (DV). Hazelnuts are also good, with 1 ounce containing nearly 7 international units, just under 23 percent of the DV. And some breakfast cereals are fortified with vitamin E.

Repairing the Damage

Even though the antioxidant vitamins can help protect dopamine-producing cells, they can't repair damage that has already been done. Preliminary evidence, however, suggests that getting more niacin in your diet may help bring these cells up to speed.

Like vitamins C and E, nicotinamide, a form of niacin found in meats, grains, fish, and legumes, is an antioxidant that can help stop damage from free radicals. More important, it appears to protect enzymes in the brain that are needed to repair damaged cells. Theoretically, getting more of this vitamin could allow the brain to begin producing more dopamine, says Dr. Adams.

The research is very new, so it's not yet certain how much niacin you might need to help keep the brain healthy, Dr. Adams says. Until more studies are done, he recommends getting the DV of 20 milligrams of niacin. This is especially important for people between the ages of 60 and 65, since folks in this age group frequently don't get enough niacin, and they're also the ones most at risk for Parkinson's disease.

Many foods are high in niacin. A 3-ounce serving of fresh tuna, for example, has more than 10 milligrams of niacin, about 5 percent of the DV. The same amount of white turkey meat has over 5 milligrams, approximately 27 percent of the DV, and a serving of flank steak has more than 4 milligrams, nearly 22 percent of the DV. You can also get niacin in legumes. A half-cup of lentils, for example, contains 1 milligram of niacin, 5 percent of the DV.

Fabulous Favas

For years, people with Parkinson's disease have traded stories about getting relief by eating fava beans. Research now suggests that they might be on to something.

Fava beans (also known as broad beans) contain a compound called levodopa, which is the active ingredient in medicines used to treat Parkinson's disease. The body converts the levodopa in fava beans into dopamine, the chemical the brain needs to communicate with muscles, Dr. Tangney says. A half-cup of fava beans contains about 250 milligrams of levodopa, the same amount that you'd get in one pill.

One study found that people eating large amounts of fava beans—approximately 10 ounces a day—got about the same benefits as they did when taking medication, Dr. Tangney says.

But if you're already taking levodopa, talk to your doctor before feasting on favas, Dr. Tangney adds. Having even a half-cup of beans in addition to your regular medication could overload your system with dopamine, causing the chemical to work less effectively.

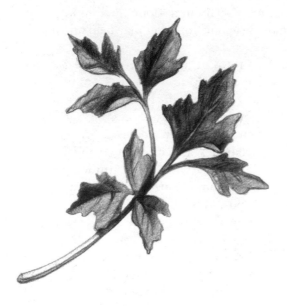

PARSLEY
MORE THAN A GARNISH

HEALING POWER

CAN HELP:
Relieve urinary tract infections

Prevent birth defects

Ease premenstrual discomfort

There's probably no other green as universally recognized as parsley. Each year, tons of this aromatic leaf are placed upon dinner plates worldwide, only to be scraped away with the leftovers. To most, parsley's purpose is merely to garnish, along with a slice of orange or lemon, an otherwise brown-looking entrée. But parsley's original intent upon the dinner plate was for a much nobler cause. Parsley is nature's original breath freshener, and it's also a delicious way to cleanse the palate.

Today the strength of these sprigs supersedes sweet-smelling breath. Eaten as a food rather than a garnish, parsley has earned a reputation as a natural healer.

URINARY RELIEF

Parsley's healing magic can be found in two compounds it contains, myristicin and apiol, that can help increase the flow of urine, says Varro E. Tyler, Ph.D., professor emeritus of pharmacognosy at Purdue University School of Pharmacy in West Lafayette, Indiana. Passing more urine helps remove infection-causing bacteria from the urinary tract.

This same diuretic action can also help prevent premenstrual bloating. Nibbling parsley in the days before menstruation can help increase urine flow, thus removing excess fluids from the body before they cause discomfort.

A Natural Multivitamin

Even though parsley is generally used in small amounts, it has as much healing power, tablespoon for tablespoon, as many of the more healthful foods.

For example, a half-cup of fresh parsley contains 40 milligrams of vitamin C, 66 percent of the Daily Value (DV). That's more than half the amount found in a whole orange.

Parsley is also a good source of folate, with a half-cup containing 46 micrograms, more than 11 percent of the DV. You need folate, a B vitamin, for producing red blood cells and helping to prevent birth defects.

Getting the Most

Favor it fresh. While dried parsley isn't a nutritional slouch, fresh is much better. "It may retain more of the healing volatile oil than the dried herb," says Dr. Tyler.

In the Kitchen

Even though fresh parsley is readily available in supermarkets, it's often in short supply at home. The reason for this is that parsley is somewhat perishable and doesn't always last long enough to use for a second meal.

To keep parsley fresh and available, here's what you need to do:

Keep it cold. Parsley will wilt within hours when stored at room temperature, so it's important to get it into the refrigerator as soon as possible.

Store it with care. Wash the parsley when you get it home from the store, discarding any bad leaves or stems. Then dry it, wrap it in a moist paper towel, and store it in a loosely closed plastic bag in the crisper drawer of the refrigerator.

Let it drink. Another way to keep parsley fresh is to stand the bunch in a drinking glass filled halfway with water, with a moist paper towel wrapped around the leaves to prevent them from wilting.

Make it a main ingredient. Even though parsley is best known as a culinary herb, you'll get more of its healing benefits by using it as a main ingredient. The Lebanese salad called tabbouleh, for example, typically calls for up to 1 cup of chopped fresh parsley. Or you can add half a bunch to a garden salad. Using whole sprigs will provide a pleasant texture, along with a celery-like flavor. Italian flat-leaf parsley has a stronger flavor than curly parsley.

Store it well. Since it's easier to store dried parsley than fresh, most cooks have a small bag or bottle stored in the kitchen pantry. To prevent dried parsley from giving up its benefits, it should be stored in a cool, dry place, preferably in an airtight opaque container.

Parsley-Garlic Topping

1½ **cups tightly packed flat-leaf parsley leaves**

1 **tablespoon grated lemon rind**

1 **clove garlic, minced**

1 **tablespoon fresh lemon juice**

Per 3 tablespoons

calories	**61**
total fat	**0.8 g.**
saturated fat	**0 g.**
cholesterol	**0 mg.**
sodium	**97 mg.**
dietary fiber	**5.2 g.**

In a food processor, combine the parsley, lemon rind, and garlic. Process until the parsley is minced. Add the lemon juice and process briefly to mix. Serve immediately.

Makes ¾ cup

Cook's Note: Sprinkle the topping on grilled fish or chicken. Or toss with cooked pasta or potatoes.

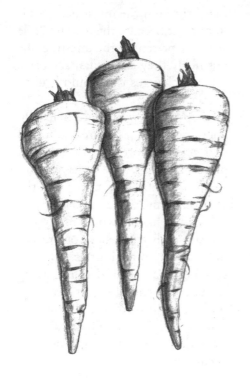

PARSNIPS
A PARTNER AGAINST STROKE

HEALING POWER

CAN HELP:
Prevent colon cancer

Lower the risk
of heart disease

Stabilize blood sugar
levels

Decrease the risk of stroke

Protect against
birth defects

Parsnips might as well be called Pursed Lips for the reaction that these strong-tasting, oddly sweet vegetables often get. And they certainly won't win any awards for Best-Looking Vegetable in Show. They look like carrots that have seen a ghost.

But despite parsnips' strong flavor and pale appearance, their nutritional profile is quite attractive. A member of the parsley family, parsnips are good sources of folate, fiber, and phenolic acids, which have been shown in laboratory studies to help block cancer.

FABULOUS FIBER

Whenever experts compile their "A" lists for healing substances, they put dietary fiber near the top. And parsnips are an excellent source. One cup of cooked parsnips contains nearly 7 grams, 28 percent of the Daily Value (DV).

A little more than half of the fiber in parsnips is the soluble kind, which means that it becomes gel-like in the digestive system. This helps block the intestine from absorbing fats and cholesterol from foods. At the same time, it dilutes bile acids in the intestine, which can prevent them from causing cancer. Parsnips also contain insoluble fiber, which speeds the rate at which stools

IN THE KITCHEN

Parsnips cook up like carrots, except they don't take as much time. What's more, they're prepared in similar ways—that is, they can be mashed, pureed, or served in chunks.

To a greater degree than carrots, however, parsnips are a vigorous vegetable. It's not uncommon for them to grow quite large, sometimes up to about 20 inches long. Large parsnips tend to have a strong flavor that many people find disagreeable. "Look for small or medium parsnips," advises Marilyn A. Swanson, R.D., Ph.D., professor and head of the department of nutrition and food science at South Dakota State University in Brookings. "They have a better flavor and texture." Parsnips measuring about 8 inches in length are the most tender.

move through the intestine. This is important because the less time bile acids are present in the intestine, the less likely they are to damage cells, causing changes that could lead to cancer.

In a review of more than 200 scientific studies, researchers found that getting more dietary fiber can protect against a wide variety of cancers, including cancer of the stomach, pancreas, and colon.

Fiber has shown similarly impressive ability to relieve or prevent many other conditions as well. Researchers have found that getting enough fiber in the diet can help prevent hemorrhoids and other intestinal conditions. Fiber can also curb the blood sugar swings that occur with diabetes.

STROKE PREVENTION

Some nutrition experts say that too little folate is our number one nutritional deficiency, particularly among younger folks, who often eat large amounts of fast food that's largely devoid of vitamins. Parsnips are a good source of folate, with 1 cup containing 91 micrograms, 23 percent of the DV.

Getting enough folate has been shown to prevent certain birth defects. It's also strongly suspected of reducing the risk of stroke. Folate decreases blood levels of homocysteine, a chemical that may jam up the arteries and stop blood flow.

Researchers in the Framingham Health Study found that men who ate the most produce had a 59 percent lower stroke rate than those who ate the least. Even those who ate just a little more produce reaped substantial benefits. The study found that folks who helped themselves to an extra three servings of fruits and vegetables a day lowered their risk of stroke by 22 percent.

Obviously, unless you truly have a passion for parsnips, it's unlikely that you'll ever eat three or more servings a day. But eating just a half-cup will provide not only fiber and folate but also 280 milligrams of potassium, 8 percent of the DV. This will go a long way toward keeping your arteries in the swim.

THE ACID TEST

Along with carrots and celery, parsnips are members of the umbelliferae family. Foods in this family contain a number of natural compounds called phytonutrients, which have been shown in laboratory studies to block the spread of cancer cells. Chief among these are compounds called phenolic acids. What phenolic acids do is attach themselves to potential cancer-causing agents in the body, creating a bigger molecule—so big that the body can't absorb it.

Research has shown that members of the umbelliferae family can also fight cancer by inhibiting tumor growth.

The research is still preliminary, so it's not yet certain how effective parsnips are at blocking cancer. In the meantime, go ahead and enjoy parsnips for all the fiber and folate they contain.

Getting the Most

Trim the greens. Before storing parsnips in the refrigerator, snip the greens from the top. Otherwise, the greens will draw moisture and nutrients from the root itself, according to Densie Webb, R.D., Ph.D., co-author of *Foods for Better Health*.

Keep them cold. Although some root vegetables keep well at room temperature, parsnips should be kept in the refrigerator or root cellar. "Keeping them cold and humid will keep them from drying out and losing some of their nutritional value," says Susan Thom, R.D., a resource spokesperson for the American Dietetic Association and a nutrition consultant in Brecksville, Ohio.

Stock up ahead of time. Parsnips will keep for a couple of weeks when stored in the refrigerator in a perforated or loosely closed plastic bag. "The longer you keep them in storage, the sweeter they get," says Thom.

Boil before peeling. Some of the nutrients in parsnips are water-soluble and are quickly lost during cooking. "They're fragile in boiling water—some of those vitamins float away," says Anne Dubner, a spokeswoman for the American Dietetic Association and a nutrition consultant in Houston.

In fact, you can lose almost half the water-soluble nutrients by cooking peeled parsnips. The solution, of course, is to cook them unpeeled. Once they're tender, let them cool, then scrape or peel the skin away.

Mashed Parsnips with Sour Cream

1   pound parsnips
⅓   cup nonfat sour cream
⅛   teaspoon salt
⅛   teaspoon ground allspice

Per serving

calories	**99**
total fat	**0.3 g.**
saturated fat	**0 g.**
cholesterol	**0 mg.**
sodium	**91 mg.**
dietary fiber	**4.3 g.**

Trim about ½″ from the top and bottom of each parsnip. Scrub the parsnips well but do not peel.

Bring a large saucepan of water to a boil over high heat. Add the parsnips. Cover, reduce the heat to medium-low, and cook for 25 to 30 minutes, or until very tender. Test for doneness by inserting the tip of a sharp knife into a parsnip.

Remove the parsnips with tongs and place on a clean work surface. Set the cooking water aside.

Using a paper towel to protect your fingers, hold each parsnip by the end and scrape off the skin with a small paring knife or vegetable peeler. Discard the skin. Place the parsnips in a large bowl.

Add the sour cream, salt, allspice, and 2 tablespoons of the reserved cooking liquid. With a potato masher or fork, coarsely mash the parsnips. Add 1 to 3 more tablespoons of cooking liquid if necessary to make the mixture smooth and creamy.

Makes 4 servings

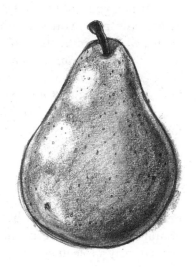

Pears
The Cholesterol-Fighting Fruit

Healing Power
Can help:
Lower cholesterol

Improve memory
and alertness

Keep bones strong

When it comes to good health, you would think that pears would have more in common with apples and oranges than with a bowl of beans. But as it turns out, pears (along with beans) contain a type of dietary fiber that is very effective for lowering cholesterol.

Pears contain lignin, an insoluble fiber that helps usher cholesterol out of the body. Lignin acts like Velcro, trapping cholesterol molecules in the intestine before they get absorbed into the bloodstream. And because lignin can't pass through the intestinal wall, it goes into the stool, taking cholesterol along with it, explains Mary Ellen Camire, Ph.D., associate professor and chair of the department of food science and human nutrition at the University of Maine in Orono. "Because of the lignin, eating pears on a regular basis can have a big impact on lowering cholesterol," she says. "There aren't many fruits that measure up to the lignin in pears."

The insoluble fiber in pears serves another useful purpose. Insoluble fiber, as the name suggests, doesn't dissolve in the intestine. What it does, however, is absorb large amounts of water. This causes stools to pass more easily and quickly through the digestive tract, which helps prevent constipation and hemorrhoids and also reduces the risk of colon cancer.

Pears contain another type of fiber, called pectin, which is the same stuff you add to jellies and jams to help them jell. Pectin is a soluble fiber, meaning that it

In the Kitchen

With more than 5,000 varieties of pears worldwide, you could eat a different one every day for years and never have the same taste twice. Here are a few of the pears you're most likely to find in neighborhood markets.

Anjou. These pears have a yellow-green skin and are usually available in winter. They're sweet and very juicy and make a pleasant addition to salads.

Bartlett. Available during the summer and early fall, Bartletts, have yellow-green skin and a sweet and juicy flesh. They can be eaten as a snack or peeled and cooked.

Bosc. Bosc pears have a slender neck, russeted yellow skin, and a sweet-tart flavor. The flesh is firm, making them a good choice for poaching. They can even be grated, adding a sweet accent to oatmeal or dry cereal.

Comice. With a color range from greenish yellow to yellow brushed with red, Comice pears have melt-in-your-mouth texture and a sweet fragrance. Because they're so soft and lush, they're frequently served as a dessert fruit.

dissolves in the intestine, forming a sticky, gel-like coating. As with lignin, pectin binds to cholesterol, causing it to be removed in the stool.

When you add up all the fiber in a single pear, you get about 4 grams, which is more than you'd get in a serving of Common Sense Oat Bran cereal or even a bran muffin. Eating just two pears will provide about 32 percent of the Daily Value for fiber.

Saving Minerals

We don't usually think of pears as being "bone food," but they contain a mineral, boron, that appears to play a role in keeping bones strong.

Boron wasn't considered essential for a healthy diet until very recently. Researchers have since discovered that getting enough boron can help prevent the loss of calcium in postmenopausal women. This is important because these women have a high risk of osteoporosis, the bone-thinning disease that's caused by a gradual loss of minerals from the body.

What's good for the bones is also good for the brain. In tests of memory, perception, and attention, people low in boron did not perform as well as when they had higher amounts. And a study done by researchers at the U.S. Department of Agriculture found that reflexes and mental alertness improved when people were given additional boron.

It doesn't take a lot of boron to get the benefits. Just 3 milligrams a day has been shown to help prevent the loss of calcium and keep the mind strong. While it's unlikely that you would ever get all your boron from pears—one pear contains a little more than 0.3 milligram—having at least five servings a day of a variety of fruits and vegetables, including pears, will provide all the boron your body needs.

Getting the Most

Keep it clothed. Most of a pear's fiber is in the peel. By eating pears with the skin on, you'll get the full complement of fiber, along with the cholesterol-lowering benefits, Dr. Camire says.

Fresh is better. While canned pears are convenient, they don't provide anywhere near the benefits of fresh, says Donald V. Schlimme, Ph.D., professor of nutrition and food science at the University of Maryland in College Park. For one thing, canned pears have been peeled, so they have lost most of their healing fiber. In addition, they may lose large amounts of nutrients during the canning process.

This isn't to say that you don't gain anything from canned pears. You do, although you probably don't want it. A serving of canned pears packed in heavy syrup delivers 25 percent more calories more than its fresh counterpart, Dr. Schlimme says.

PEAR AND SMOKED TURKEY SALAD

4 **Anjou or Bartlett pears**

2 **ounces thinly sliced smoked turkey breast**

2 **tablespoons rice vinegar or white-wine vinegar**

4 **teaspoons olive oil**

1 **tablespoon honey**

2 **tablespoons minced fresh basil**

Ground black pepper

PER SERVING
calories	**190**
total fat	**5.3 g.**
saturated fat	**0.7 g.**
cholesterol	**4 mg.**
sodium	**151 mg.**
dietary fiber	**5 g.**

Quarter the pears lengthwise and remove the cores. Cut each quarter in half lengthwise. Arrange the pears decoratively on a platter, alternating occasionally with strips of smoked turkey.

In a small bowl, combine the vinegar, oil, and honey. Whisk until smooth. Add the basil and stir to mix. Spoon the dressing evenly over the pears and turkey. Season lightly with the pepper.

Makes 4 appetizer servings

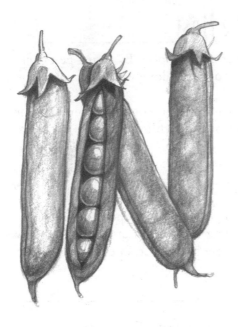

PEAS
LITTLE GREEN CANCER TRAPS

HEALING POWER
CAN HELP:
Relieve cold symptoms

Prevent cancer
and heart disease

Thanks to peas and an Austrian monk named Gregor Johann Mendel, we now have the science of genetics. Mendel found that when he bred two different peas together, their offspring had the features of both "parents." He concluded that physical characteristics could be passed down from generation to generation—not only in plants but in people as well.

Peas are more than an interesting scientific footnote, however. Researchers have found that they contain a powerful compound that can help prevent healthy cells from becoming cancerous. In addition, peas contain substances that can help lower cholesterol and ease symptoms of the common cold.

IT'S HEALTHY BEING GREEN

The cancer-fighting compound in peas is called chlorophyllin, which is the pigment responsible for giving them their shiny green hue. Chlorophyllin (which is related to chlorophyll, the substance that allows plants to convert sunlight into food) has a special molecular shape that allows it to grab cancer-causing chemicals in the body. "When you eat peas, the chlorophyllin attaches to carcinogens and helps prevent them from being absorbed," says Mary Ellen Camire, Ph.D., associate professor and chair of the department of food science and human nutrition at the University of Maine in Orono.

Researchers haven't pinned down exactly how many peas you'd have to eat to get the most benefits from chlorophyllin, Dr. Camire says. You can't go wrong, however, by including them on your menu as often as possible, along with other bright, green vegetables. After all, the greener a vegetable is, the more chlorophyllin it contains.

Helping Your Heart

Doctors have known for a long time that getting more dietary fiber is one of the best ways to lower cholesterol, and with it the risk for heart disease and other serious conditions. Green peas are an excellent source of fiber, with more than 4 grams in each half-cup serving.

Inside the intestine, the fiber in peas binds with bile, a digestive fluid produced by the liver, and traps it inside the stool. Since bile is very high in cholesterol, removing it from the body will automatically help bring cholesterol levels down.

Research suggests that eating peas can also bring down levels of triglycerides, blood fats that play a role in heart disease. A study in Denmark, for example, found that when people were given small amounts of pea fiber in addition to their usual diets, total tryglyceride levels fell almost 13 percent within two weeks.

Pods of Good Health

Peas have always been a favorite in school cafeterias—not because they're fun to flip off a fork but because they contain an abundance of disease-fighting vitamins. A half-cup of green peas, for example, contains more than 11 milligrams of vitamin C, almost 19 percent of the Daily Value. This is important because getting enough vitamin C in the diet has been shown to reduce the risk of cancer and heart disease. And when you have a cold, getting extra vitamin C will make the symptoms just a little more bearable.

Getting the Most

Fresh is finer. Peas shucked right out of the pod have more vitamin C than those that come in a can because canned peas lose many of their nutrients during processing, says Donald V. Schlimme, Ph.D., professor of nutrition and food science at the University of Maryland in College Park.

Visit the freezer case. Fresh peas can be hard to come by at certain times of the year, but frozen peas are always available. While they lack some of the crispness of fresh, they're just as good for you because freezing keeps most of the nutrients, especially vitamin C, intact.

Shuck the pods. Even though edible-podded peas (such as sugar snap peas) contain large amounts of vitamin C, the peas themselves contain most of the fiber, folate, niacin, phosphorus, riboflavin, thiamin, and vitamin A. To get the most nutritional bang for your buck, it's better to eat a half-cup of peas than an equal serving of peas in the pod, Dr. Camire says

Turn on the steamer. Whether you're using fresh or frozen peas, it's best to heat them by steaming rather than boiling. Boiling leaches nutrients out of peas into the cooking water. In addition, the high heat used in boiling may destroy some of the nutrients, particularly the vitamin C. If you don't have a steamer, heating them quickly in the microwave is a good alternative.

BUTTERED PEAS WITH CHIVES AND TARRAGON

1   **bag (16 ounces) frozen peas**
¼   **cup water**
2   **teaspoons unsalted butter**
1   **tablespoon minced fresh chives**
2   **teaspoons minced fresh tarragon**
⅛   **teaspoon salt**

In a medium saucepan, combine the peas and water. Cover and cook over medium heat for 3 minutes, or just until the peas are hot and bright green. Drain the peas through a fine sieve. Return to the saucepan. Add the butter, chives, tarragon, and salt. Stir or toss to mix. Serve immediately.

Makes 4 servings

PER SERVING

calories	**103**
total fat	**2.3 g.**
saturated fat	**1.3 g.**
cholesterol	**5 mg.**
sodium	**159 mg.**
dietary fiber	**6.1 g.**

PECTIN
STAY WELL WITH GEL

The next time you sit down to breakfast, spread a little jam on a piece of toast. Then take a bite from a succulent pear. Even though their tastes and textures are totally different, these foods actually have something in common, and that something is very good for your health.

Jellies and jams, along with legumes, fruits, vegetables, and a variety of grains, contain pectin, a type of dietary fiber that acts as a natural thickener. Food manufacturers often use pectin as a binding agent in jellies and jams. Nature, as it turns out, uses pectin in much the same way.

Because pectin is a soluble fiber, it dissolves in the body, creating a sticky gel inside the intestine. The gel binds to potentially harmful substances, preventing them from being absorbed. At the same time, it causes nutrients to be absorbed a little more slowly. Both of these factors make pectin a key player in preventing a number of conditions, from heart disease and diabetes to weight gain.

TRAPPING THE FAT

The biggest health threat that Americans face is heart disease, and one of the leading causes of heart disease is high cholesterol. The danger from cholesterol is so great, in fact, that doctors estimate that for every 1 percent that you lower your cholesterol, you reduce the risk of heart disease by 2 percent.

Getting more pectin in your diet is an excellent strategy for lowering cholesterol, says Beth Kunkel, R.D., Ph.D., professor of food and nutrition at Clemson University in South Carolina. Because pectin dissolves into a gel, molecules of fat and cholesterol get trapped before they make it into your bloodstream. And because pectin itself isn't absorbed, it goes out of the body in the stool, taking the fat and cholesterol with it.

Pectin helps lower cholesterol in yet another way. Because it isn't digested, bacteria in the intestine start gobbling it up. In the process, they release chemicals that travel to the liver, interrupting the production of cholesterol, says Michael H. Davidson, M.D., president of the Chicago Center for Clinical Research. Research has shown that people who get about 6 grams of pectin a day—approximately the amount in 3 cups of grapefruit sections—can lower their

In the Kitchen

Pectin, whether it comes in a plastic package or ready-wrapped in nature's own fruit, is what makes it possible for jellies, jams, and preserves to jell. Here are a few pectin pointers for the next time you're making your own.

- Some fruits, like apples and gooseberries, are naturally high in pectin and will jell without the addition of commercial pectin.
- Blueberries and peaches contain very little pectin. To help them jell, you'll probably need to add liquid or powdered pectin.
- Another way to promote jelling is to combine low-pectin fruits with those that are higher in pectin. Apples are a common addition to jams, not just for their flavor but also because of their high pectin content.

cholesterol by at least 5 percent.

While grapefruit is a good source of pectin, with 1 gram in a 4-ounce serving of sections, it's not the only one. Apples, bananas, peaches, and other fruits all contain pectin. So do vegetables and legumes. In fact, virtually all plant foods contain healthful amounts of pectin.

Smoother Digestion

People who are trying to lose weight are often advised to eat more fruits, legumes, and other pectin-rich foods. There's a good reason for this. When pectin dissolves in the stomach, it gradually expands, taking up more room. At the same time, it slows the absorption of sugars and nutrients into the bloodstream. This helps you feel more satisfied even when you haven't had a lot to eat.

"Pectin helps to give you that feeling of fullness, so you don't need to eat as much," says Barbara Harland, Ph.D., professor of nutrition at Howard University in Washington, D.C. "One of the most important things for losing weight and keeping it off is getting more fiber, including pectin."

Getting more pectin can be especially important for people with diabetes, who must do everything they can to keep their blood sugar levels steady. Since pectin slows the rate at which sugars are absorbed, it can prevent the sudden surges of glucose (blood sugar) that can damage the nerves, eyes, and vital organs in people with diabetes, Dr. Harland says.

Phytonutrients
Beyond Vitamins and Minerals

Somewhere in China, a 12-year-old girl sits down to her evening meal of tofu-scallion soup, a bowl of rice, green tea, and a stir-fry containing bok choy, snow peas, and eggplant.

Across the globe in the United States, a girl the same age dines on a burger and fries and washes it down with a frosty cola.

If both girls continue their culinary courses, the girl in China will be about half as likely to get cancer during her lifetime as her American counterpart.

Now let's sail across the ocean to Finland, where two men are sitting down to their dinner of meat, potatoes, and good beer. One of the men routinely eats an apple a day, along with ⅛ cup of onions and four cups of tea. As a result, he's less likely to die of heart disease than his fellow Finn, who sticks to the main course.

What is going on here?

That is a question scientists have asked themselves since Hippocrates first proclaimed, "Let food be thy medicine." What does diet have to do with disease?

More than we ever imagined. We've known for a long time that we need vitamins and minerals from foods to maintain good health and to prevent malnutrition and diseases such as rickets and scurvy. But research is revealing that the essential nutrients we all know about, such as vitamins A through E, are just the beginning: Hidden within plant foods are hundreds of compounds that are taking the diet-disease connection to an exciting new level. It appears likely that some of these previously unknown compounds will fight not only deficiency-type diseases such as anemia but also elusive, age-related illnesses such as heart disease and cancer.

Health from the Garden

Researchers call these compounds phytochemicals or phytonutrients, terms that simply mean chemicals or nutrients found in plants. They're not there accidentally—they're Mother Nature's way of keeping her garden beautiful. Potent sulfur compounds in garlic and onions, for instance, act as bug repellents to keep the vegetables healthy. Vibrant pigments like beta-carotene, found in carrots and cantaloupe, put the vivid hues in the foods we eat. Other compounds protect plants from bacteria, viruses, and other natural enemies.

We aren't onions or carrots, so why should we care about this? Because nature recycles its resources. When we eat foods containing these plant-protecting compounds, they begin protecting us—not from bugs but from the forces that wreak havoc in humans, such as high cholesterol, hardening of the arteries, heart disease, certain cancers, and even aging itself.

And the research has only begun. Scientists are discovering new phytochemicals all the time, and also ways in which these compounds fight disease.

Neutralizing Free Radicals

The family of phytonutrients is a large one, and each member of this family works in different ways. Their most common weapons against disease, however, appear to be their antioxidant abilities.

Every day your body is under attack by harmful substances known as free radicals. These are oxygen molecules that, due to pollution, sunlight, and everyday wear and tear, have each lost an electron. As they attempt to regain their missing electrons, they career through your body, stealing electrons wherever they can. The molecular victims of these raids are damaged in the process and become free radicals themselves. Unless this chain reaction is stopped, the result is huge numbers of damaged molecules and, over time, irreparable damage and disease.

Here's an example. Normal cholesterol is a benign, helpful substance. But when cholesterol molecules are damaged by free radicals, they begin sticking to artery walls, causing hardened arteries and heart disease. Another example: When free radicals attack molecules in your body's DNA, the genetic blueprint that tells your cells how to function, the blueprint is damaged. This is what allows cancer to develop. Even aging, many scientists believe, is caused by free radical damage.

The phytonutrients in plants, using their antioxidant powers, can quite literally save your life. Essentially, they step between the marauding free radicals and your body's cells, offering up their own electrons. When free radicals grab these "free" electrons, they become stable again and do no further damage. Most phytonutrients are potent antioxidants.

Eliminating Toxic Wastes

Another way phytonutrients keep us healthy is by neutralizing and flushing toxic chemicals from our bodies before they have time to make us sick. They do this by manipulating enzymes known as phase-1 and phase-2 enzymes, explains Gary Stoner, Ph.D., director of the cancer chemoprevention program at the Ohio State University Comprehensive Cancer Center in Columbus.

Phase-1 enzymes are like double agents. They're created by your body and are important for normal cell function. But they have the ability to work against you, too. When cancer-causing toxins enter your system, phase-1 enzymes help make them active. Phase-2 enzymes, on the other hand, are real good guys. They seek out carcinogens and detoxify them before they do damage.

When you eat broccoli or other vegetables, some of the phytonutrients begin stomping out the enemy phase-1 enzymes while increasing the production of helper phase-2 enzymes. This process helps neutralize various cancer-causing toxins that naturally accumulate in the body.

Regulating Hormones

A third way in which some phytonutrients fend off disease is by keeping certain hormones—most notably the female sex hormone estrogen—at healthy levels.

Estrogen is a good news–bad news kind of hormone. When it's produced at normal levels, it helps control everything from menstruation to childbirth. At the same time, it helps keep artery-clogging cholesterol in check, thus preventing heart disease. When estrogen levels rise, however, they can stimulate hormone-related cancers like those of the breast and ovaries, says Leon Bradlow, Ph.D., director of biochemical endocrinology at the Strang Cancer Research Laboratory in New York City.

There are several ways in which phytonutrients keep estrogen at its proper levels. For example, a class of phytonutrients called isoflavones are extremely similar to natural estrogen. When we eat foods containing isoflavones, these faux hormones bind to the body's estrogen receptors, leaving the real hormone with nowhere to go but out.

Although estrogen is often referred to as if it were one hormone, in fact there are different forms. One kind of estrogen, called 16-alpha-hydroxyestrone, has been linked to breast cancer. Another form, 2-hydroxyestrone, appears to be harmless. Certain phytonutrients are able to increase levels of the harmless form of estrogen while decreasing levels of the dangerous kind, says Dr. Bradlow.

Eating Your Medicine

As you can see, phytonutrients put up a variety of powerful defenses. Indeed, their potential is staggering. As with vitamins and minerals before them, scientists foresee a day when many of these compounds will be used for treating disease in the hospital and for preventing it at home.

"People used to get beriberi, a vitamin-deficiency disease marked by a decline in neuromuscular coordination, because they weren't getting enough thiamin in their diets," says Dr. Bradlow. "We started enriching our bread with thiamin, and now nobody gets beriberi anymore. In the same way, it may be possible to develop high-phytochemical-yielding strains of vegetables so that they can be used therapeutically against diseases like cancer and heart disease."

In the meantime, researchers stress that there is only one way to get the phytonutrients your body needs: You must eat them in the packages Mother Nature provides, that is, fruits, vegetables, and grains, getting at least five to nine servings a day.

While little is known about many of these compounds, a few are already showing great promise. Let's take a look at some of the emerging stars.

ALLYLIC SULFIDES

Take a sharp knife to a fresh onion or peel a clove of garlic and you'll be introduced to some of nature's most potent phytonutrients, allylic sulfides. These compounds, known for their power to bring tears to your eyes, may also have the power to prevent heart disease and cancer.

Allylic sulfides are a class of phytonutrients that stimulate toxin-eliminating enzymes. According to sulfide researcher Michael J. Wargovich, Ph.D., professor of medicine at the M. D. Anderson Cancer Center at the University of Texas in Houston, these compounds are particularly effective against cancers of the gastrointestinal tract.

In a study of more than 120,000 men and women in the Netherlands, researchers looked at the amounts of sulfide-containing onions these Hollanders ate and compared them with the incidences of stomach cancer. The more onions people put on their plates, the lower their risks of stomach cancer.

In another study, garlic, which is a member of the onion family, showed equal tumor-squelching promise. Researchers gave one group of mice large amounts of garlic every day for two weeks; another group received no garlic. When the animals were exposed to cancer-inducing chemicals, the group that received the garlic developed 76 percent fewer tumors than those given only their normal food.

Allylic sulfides also have the unique ability to keep cholesterol and other blood fats, known as triglycerides, from causing health-threatening blood clots and hardening of the arteries.

In one study, researchers loaded volunteers' diets with more butter and lard than you'd find in a French bakery, then watched their cholesterol climb and their blood coagulate. Then they gave the same volunteers a sulfide-packed onion extract. Not only did it prevent the fat-induced rise in cholesterol; it also increased the volunteers' ability to dissolve clots.

CAROTENOIDS

Carotenoids are the phytonutrients you can thank for adding bright, colorful hues to your salad. This class of about 600 red and yellow plant pigments, which includes beta-carotene, gives the deep reds to tomatoes and the vibrant oranges to carrots and cantaloupes. Carotenoids are also prevalent in dark-green, leafy vegetables like spinach—only you can't see them because the green chlorophyll in these plants overpowers the lighter carotene pigments.

Carotenoids are powerful antioxidants, making them prime fighters against heart disease and cancer. "There are good, clear associations between eating a lot of beta-carotene-packed foods and low levels of heart disease and cancer," says carotenoid researcher Dexter L. Morris, M.D., Ph.D., vice chairman and associate professor in the department of emergency medicine at the University of North Carolina School of Medicine at Chapel Hill. "But some of those benefits may be from some other carotenoid in fruits and vegetables that we have not even begun to study yet."

Research has shown promising results for a number of carotenoids, particularly lycopene (found in tomatoes), lutein (found in vegetables such as spinach and kale), and zeaxanthin (found in green, leafy vegetables).

In one study, researchers found that people in northern Italy who ate seven or more servings of raw tomatoes every week had a 60 percent lower chance of developing colon, rectal, and stomach cancer than those who ate only two servings or less. And since lycopene, the active ingredient in tomatoes, stands up to heat and processing, it appears likely that even ketchup and tomato sauce provide similar benefits.

Finally, Harvard researchers looking at green, leafy vegetables, especially spinach, had quite an eye-opener. They found that people eating the most lutein and zeaxanthin—two carotenoids found in these vegetables—had a 43 percent lower risk of macular degeneration than those eating the least. Macular degeneration is the leading cause of irreversible vision loss in people over 50.

FLAVONOIDS

You've probably heard of the French Paradox—the unfair fact that even though our lard-loving French allies down a diet loaded with culinary no-no's, they die of heart disease 2½ times less often than we do.

The reason, researchers believe, may lie in a group of phytonutrients called flavonoids. Like carotenoids, flavonoids add color—specifically reds, yellows, and blues—to the foods we eat. (Also as with carotenoids, these colors often are masked by chlorophyll in the plants.)

Present in the largest quantities in apples, onions, celery, cranberries, grapes, broccoli, endive, green and black teas, and red wines, flavonoids are powerful antioxidants, making them sturdy defenders against heart disease and cancer.

Their antioxidant prowess isn't the only thing that makes flavonoids the darling of every Frenchman's heart. They also act like Teflon coating for the millions of tiny disks in your blood called platelets. They keep the platelets from clumping together in the bloodstream and forming clots, which helps prevent heart attacks.

In one study, Dutch scientists examined the eating patterns of 805 men ages 65 to 84. They found that those who got the least flavonoids in their diets were

Phytonutrients at a Glance

Here's a guide to the most potent phytonutrients and the foods with the highest amounts, plus the best ways to prepare the foods to unlock their healing potential.

Phytonutrient	Food Source
Allylic sulfides	Garlic and onions
Carotenoids	Broccoli, cantaloupes, carrots, greens, and tomatoes
Flavonoids	Apples, broccoli, citrus fruits, cranberries, endive, grape juice, kale, onions, and red wines
Indoles and isothiocyanates	Broccoli, cabbage, cauliflower, and mustard greens
Isoflavones	Chickpeas, kidney beans, lentils, and soybeans
Lignans	Flaxseed
Monoterpenes	Cherries and citrus fruits
Phenolic compounds	Almost all cereal grains, fruits, green and black teas, and vegetables
Saponins	Asparagus, chickpeas, nuts, oats, potatoes, soybeans, spinach, and tomatoes

32 percent more likely to die from heart attacks than those who ate the most.

It didn't take many flavonoids to get the benefits. The high-flavonoid group had the equivalent of four cups of tea, ½ cup of apple, and ⅛ cup of onions a day.

Indoles

Broccoli, cabbage, and other cruciferous vegetables have a bitter taste that bugs don't like. The phytonutrient responsible for this clever bit of plant pro-

Disease Prevention

Raise good high-density lipoprotein (HDL) cholesterol; lower blood fat, or triglyceride, levels; prevent heart disease; stimulate enzymes that suppress tumor growth

Antioxidant action; prevent heart disease and certain cancers

Antioxidant action; prevent blood clotting and heart disease

Stimulate cancer-preventing enzymes; lower levels of harmful estrogen

Lower levels of harmful estrogen; prevent certain cancers

Antioxidant action; lower levels of harmful estrogen; may prevent certain cancers

Prevent cancer by blocking certain cancer-causing compounds

Antioxidant action; activate cancer-fighting enzymes

Bind with and flush out cholesterol; stimulate immunity; prevent heart disease and certain cancers

Preparation Hints

Chop or crush to release the phytonutrients.

Eat with meat or foods that contain oil. Your body absorbs carotenoids better with a little fat.

Eat pulpy parts of citrus fruits and keep the skin on apples for the most flavonoids.

Microwave or steam lightly to preserve the phytonutrients.

Isoflavones hold up through processing, so you can save time and buy canned beans.

The recommended amount for optimum benefits is 1 to 2 heaping tablespoons of flaxseed.

Though most of the monoterpenes are found in the citrus peel, you can also get them by drinking the juice.

These ubiquitous phytonutrients are pretty hardy. Just eat a wide variety of fresh fruits and vegetables.

The richest sources are soybeans and chickpeas.

tection is called indole-3-carbinol. In humans this compound plays a role in regulating hormones, which may be useful in preventing breast cancer.

Indole-3-carbinol has been shown to knock down levels of harmful forms of estrogen while increasing more-benign forms of the hormone. Dr. Bradlow and colleagues at Strang Cancer Research Laboratory found that when women took 400 milligrams of this compound a day—the amount found in about half a head of cabbage— their levels of the harmless estrogen increased dramatically.

In fact, they had the same levels as those found in marathon runners, which is quite a feat, since vigorous exercise has been shown to have a strong positive effect on estrogen levels.

"Indole-3-carbinol (I3C) may also work against cervical cancer," says Dr. Bradlow, who foresees a day when women will be able to take an I3C supplement to help prevent breast and other hormone-related cancers.

ISOFLAVONES

Asian women have breast cancer rates five to eight times lower than those of American women. One of the reasons, say experts, may be all the soy foods in their diet.

Soybeans and foods made from them, like tofu and tempeh, along with kidney beans, chickpeas, and lentils, contain compounds called isoflavones—most notably genistein and daidzein. Like indoles, these may act as estrogen regulators in the body and therefore may help lower the risk of hormone-based cancers.

In a landmark study of nearly 143,000 women in Japan that spanned 17 years, researchers found that women eating the most miso (a soybean-based broth) had the lowest incidences of breast cancer.

Although more research needs to be done, it's possible that these compounds may eventually be used as an alternative to hormone replacement therapy and also to help prevent and treat heart disease and cancer, says Stephen Barnes, Ph.D., professor of pharmacology and toxicology at the University of Alabama at Birmingham.

ISOTHIOCYANATES

Isothiocyanates, sometimes called mustard oils, protect cruciferous vegetables by leaving invading insects with a bitter taste in their mouths. Like indoles, isothiocyanates, which are found in broccoli, brussels sprouts, and cabbage, show promise for helping to prevent cancer.

So far, sulforaphane, a compound abundant in broccoli, has been crowned the leading isothiocyanate for its cancer-blocking ability in laboratory tests. In one study, researchers at Johns Hopkins University in Baltimore exposed laboratory animals to a powerful cancer-causing agent. In animals given high doses of sulforaphane, only 26 percent developed breast tumors, compared with 68 percent of the group that didn't get the compound.

Isothiocyanates may be particularly effective against the damaging effects of cigarette smoke, says Stephen Hecht, Ph.D., professor of cancer prevention at the University of Minnesota Cancer Center in Minneapolis.

In a laboratory study, a compound called phenethylisocyanate, found in watercress, was able to reduce by 50 percent the rate of lung cancer in rats exposed to carcinogens found in tobacco smoke. Human trials have revealed similar results, says Dr. Hecht.

LIGNANS

Like isoflavones, lignans are plant estrogens that help keep levels of human estrogen in check. Found in flaxseed, lignans have been shown in a laboratory study to help prevent breast cancer from getting started. Indeed, one study found that flaxseed was able to reduce the growth of tumors in rats by more than 50 percent.

In addition, studies suggest that the lignans in flaxseed can help lower cholesterol. In one study, people who were given two flaxseed muffins a day saw their harmful low-density lipoprotein (LDL) cholesterol drop 8 percent.

The studies are preliminary, but research suggests that getting 1 to 2 heaping tablespoons of ground flaxseed a day—sprinkled on cereal or baked into bread—may be enough to provide protection.

MONOTERPENES

If you've ever polished furniture, you've likely smelled the "lemony" odor of limonene, a phytonutrient that scientists say may be yet another important warrior in the battle against cancer.

Large doses of limonene, which is found primarily in orange peels and citrus oils, have actually shrunk breast tumors in laboratory animals. This fragrant phytonutrient has also prevented tumors from developing when breast tissue is exposed to high doses of cancer-causing chemicals. In laboratory studies, limonene has been shown to reduce tumor production by 55 percent.

Unlike other cancer-preventing phytonutrients, limonene works by blocking proteins that are known to promote cell growth in various cancers. Limonene may be the reason that people who eat a lot of oranges and other citrus fruits appear to have a reduced risk of cancer.

A monoterpene that is found in cherries, called perillyl alcohol, has been shown to prevent cancers of the breast, lung, stomach, liver, and skin in preliminary animal studies at Indiana University School of Medicine in Indianapolis. But more research needs to be done before scientists know how effective this compound is in people.

"Perillyl alcohol has been very promising in clinical trials," says Charles Elson, Ph.D., professor of nutritional sciences at the University of Wisconsin in Madison. "We're not just showing that this compound fights cancer, meaning that it neutralizes cancer-causing toxins. We're also showing that it is effective in animals with existing tumors."

PHENOLIC COMPOUNDS

Almost all fruits, vegetables, cereal grains, and green and black teas are rich in phytonutrients called phenolic compounds, or polyphenols. These compounds fight cancer on two fronts. They stimulate protective enzymes while squelching harmful ones, and they're also heavy-duty antioxidants.

Particularly active polyphenols include ellagic acid from strawberries, green tea polyphenols, and curcumin, the yellow coloring in the spice turmeric, says Dr. Stoner.

In one study, researchers at the University of Scranton in Pennsylvania found that of 39 antioxidants found in food, polyphenols from tea showed the greatest prowess at controlling free radicals.

SAPONINS

Perhaps the most common phytonutrients are the molecules called saponins. You can find saponins in a wide variety of vegetables, herbs, and legumes, including beans, spinach, tomatoes, potatoes, nuts, and oats. Soybeans alone harbor 12 different kinds of saponins.

Studies show that people who eat saponin-rich diets have consistently lower rates of breast, prostate, and colon cancers, says A. Venket Rao, Ph.D., professor of nutrition at the University of Toronto.

Unlike other cancer-fighting phytonutrients, however, saponins possess a unique array of weapons. One way that they help prevent cancer is by binding with bile acids, which over time may metabolize into cancer-causing compounds, and eliminate them from the body, says Dr. Rao. They also stimulate the immune system so that it's better able to detect and destroy precancerous cells before they develop into full-blown cancer.

Perhaps most important, saponins have a special ability to target the cholesterol found in cancer cell membranes. "Cancer cells have a lot of cholesterol in their membranes," Dr. Rao explains, "and saponins selectively bind to these cells and destroy them."

Not surprisingly, this ability to bind to cholesterol is helpful for lowering total cholesterol as well. Certain saponins bind to cholesterol in the intestinal tract, making the cholesterol unavailable for absorption. This, in turn, could lower your risk of heart disease, Dr. Rao says.

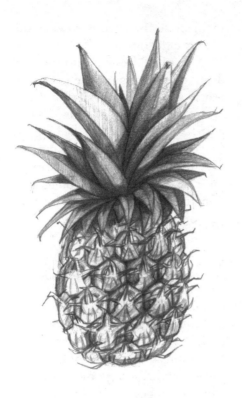

PINEAPPLE
A TROPICAL CHAMP

HEALING POWER
CAN HELP:

Keep bones strong

Improve digestion

Relieve cold symptoms

Lower the risk of cancer and heart disease

When King Louis XIV of France was first presented with a pineapple—the most exotic and sought-after fruit in seventeenth-century Europe—he immediately took a huge bite. Unfortunately, His Greediness hadn't given his servants a chance to peel it, so he cut his royal lips on the prickly rind. This episode put an end to the royal cultivation of pineapple in France until Louis XV took the throne in 1715.

The pineapple-punctured potentate didn't know what he was missing. Stripping a pineapple of its spiny hide (or at least opening a can of the stuff) is well worth your time. Not only is pineapple a rich source of vitamin C, it also contains substances that keep bones strong and promote digestion.

A JUICY BONE-BUILDER

You know that you need calcium to prevent osteoporosis, the bone-thinning disease that primarily affects postmenopausal women. What you may not know is that your bones need manganese as well.

The body uses manganese to make collagen, a tough, fibrous protein that helps build connective tissues like bone, skin, and cartilage. Research has shown that people deficient in manganese develop bone problems similar to osteoporosis. One study found that women with osteoporosis had lower levels of

In the Kitchen

With its tough skin and sharp edges, the pineapple doesn't give up its sweetness easily. To choose the best fruit and get to the "heart of gold" inside, here's what you need to do.

Buy it firm. Find a fruit that's plump and firm. Avoid pineapples that are bruised or have soft spots. Surprisingly, shell color is not always a reliable indicator of ripeness. The stem end should have a sweet, aromatic fragrance and not smell fermented.

Look for freshness. The leaves on pineapple should be crisp and deep-green, without yellowed or browned tips. Don't bother testing the fruit by pulling a leaf from the crown. Contrary to popular wisdom, a leaf that comes off easily doesn't indicate that the fruit is ripe.

Reveal the fruit. When you get the pineapple home, cut off the top and bottom ends, then place it on its side in a shallow dish to catch the juices as you slice it. Cut it into $1/2$-inch slices and trim away the rind. Then use a sharp knife—or better yet, a small cookie cutter—to remove the tough core.

manganese than women who did not have the disease.

"Eating fresh pineapple or drinking pineapple juice is a good way to add manganese to your diet," says Jeanne Freeland-Graves, Ph.D., professor of nutrition at the University of Texas in Austin. A cup of fresh pineapple chunks or pineapple juice will give you over 2 milligrams of manganese, more than 100 percent of the Daily Value (DV).

Sweeten Your Digestion

Pineapple has a centuries-old reputation for relieving indigestion, and there may be good reasons for that. Fresh pineapple contains bromelain, an enzyme that helps digestion by breaking down protein. This might be important for some older people who have low levels of stomach acid, which is needed for protein digestion.

Even if you love pineapple, of course, it's unlikely you'd eat it after every meal. But if you are older and have frequent indigestion, adding a few pineapple slices to your dessert plate might help keep your stomach calm, says Joanne Curran-Celentano, R.D., Ph.D., associate professor of nutritional sciences at the University of New Hampshire in Durham.

A Great Source of Vitamin C

Few nutrients get as much attention as vitamin C, and for good reason. This vitamin is a powerful antioxidant, meaning that it helps thwart free radicals, unstable oxygen molecules that damage cells and contribute to the development of cancer and heart disease. In addition, the body uses vitamin C to make collagen, the "glue" that holds tissue and bone together. And when you have a cold, the first thing you probably reach for is vitamin C. It reduces levels of a chemical called histamine, which causes such cold symptoms as watery eyes and runny noses.

While pineapples aren't as rich in vitamin C as oranges or grapefruits, they're still excellent sources. One cup of pineapple chunks, for example, contains about 24 milligrams of vitamin C, 40 percent of the DV. Juice is even better. A glass of canned pineapple juice contains 60 milligrams, 100 percent of the DV.

Getting the Most

Buy it fresh. Canned pineapple is convenient, but when you're eating it to soothe an upset stomach, the fresh fruit is best because the intense heat used in canning destroys the bromelain, says Dr. Taussig.

Try a new variety. The next time you're at the store, look for a "Gold" pineapple. Imported from Costa Rica, this variety is exceptionally sweet, and it has more than four times the vitamin C found in other varieties.

Have some juice. Canned pineapple juice is an excellent way to get your DV of vitamin C. In fact, 4 ounces of pineapple juice contain more vitamin C than the same amount of apple, cranberry, or tomato juice.

PINEAPPLE WITH ALMOND CREAM TOPPING

1 **large pineapple, peeled**
²/₃ **cup 1% cottage cheese**
1 **tablespoon sugar**
¼ **teaspoon vanilla**
¼ **teaspoon almond extract**

PER SERVING

calories	**98**
total fat	**0.9 g.**
saturated fat	**0.3 g.**
cholesterol	**2 mg.**
sodium	**153 mg.**
dietary fiber	**1.4 g.**

Cut the pineapple crosswise into 8 slices. Use a knife or small cookie cutter to remove the center core from each slice. Place 4 of the slices on dessert plates. Cut the remaining slices into small chunks.

In a blender or food processor, combine the cottage cheese, sugar, vanilla, and almond extract. Process until smooth and creamy.

Place a dollop of the cream topping in the center of each pineapple slice. Scatter the pineapple chunks around the sliced pineapple.

Makes 4 servings

Cook's Note: Some supermarkets sell pineapples already peeled, with or without the center core still in place. If the core is there, simply slide it out and discard before using.

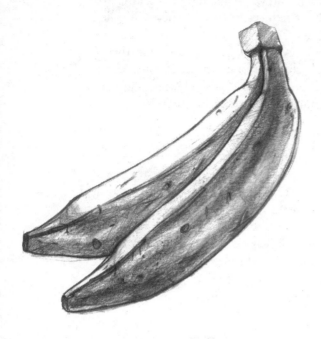

PLANTAINS
ULCER PROTECTION IN A PEEL

HEALING POWER
CAN HELP:
Lower blood pressure

Prevent and treat ulcers

Prevent constipation

Decrease the risk
of heart disease

It looks like a banana. It feels like a banana. But peel back the skin and take a bite, and you'll know it's no banana.

Though people often bunch them in the same category, comparing bananas and plantains is a bit like comparing, well, apples and oranges.

First, you can't eat plantains raw—it would be like taking a bite of uncooked potato. (Plantains are often called cooking bananas.) Second, taste isn't all that separates bananas from plantains. Plantains also pack different nutrients inside their green peels.

KEEPING YOUR PUMP PRIMED

Ounce for ounce, plantains contain more potassium than their yellow-skinned cousins, the bananas. That means that if your blood pressure has been climbing to new heights and you need to bring it down, a plateful of plantain chips is a step in the right direction.

One cup of sliced, cooked plantain delivers a potassium lode of 716 milligrams, or about 20 percent of the Daily Value (DV). Potassium has been well-established as a key mineral for heart disease prevention.

Studies have shown that people who don't get enough potassium in their diets are at much higher risks of high blood pressure, heart attacks, and strokes.

A study conducted by scientists at the University of Naples in Italy found that eating three to six servings a day of potassium-rich foods such as plantains allowed many people to reduce or even eliminate their need for blood pressure medication.

At the same time, a potassium-rich diet reduces the risk of stroke significantly—by up to 40 percent in some cases, say researchers from the University of California, San Diego, and the University of Cambridge School of Medicine in England.

Plantains can also keep your ticker in tip-top shape by helping to keep your arteries plaque-free, according to researchers. This is because potassium-rich foods like plantains appear to help prevent the body's low-density lipoprotein (LDL) cholesterol from oxidizing, the process that makes it stick to the artery walls. This may be a good defense against atherosclerosis, or hardening of the arteries, says David B. Young, Ph.D., professor of physiology and biophysics at the University of Mississippi Medical Center in Jackson.

"Studies show that you can get a significant impact from relatively small changes," says Dr. Young. "But you can never eat too many potassium-rich foods, especially since so much of our modern diet is overprocessed, so it's high in sodium and depleted of potassium."

One last word about blood pressure: One cup of cooked plantains delivers about 49 milligrams of magnesium, or more than 12 per-

IN THE KITCHEN

Like potatoes, plantains are extremely easy to work with. In fact, you can use plantains in almost exactly the same ways you use potatoes: mashed, sautéed, or baked. Their mild flavor works well in omelets, soups, and stews.

Here's some expert advice on the easiest ways to choose and prepare your plantains.

Choose your color. Like bananas, plantains change color from green to yellow to black when ripening. Even though all plantains need to be cooked before eating, the ripe, black ones are sweeter than their greener counterparts. Which you choose is a matter of taste.

Peel and simmer. When cooking plantains, first peel them as you would a banana. Remove and discard the long, fibrous strings that run alongside the vegetable. Cut into 1- or 2-inch pieces, then steam for 10 minutes. When the plantains are tender, they can be mashed or sautéed. Or simply drizzle them with a little olive oil and serve.

Cook them gently. While plantains must be cooked until tender, you don't want to cook them too long. When overcooked, they release a compound that causes a bitter taste. In fact, when adding plantains to stews, omelets, or other dishes, it's best to add them late in the cooking process to prevent the taste from turning.

cent of the DV. This is another mineral that can help keep blood pressure in check, especially among people who are sensitive to sodium.

Quenching the Flames

In India, if you go to a doctor's office clutching your stomach, you're more likely to walk out with a bag of plantain powder than a bottle of Tagamet.

Experts aren't sure how they do it, but plantains are known for their ability to both prevent and treat ulcers as well as to quell digestive upset such as flatulence and indigestion.

"There seems to be a compound in plantains that forms a protective coating on the walls of the stomach," says Robert T. Rosen, Ph.D., associate director of the Center for Advanced Food Technology at Cook College of Rutgers University, in New Brunswick, New Jersey. "But we need more research before we know exactly how it works or how much plantain is needed for the effect."

More Filling, Fewer Calories

Although they're not one of the best food sources of fiber, plantains have the distinction of being among the top foods to offer a gram of fiber for the fewest calories. To get about 1 gram of fiber, all you need is ⅒ cup of boiled, mashed plantain, for the small price of 58 skinny calories.

Serve yourself 1 cup of this starchy fruit and you'll have almost 5 grams of fiber, nearly 20 percent of the DV. Fiber has been shown to help reduce cholesterol and prevent a variety of digestive problems such as constipation and hemorrhoids.

Immunity Booster

On top of all its other disease-fighting abilities, the plantain also is filled with nutrients that strengthen the immune system. This means you'll be better able to stave off whatever illnesses come your way.

For example, 1 cup of cooked, sliced plantain contains almost 17 milligrams of vitamin C, or more than 28 percent of the DV. Vitamin C is perhaps the best known of the infection-fighting, immunity-building vitamins.

That same cup of sliced plantain also delivers 40 micrograms of folate, 10 percent of the DV; 0.4 milligram of vitamin B_6, 20 percent of the DV; and 1,400 international units of vitamin A, 28 percent of the DV.

The benefits? Folate promotes normal tissue growth and may protect against cancer, heart disease, and birth defects. Vitamin B_6 is essential to keep your nervous system working in peak condition and to increase immunity. Vitamin A also bolsters immunity, as well as safeguarding against impaired night vision and vision problems associated with aging, like macular degeneration.

Getting the Most

Go for the green. When you're eating plantains to prevent ulcers or to speed the healing of an ulcer you already have, experts advise choosing those that are green and unripe because they're thought to contain more of the healing enzymes than fruits that are a ripe yellow or black.

PLANTAINS WITH GARLIC AND THYME

2	**large green plantains**
2	**cups water**
1½	**teaspoons dried thyme**
1	**teaspoon paprika**
¼	**teaspoon salt**
4	**teaspoons olive oil**
3	**cloves garlic, minced**

PER SERVING

calories	**137**
total fat	**4.9 g.**
saturated fat	**0.8 g.**
cholesterol	**0 mg.**
sodium	**138 mg.**
dietary fiber	**2 g.**

Cut the tips off both ends of the plantains and discard. Run a knife lengthwise down a "seam" of each plantain. Peel off and discard the skin. Cut into ⅛"-thick slices.

In a large no-stick skillet over medium heat, bring the water to a boil. Add the plantains. Cover and simmer for 15 minutes, or until tender. Test for doneness by inserting the tip of a sharp knife into a slice.

With tongs or a slotted spoon, remove the plantains to paper towels to drain. Pour off the liquid from the skillet and wipe the skillet with paper towels.

In a large bowl, combine the thyme, paprika, and salt. Add the plantain slices and toss with your hands to coat.

Add the oil to the skillet and warm over medium-high heat. Add the plantain slices and spread them evenly in the skillet. Cook for 2 to 3 minutes, or until the plantains are golden on the bottom. Turn. Scatter the garlic over the plantains. Cook for another 2 to 3 minutes, or until golden on the bottom. Toss gently to coat with the garlic.

Makes 4 servings

Cook's Note: The plantains may be easier to peel if you cut them in half through the middle crosswise.

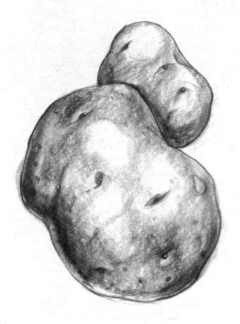

POTATOES
OUR SUPER STAPLE

HEALING POWER
CAN HELP:
Prevent cancer

Control high blood
pressure and diabetes

Early in the history of the New World, in the Andes mountains of Peru and Bolivia, the people had a thousand names for the potato. It was that important.

In the 4,000 or so years since, the starchy tuber's reputation has peaked and dipped. The Spanish conquistadors thought the new root captivating enough to take back to the Old World. (Within a few years, potatoes became standard fare on Spanish ships because they prevented scurvy.) Once the potato arrived in Europe, though, its fortunes sagged, not because of any shortcomings of its own but because of its kinship with the deadly nightshade family, plants that had the reputation for being toxic. Potatoes were feared rather than appreciated.

Eventually, though, both botanists and diners alike learned the whole story. Potatoes aren't remotely dangerous. Plus, they're a super food staple, making them the world's number one vegetable crop. In fact, it's not uncommon for people to eat potatoes, cooked in a variety of ways, with every meal.

"The potato has a little bit of almost everything," says Mark Kestin, Ph.D., chairman of the nutrition program at Bastyr University and affiliate assistant professor of epidemiology at the University of Washington, both in Seattle. "You could get many of your nutritional needs met from potatoes, if you had to," he adds.

Peel Power

A potato's healing abilities start in the peel, which contains an anticarcinogenic compound called chlorogenic acid, says Mary Ellen Camire, Ph.D., associate professor and chair of the department of food science and human nutrition at the University of Maine in Orono. In laboratory studies, this particular acid has been shown to help the fiber in potatoes absorb benzo(a)pyrene, a potential carcinogen found in smoked foods such as grilled hamburgers. "The acid in the food reacts with the carcinogen by basically binding it up and making too big a molecule for the body to absorb," she explains. "In our laboratory study, it prevented the carcinogen from being absorbed almost completely."

Slashing the Pressure

We don't normally think of potatoes as being high in potassium, but in fact, a baked 7-ounce spud contains more than twice the potassium of one medium-size banana. One baked potato with the skin will give you about 1,137 milligrams of potassium, almost a third of the Daily Value (DV).

Potassium is important because it seems to calm the spiking effect that salt has on blood pressure. For some people, increasing potassium in their diets by eating potatoes could reduce the need for blood pressure medication, notes pharmacist Earl Mindell, R.Ph., Ph.D., professor of nutrition at Pacific Western University in Los Angeles and author of *Earl Mindell's Food as Medicine*. In one study of 54 people with high blood pressures, half added potassium-rich foods like potatoes to their diets, while the other half continued to eat their normal fare. By the end of the study, Dr. Mindell says, 81 percent of the potato-eaters were able to control their blood pressures with less than half the medication they had used previously.

Blood Sugar Savior

We don't think of vitamin C as affecting our blood sugar, but there's emerging evidence that this powerful antioxidant vitamin, well-known for helping prevent heart disease, may be of help to people with diabetes. On top of this, vitamin C may also be effective in diminishing the damage to proteins caused by free radicals, dangerous oxygen molecules that damage tissues in the body.

In one study, researchers in the Netherlands found that men eating healthy diets, which were high not only in potatoes but also in fish, vegetables, and legumes, appeared to have a lower risk for diabetes. It's not yet clear what the protective mechanism is, but researchers speculate that antioxidants, including vitamin C, may play a role in keeping excess sugar out of the bloodstream. One

IN THE KITCHEN

Potatoes aren't all created equal. Some taste better baked, while others are good for soups or salads. A third type, the all-purpose potato, has been "designed" both for baking and steaming. The next time you're at the supermarket, here's what to look for.

Waxy potatoes. Known as round whites or round reds, waxy potatoes are low in starch and high in moisture. They keep their shape well during cooking, making them a good choice for soups, stews, and salads.

Starchy potatoes. The russet potato is a common type of starchy spud. It has a mealy, floury interior, which works well for mashing or baking.

All-purpose potatoes. Spuds like long whites are great to keep on the shelf because they can be prepared any way—baked, boiled, or steamed.

7-ounce potato contains about 27 milligrams of vitamin C, about 45 percent of the DV.

Because potatoes are high in complex carbohydrates, they're also good for people who already have diabetes. Complex carbohydrates must be broken down into simple sugars before they're absorbed into the bloodstream. This means that the sugars enter the bloodstream in a leisurely fashion rather than pouring in all at once. This, in turn, helps keep blood sugar levels stable, which is a critical part of controlling the disease.

Further, potatoes can be key players in helping people with diabetes keep their weight down, an important benefit since being overweight makes it more difficult for the body to produce enough insulin, the hormone that helps transport sugars out of the bloodstream and into individual cells. At the same time, being overweight makes the insulin that the body does produce work less efficiently. What potatoes do is keep you full so that you're less likely to be hungry later on.

In a study of 41 hungry students at the University of Sydney in Australia, researchers found that spuds filled them up more than other foods, while at the same time delivering fewer calories. On a satiety scale that measured white bread at 100, oatmeal at 209, and fish at 225, potatoes were way ahead at 323.

Getting the Most

Keep the peel. To take advantage of potatoes' cancer-fighting abilities, you really have to eat the peel, says Dr. Camire. This can be particularly important when eating grilled foods, which leave small amounts of cancer-causing substances on the food. It would be nice if you could get a fast-food burger on a potato-peel bun, says Dr. Camire. "That would help absorb the carcinogens from the grilling," she says.

A more practical solution is simply to add a baked potato or potato salad (with the peel) to your plate whenever you eat a grilled hamburger, a hot dog, or other smoky foods.

Cook them carefully. Although boiling is one of the most popular cooking methods for potatoes, it's perhaps the worst choice for preserving nutrients, since vitamin C and some B vitamins are pulled out of the potatoes and into the cooking water. In fact, boiling potatoes can result in losing about half the vitamin C, a quarter of the folate, and 40 percent of the potassium, says Marilyn A. Swanson, R.D., Ph.D., professor and head of the department of nutrition and food science at South Dakota State University in Brookings.

If you do boil potatoes, you can recapture some of the nutrients by saving the cooking water and adding it to other foods such as soups and stews.

Baking and steaming do a good job of tenderizing potatoes, while at the same time preserving more of their nutrients. "Microwaving is your first choice," says Susan Thom, R.D., a resource spokesperson for the American Dietetic Association and a nutrition consultant in Brecksville, Ohio.

Prepare them late. Busy cooks have traditionally peeled and sliced potatoes ahead of time, then submerged them in water to keep them from darkening. This may keep potatoes looking fresh, but it also strips valuable nutrients. "You lose some of the soluble vitamins in the water," says Mona Sutnick, R.D., a nutrition consultant in Philadelphia and a spokesperson for the American Dietetic Association.

BARBECUE OVEN FRIES

4	medium baking potatoes
2½	tablespoons ketchup
4	teaspoons canola oil
2	teaspoons Worcestershire sauce
2	teaspoons cider vinegar
⅛	teaspoon salt

PER SERVING
calories	**185**
total fat	**4.7 g.**
saturated fat	**0.3 g.**
cholesterol	**0 mg.**
sodium	**218 mg.**
dietary fiber	**3 g.**

Preheat the oven to 425°F. Coat a baking sheet with no-stick spray.

Scrub the potatoes and pat dry with paper towels. Cut each potato lengthwise into 5 or 6 slices, then stack the slices and cut at ¼" intervals to make french fries.

In a large bowl, combine the ketchup, oil, Worcestershire sauce, vinegar, and salt. Add the potatoes. Toss to coat.

Spread the potatoes evenly on the baking sheet. Bake for 20 minutes. Turn the potatoes. Bake for 10 to 15 minutes, or until tender and golden. Test for doneness by inserting the tip of a sharp knife in a potato.

Makes 4 servings

Microwaved Potatoes
with Marinated Shrimp

4   **large baking potatoes**

12   **ounces peeled deveined and cooked shrimp**

2½ **tablespoons extra-virgin olive oil**

2   **tablespoons fresh lemon juice**

2   **teaspoons dried basil**

¼ **teaspoon salt**

Per serving

calories	**340**
total fat	**9.3 g.**
saturated fat	**1.4 g.**
cholesterol	**121 mg.**
sodium	**287 mg.**
dietary fiber	**4.6 g.**

Scrub the potatoes and pat dry with paper towels. With a fork, pierce each in 3 or 4 places. Arrange the potatoes, spoke fashion, in the microwave on a paper towel. Microwave on high power for 10 minutes. Turn the potatoes and rotate from the front to the back of the microwave (if your oven does not have a carousel.) Microwave for 8 to 10 minutes, or until the potatoes are tender. Test for doneness by inserting the tip of a small sharp knife in a potato. Let the potatoes stand for 5 minutes.

Meanwhile, place the shrimp in a medium bowl. Add the oil, lemon juice, basil, and salt. Set aside for 10 minutes to allow the flavors to blend.

Cut the potatoes lengthwise down the center and squeeze to open. Spoon the shrimp mixture over them.

Makes 4 main-dish servings

Cook's Note: If desired, mince a clove of garlic and add to the shrimp mixture.

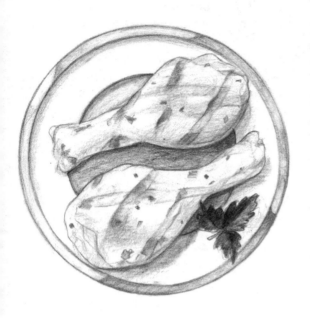

POULTRY
BIRDS FOR STRONG BLOOD

HEALING POWER
CAN HELP:
Prevent iron-deficiency anemia

Prevent vision loss

Maintain a healthy nervous system

Prevent energy and memory problems

Keep immunity strong

Americans have long considered poultry to be a sign of prosperity. During the Depression, Franklin Delano Roosevelt promised a chicken in every pot. And every Thanksgiving we gather around a dressed turkey and show appreciation for our blessings.

A bird on the table is more than just a symbol, however. Properly prepared, poultry is an important part of a healthful diet. Without the skin, poultry not only is a low-fat alternative to fattier meats like beef and pork but also provides a host of disease-fighting, energy-boosting vitamins and minerals that are difficult to get from plant foods alone.

Of course, there is one caveat: That healthy piece of poultry may become a permanent part of your waistline unless you remove the skin before taking a bite. This is particularly true when buying fast food or the rotisserie birds served at popular chain restaurants. For example, researchers found that a half-chicken platter at Boston Market rivaled a Big Mac, served with large fries and a chocolate milkshake, in fat, sodium, and calories.

A B VITAMIN BOOST

Most of us understand the importance of getting our daily fill of the vitamin all-stars, like vitamins C and E and beta-carotene. But ask someone what the B vi-

In the Kitchen

Chefs agree that the trick to making perfect poultry is to cook the bird in the skin. The melting fat from skin acts like a natural baste, keeping the meat flavorful and moist during the long cooking process.

"Poultry can be horribly dry when you cook it without the skin," says Susan Kleiner, R.D., Ph.D., owner of High Performance Nutrition in Mercer Island, Washington. "And studies show that as long as you remove the skin when it's done cooking, the fat content of the poultry is about the same as if you had removed it beforehand."

tamins are good for, and you'll likely get a blank stare.

That's because these unsung heroes of the vitamin world don't directly prevent major health problems like heart disease and cancer—though they certainly may lend a helping hand. Mostly, they're maintenance workers; in a lot of little ways, they keep our minds and bodies working smoothly. Take away the B vitamins and you'd find yourself fumbling through life, depressed, confused, anemic, and nervous—or worse.

Luckily, poultry is bursting with three essential B vitamins: niacin, vitamin B_6, and vitamin B_{12}.

Depending on the part of the bird you pick, chicken and turkey provide between 16 and 62 percent of the Daily Value (DV) of 20 milligrams for niacin. (Chicken breast is at the high end of the scale, and turkey dark meat is at the low end.) Studies show that it may reduce cholesterol and cut the risk for heart attacks.

Poultry also contains 0.3 microgram of vitamin B_{12}, 5 percent of the DV. Vitamin B_{12}, which is found almost solely in animal foods, is essential for healthy brain function. Get too little B_{12} and you may find yourself feeling fatigued and experiencing memory loss and other neurological problems.

Another B vitamin, B_6, is critical for maintaining immunity. It's also necessary for making red blood cells and maintaining a healthy nervous system. Poultry provides between 0.2 and 0.5 milligram of vitamin B_6, 10 to 25 percent of the DV.

Metal for Your Mettle

When knights went into battle, they donned suits of armor to make them stronger. Though none of us are jousting these days, we still need iron for the everyday battles of life. We just need to eat it, not wear it.

Iron is one of the most important nutrients for maximum energy and vitality. Yet many of us, especially women, fall short of the 15 milligrams needed each day, says Susan Kleiner, R.D., Ph.D., owner of High Performance Nutrition in Mercer Island, Washington.

You can get between 5 and 16 percent of the iron you need each day by

Take Flight on the Wild Side

Have you eaten so much chicken that you're starting to resemble Frank Purdue? Maybe it's time to leave the pedestrian poultry behind and take flight with some birds of a different feather. Although they tend to be higher-priced, birds like pheasant and quail add variety to your diet while providing the same nutritional benefits as chicken or turkey.

Here's how two of the less common varieties of poultry add up. All nutritional information is based on 3-ounce servings, and the percentages of the Daily Values (DV) or, in the case of iron, the Recommended Dietary Allowance (RDA), are given.

Pheasant		**Quail**	
Calories	113	Calories	123
Fat	3 grams	Fat	4 grams
Calories from fat	25 percent	Calories from fat	31 percent
Iron	1 milligram (10 percent of RDA for men and 7 percent for women)	Iron	4 milligrams (40 percent of RDA for men and 27 percent for women)
Niacin	6 milligrams (30 percent of DV)	Niacin	8 milligrams (40 percent of DV)
Vitamin B_6	0.6 milligram (30 percent of DV)	Vitamin B_6	0.5 milligram (25 percent of DV)
Vitamin B_{12}	0.7 microgram (12 percent of DV)	Thiamin	0.3 milligram (20 percent of DV)
Zinc	0.8 milligram (5 percent of DV)	Zinc	3 milligrams (20 percent of DV)
Riboflavin	0.1 milligram (8 percent of DV)	Riboflavin	0.3 milligram (18 percent of DV)
Vitamin C	5 milligrams (6 percent of DV)	Vitamin C	7 milligrams (12 percent of DV)

eating a piece of poultry. About 3 ounces of chicken leg or white-meat turkey breast provides 1.2 milligrams of iron, 8 percent of the Recommended Dietary Allowance (RDA) for women. Three ounces of roasted turkey dark meat will give you 2.0 milligrams, 13 percent of a woman's RDA.

Food Alert
Infection Protection

Poultry is packed with more than essential vitamins and minerals. It's also a playground for microorganisms, particularly salmonella, a type of bacteria that can cause food poisoning.

There's no way to eliminate bacteria entirely, but there are ways to keep your poultry safe and healthy. Here's what experts advise.

Clean up frequently. When you're working with raw poultry, bacteria readily pass from the bird to cutting boards and utensils—and back to you. To prevent bacteria from multiplying, scrub your tools and work area thoroughly and often, using soap and warm water.

Keep it cold. Since salmonellae breed rapidly at room temperature, experts recommend defrosting poultry in the refrigerator, not on the countertop. The same goes for marinating your bird: Do it in the refrigerator, not on the counter. In addition, never reuse poultry marinade, because it's often contaminated after prolonged contact with the bird, experts say.

Cook it clear. To kill all the bacteria, it's important to cook poultry thoroughly, say experts. When you slice the meat, it should be completely white, or brown if it's dark meat, with no signs of pink. The same goes for the juices. If you press on the meat, the juices should be clear, not pink. To assure safety, use a meat thermometer to check the bird for an internal temperature of 140°F.

Although iron abounds in fortified cereals, tofu, beans, and other nonmeat foods, it's not always easy for the body to absorb. By contrast, the iron in poultry (called heme iron) is easily absorbed, says Dr. Kleiner. Your body can absorb up to 15 percent more heme iron than nonheme iron, she explains. Plus, when you eat heme iron, it helps your body absorb nonheme iron. That way, you get the most iron from all your food, says Dr. Kleiner.

In the Pink with Zinc

In order to stay in the pink—free from infections, colds, and other health problems that keep us home in bed watching bad daytime TV—we need strong immune systems. Getting enough zinc in the diet is critical for immunity because our infection-fighting cells require adequate stores of this trace mineral to do their job.

In addition, studies show that getting enough zinc can help slow the progression of a prevalent eye disorder called macular degeneration, which can cause irreversible vision loss, especially among the elderly.

As with iron, zinc is found in foods besides meat, like whole grains and wheat germ—but again, your body has a harder time absorbing it from plant foods than from meats, says Dr. Kleiner. "Women especially are at risk for not getting enough zinc," she says.

Eating poultry will help keep your zinc supply at the necessary levels, Dr. Kleiner says. Most poultry provides 6 to 25 percent of the 15 milligrams of zinc you need each day.

Getting the Most

Grab a drumstick. Lots of people pick around the dark meat of their poultry because it's higher in fat. And that's true, concedes Dr. Kleiner, but it's also a lot higher in minerals and, therefore, worth digging into occasionally.

"If you've removed the skin, you've removed the mother lode of fat anyway," she says, "and a lot of the iron and zinc are in the dark meat."

WESTERN-STYLE DRUMSTICKS

8   chicken drumsticks
1   tablespoon paprika
1   tablespoon Worcestershire sauce
2   teaspoons packed light brown sugar
1/2 teaspoon ground red pepper
1/2 teaspoon onion powder
1/4 teaspoon celery seeds

PER SERVING
calories	**167**
total fat	**5.3 g.**
saturated fat	**1.4 g.**
cholesterol	**82 mg.**
sodium	**127 mg.**
dietary fiber	**0.4 g.**

Preheat the broiler. Coat the broiler pan with no-stick spray. Loosen the skin on each drumstick but do not remove.

In a small bowl, combine the paprika, Worcestershire sauce, brown sugar, pepper, onion powder, and celery seeds to make a thick paste. Smear evenly over the meat of the drumsticks, under the skin. Pull up the skin to cover as much of the drumstick as possible. Place the drumsticks on the broiler pan.

Broil 6" from the heat for 8 to 10 minutes per side, or until the drumsticks are no longer pink in the center. Test for doneness by inserting the tip of a sharp knife in the thickest part of a drumstick. Remove the skin before serving.

Makes 4 servings

Turkey Cutlets with Oregano and Lemon

1 pound turkey breast cutlets

3 tablespoons unbleached all-purpose flour

1/8 teaspoon salt

3/4 teaspoon teaspoon dried oregano

1 tablespoon olive oil

2 cloves garlic, minced

1/4 cup defatted reduced-sodium chicken broth

3 tablespoons fresh lemon juice

Per serving

calories	**184**
total fat	**4.6 g.**
saturated fat	**0.8 g.**
cholesterol	**77 mg.**
sodium	**124 mg.**
dietary fiber	**0.3 g.**

Rinse the turkey and pat dry.

On a plate, combine the flour, salt, and 1/2 teaspoon of the oregano. Mix with a fork. Place the turkey cutlets in the flour mixture, turning to dust both sides evenly. Shake off the excess.

Warm the oil in a large no-stick skillet over medium-high heat. Add the cutlets in a single layer and cook for 2 to 3 minutes per side, or until golden and cooked through. Check for doneness by inserting the tip of a sharp knife into a cutlet. Remove the turkey to a clean plate.

Add the garlic to the skillet and cook for 10 to 12 seconds, or until fragrant. Add the broth, lemon juice, and the remaining 1/4 teaspoon oregano. Cook, stirring, for 2 to 3 minutes, or until hot. Pour over the turkey.

Makes 4 servings

PREMENSTRUAL PROBLEMS
FOODS FOR MONTHLY DISCOMFORT

There's probably not a woman in the country who doesn't know what "PMS" means. Yet these three letters describe a condition that's as misunderstood as it is common.

PMS, or premenstrual syndrome, is believed to affect between one-third and one-half of American women of childbearing age. There are more than 150 symptoms that may occur in women with PMS, including anxiety, breast tenderness, and food cravings. Some women get only one or two symptoms, while others are plagued by a dozen. Discomfort usually begins 10 days to two weeks before menstruation and eases when menstruation begins.

Doctors used to believe PMS was "all in your head." They don't think that any more. But they still aren't sure exactly what causes the dizzying array of physical and emotional problems. A variety of factors are probably involved, including swings in hormones (estrogen and progesterone), blood sugar, and the brain chemical serotonin.

Even though there's still a lot of mystery surrounding this condition, one thing is clear: What you eat can make a big difference in how you feel before your period. Here are some nutritional strategies for easing the discomfort.

CALMING CARBOHYDRATES

One of the most common symptoms of PMS is the urge to binge on sugary foods, which, in turn, can lead to weight gain as well as depression and mood swings.

It's not surprising that the sweet tooth often wakes up at a woman's time of the month. In women with PMS, that's when the body's blood sugar level is often low, explains Susan M. Lark, M.D., director of the PMS and Menopause Self-Help Center in Los Altos, California, in her book *The PMS Self-Help Book*. It's not certain why this occurs, although it appears that insulin, which moves

Smart Swaps

There are many foods (and substances in foods) that can aggravate premenstrual pain. The problem, for many women, is how to go an entire week or more without enjoying their usual favorites. Here are some of the more-common culprits, along with some satisfying alternatives.

- Breast tenderness and increased irritability and anxiety can be caused by caffeine. Try caffeine-free colas or decaffeinated coffee, or coffee substitutes such as Postum.
- Too much salt can cause the body to retain fluids, increasing bloating and breast tenderness. Try flavoring foods with additional herbs, spices, or nonsalt seasonings, such as Mrs. Dash, and use low-salt canned and processed foods.
- Chocolate can often aggravate mood swings and breast tenderness. Use unsweetened carob instead.

glucose out of the bloodstream into individual cells, works more efficiently as menstruation approaches. With less glucose circulating in the bloodstream, there's less available to the brain. The brain, noting that it's low on fuel, lets the body know that it needs more, which, in body talk, loosely translates as "I need cookies!"

To quiet your body's clamor for sugar without raiding the cookie jar, it's helpful to eat complex carbohydrates. Because they're absorbed more slowly than the sugars in sweets, they help stabilize your blood sugar. And that, in turn, controls sugar cravings.

Another way in which complex carbohydrates ease premenstrual discomfort is by increasing the brain's level of serotonin, a calming chemical that regulates mood and sleep. In a small study conducted at the Massachusetts Institute of Technology in Cambridge, women with PMS reported that eating a carbohydrate-rich meal lightened their premenstrual depression, tension, and sadness and made them feel more calm and alert.

Some doctors recommend that women with premenstrual discomfort eat a small amount of pasta, cereal, or whole-grain bread every 3 hours, which will help keep blood sugar from falling too low. In one study, 54 percent of women who consumed a starch-based mini-meal such as bread, crackers, or cereal every 3 hours had less premenstrual discomfort.

For some women, however, it's important to avoid wheat during this time. Wheat contains gluten, a protein that tends to increase premenstrual bloating and weight gain. If this appears to be a problem for you, Dr. Lark advises that you may want to stick with rice, millet, or other nonwheat grains before your period.

There's no reason to limit yourself to bread and crackers when you're trying to get more carbohydrates. Having a bowl of whole-grain cereal, like granola or oatmeal, will keep you full while also keeping your sweet tooth under control. Rice cakes also make a good snack, particularly when topped with a little peanut butter or preserves. Dried beans are also good sources of complex carbohydrates.

Fruits and vegetables are other excellent sources of complex carbohydrates. Plus, they're low in calories, so you can eat them often without worrying about your weight. Dr. Lark particularly recommends eating root vegetables, such as carrots, turnips, and parsnips, and leafy green vegetables like collard and mustard greens, all of which are rich in magnesium and calcium—nutrients that have been shown to ease premenstrual discomfort.

While most fruits are good for women with PMS, tropical varieties like mangoes, papayas, and pineapple are unusually high in sugar. This means they can aggravate rather than relieve food cravings. As your period approaches, you may want to stick with homegrown fruits such as apples, oranges, or grapefruits.

COOKING FOR HEALTH

While there are many foods that worsen premenstrual discomfort, there are a few that make it better. Tofu, tempeh, and other foods made from soybeans can be excellent choices.

According to Susan M. Lark M.D., director of the PMS and Menopause Self-Help Center in Los Altos, California, soy foods contain compounds called phytoestrogens. These plant estrogens are similar to but weaker than the estrogen women produce naturally. Paradoxically, when you eat these compounds in soy, estrogen levels in the body decline, helping relieve the discomfort of PMS.

"PMS is much less common in Asian countries because women eat more vegetable protein like tofu and not so much animal protein," adds Guy Abraham, M.D., former professor of obstetrics and gynecology at the University of California, Los Angeles.

THE ROLE OF FAT

Just as women often crave sweets as their periods approach, many also get a hankering for high-fat foods like doughnuts, potato chips, or ice cream. Indeed, women in the throes of PMS can get as much as 40 percent of their calories from fat, says Guy Abraham, M.D., former professor of obstetrics and gynecology at the University of California, Los Angeles.

More is involved than just the extra calories. The kind of fat you eat before your period—and how much of it you eat—can affect the severity of your symptoms. The worst kind of fat, not surprisingly, is the saturated kind found in meats, whole-fat dairy foods, and many processed foods. Saturated fat causes estrogen levels to rise, which worsens virtually all PMS symptoms, says Dr. Abraham. Conversely, evidence suggests that women who eat a lot of fruit, vegetables, and whole grains but little or no meat tend to have fewer premenstrual symptoms than their carnivorous sisters.

All women, not just those with PMS, are advised to limit their consumption of fat to no more than 30 percent of total calories, with 10 percent coming from saturated fat and the rest from unsaturated fat, says Dr. Abraham.

Researchers are now looking into whether omega-3 fatty acids, fats that are found in certain types of fish and canola and flaxseed oils, may play a role in PMS. Preliminary evidence suggests that having too few omega-3's and too much linoleic acid (an unsaturated fat) in your system can lead to an overproduction of a certain type of prostaglandin. This hormone-like compound can cause menstrual cramps.

Because we get so much linoleic acid from oils such as corn and safflower, some nutritionists suggest getting more omega-3's from fish such as salmon, mackerel and tuna. You can also try using a little canola oil in cooking and using flaxseed oil in salad dressing.

In practical terms, this means using olive oil instead of butter and substituting such things as bagels and low-fat cream cheese for high-fat doughnuts and other snack foods. Even simple changes will help keep estrogen levels stable, thus easing the monthly woes.

CALCIUM FOR CRAMPS

While food cravings are a common symptom of PMS, they're by no means the only one. Many women also get headaches, cramps, and bloating. If this sounds familiar, you may want to pour an extra glass of low-fat milk, because getting more calcium before your period may reduce the symptoms.

In one study, researchers at the U.S. Department of Agriculture Human Nutrition Research Center in Grand Forks, North Dakota, put some women on a low-calcium diet (587 milligrams of calcium a day), while others got more calcium (1,336 milligrams a day). Seventy percent of the women on the high-calcium diet said they had fewer backaches and cramping, 80 percent felt less bloated, and 90 percent said they were less irritable or depressed.

Calcium works in a number of ways. It may help prevent the muscular contractions that cause cramping, says study leader James G. Penland, Ph.D. In addition, "calcium clearly has an impact on certain brain chemicals and hormones known to affect mood," he says.

Throughout your cycle, Dr. Penland says, it's a good idea to begin increasing your consumption of low-fat, calcium-rich foods such as skim or low-fat milk and low-fat yogurt. You don't need massive amounts to get the benefits.

The women on the high-calcium diet were getting just 336 milligrams more calcium a day than the Daily Value (DV) of 1,000 milligrams. That's about the amount of calcium in 1 cup of skim milk.

MAGNESIUM FOR MOOD SWINGS

Calcium isn't the only mineral that affects brain chemistry. A number of studies have found that women with PMS tend to have low levels of magnesium. Being low on magnesium can result in lower levels of dopamine, a brain chemical that, like serotonin, helps regulate mood, says Melvyn Werbach, M.D., assistant clinical professor of psychiatry at the University of California, Los Angeles, and author of *Nutritional Influences on Illness* and *Healing through Nutrition*. "A magnesium deficiency might also impair the metabolism of estrogen," another cause of premenstrual moodiness, he says.

In an Italian study, 28 women with PMS took 360 milligrams of magnesium a day. After two months they reported having less depression, bloating, cramps, and other premenstrual symptoms.

The DV for magnesium is 400 milligrams, an amount that's easy to get in food. A serving of instant oatmeal, for example, has 28 milligrams of magnesium, 7 percent of the DV. A banana has 33 milligrams, 8 percent of the DV, and a fillet of baked or broiled flounder has 49 milligrams, 12 percent of the DV. Brown rice is another great source of magnesium, with a half-cup providing 42 milligrams, 11 percent of the DV. Whole grains and green, leafy vegetables are also high in this mineral.

RELIEVE MOODINESS WITH B6

Yet another nutrient that can help stop the emotional swings of PMS is vitamin B6. In an English study, 32 women with PMS took 50 milligrams of vitamin B6 a day for three months. They reported having less depression, irritability, and fatigue. It may be that high doses of vitamin B6 bring premenstrual hormones into balance by lowering levels of estrogen and raising those of progesterone. And since vitamin B6 is used by the body to manufacture serotonin, taking supplements may help reduce depression, Dr. Werbach says.

Don't be concerned that the amount of B6 used in the study is so much higher than the DV of 2 milligrams. Taking 50 milligrams a day is entirely safe, says Dr. Werbach. If you're going to take more than that, however, it's essential to check with your doctor.

You don't have to take supplements in order to get more vitamin B6, says Dr. Werbach. A meal consisting of 3 ounces of boneless chicken breast, a baked potato with the skin, and a banana, for example, contains nearly 2 milligrams, 100 percent of the DV.

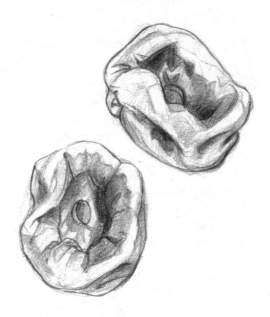

PRUNES
NATURE'S LAXATIVE

HEALING POWER

CAN HELP:
Relieve constipation

Lower cholesterol

Reduce the risk of cancer
and heart disease

Prunes have an image problem. After all, these wrinkled, purple fruits are best known as a home remedy for constipation—not exactly a sexy angle for a snazzy marketing campaign. In fact, in an effort to burnish the prune's reputation, members of the prune industry have begun to call them dried plums.

It's unfortunate that the prune's dowdy image has prevented it from being more widely enjoyed. It may not be the most glamorous fruit on the market, but it's certainly one of the healthiest.

NATURE'S LAXATIVE

Pharmacies stock dozens of medications for preventing and relieving constipation. But most of the time they really aren't necessary if you get in the habit of adding prunes to your daily diet. Prunes contain not just one but three different ingredients that work together to help keep your digestive system on track.

For starters, prunes are high in insoluble fiber, which is perhaps the key to preventing constipation. Since insoluble fiber isn't absorbed by your body, it stays in the digestive tract. And because it's incredibly absorbent, it soaks up large amounts of water, making stools larger and easier to pass. (Prunes also contain soluble fiber, the type that helps lower cholesterol and with it the risk of heart disease.) Just five prunes contain almost 3 grams of fiber, about 12 percent of the Daily Value (DV).

In addition, prunes contain a natural sugar called sorbitol. Like fiber, sorbitol soaks up water wherever it can find it, says Mary Ellen Camire, Ph.D., associate professor and chair of the department of food science and human nutrition at the University of Maine in Orono. Most fruits contain small amounts (usually less than 1 percent) of sorbitol. Prunes, however, are about 15 percent sorbitol, which explains why they're such a potent bulking agent and are often recommended for relieving constipation.

Finally, prunes contain a compound called dihydroxyphenyl isatin, which stimulates the intestine, causing it to contract. This process is essential for having regular bowel movements.

You don't need a lot of prunes to get the benefits. One daily serving—about five prunes—is all most people need to help themselves stay regular.

IN THE KITCHEN

While prunes are best known as a breakfast food, savvy chefs often use them as fat substitutes in the kitchen. Pureed prunes can be used to replace the butter, margarine, or oil in baked goods, cutting fat by as much as 90 percent, but without sacrificing the rich taste and texture that usually come from fat.

To use prunes for baking, put about 25 pitted prunes (8 ounces) in the blender, add 6 tablespoons of water, and puree. Begin by replacing 1 tablespoon of fat in the recipe with an equal amount of prune puree. Keep experimenting, replacing more and more of the fat until you get a taste and texture that's right for you. Leftover prune puree will keep for several weeks, covered, in the refrigerator.

ALL-AROUND PROTECTION

As with most fruits, prunes contain generous amounts of a variety of vitamins, minerals, and other healthful compounds. In fact, they're a concentrated source of energy because they lose water during the drying process. This means that you get a lot of value in a very small package.

One of the most healthful compounds in prunes is beta-carotene. Like vitamins C and E, beta-carotene is an antioxidant, meaning that it helps neutralize harmful oxygen molecules in the body. Prunes also contain generous amounts of potassium, a mineral that's essential for keeping blood pressure down. Studies have shown that when potassium levels decline, even for short periods of time, blood pressure rises. Prunes are a very good source of potassium, with five prunes containing 313 milligrams, about 9 percent of the DV.

Getting the Most

For vitamins, drink the juice. Although prune juice has less fiber than the whole fruit, it's a more concentrated source of vitamins. For example, five whole prunes contain more than 1 milligram of vitamin C, while a 6-ounce glass of juice contains almost 8 milligrams.

For regularity, eat the fruit. Since fiber is such an important part of digestive health, doctors recommend eating whole prunes, either fresh or canned, when you're trying to stay regular. While prune juice has also been used to help relieve constipation, it's somewhat less effective than the whole fruit.

BAKED CHICKEN WITH PRUNES

1 **pound skinless, boneless chicken breast halves**

¼ **cup red wine**

16 **pitted prunes**

1 **teaspoon minced fresh rosemary**

¼ **teaspoon salt**

Ground black pepper

PER SERVING

calories	**215**
total fat	**2.9 g.**
saturated fat	**0.8 g.**
cholesterol	**63 mg.**
sodium	**190 mg.**
dietary fiber	**3.3 g.**

Preheat the oven to 350°F.

Coat a 12″ × 8″ baking dish with no-stick spray. Arrange the chicken in the dish in a single layer.

In a small microwaveable bowl, combine the wine and prunes. Microwave on high power for 1 minute, or until the wine boils. Pour over the chicken. Sprinkle with the rosemary.

Bake for 30 minutes, or until the chicken is no longer pink in the center. Test for doneness by inserting the tip of a sharp knife in the center of a breast half. Sprinkle with the salt. Season with the pepper to taste. Stir the pan juices to combine the spices.

Makes 4 servings

PSORIASIS
FOODS TO STOP THE SCALES

You would think that the skin you have today is the same skin you had yesterday and the day before. But every day, millions of skin cells die, are shed, and then are replaced by healthy cells.

But in people with psoriasis, the body makes far too many skin cells, producing them about five times faster than average, which causes the skin to get thick and scaly. Doctors aren't sure what causes psoriasis, although it appears that the immune system may damage genetic material that tells skin cells how often to divide.

There's some evidence that eating more produce can help control psoriasis. In a study of more than 680 people, researchers at the University of Milan in Italy found that those who ate the most carrots, tomatoes, fresh fruits, and green vegetables were much less likely to get psoriasis than folks who ate less. In fact, eating just three or more servings of carrots a week reduced the risk of psoriasis by 40 percent. Those who ate seven or more servings of tomatoes a week reduced their risk by 60 percent, and those who had two servings a day of fresh fruits reduced their risk by 50 percent.

Since carrots, tomatoes, and fruits are all important sources of beta-carotene and vitamins C and E, the researchers speculate that it's the antioxidant and immune-stimulating effects of these foods that may make the difference.

HEALING OILS

For a long time, researchers have suspected that eating certain types of fish can help ease psoriasis. A British study, for example, found that people with psoriasis who ate 6 ounces of fish such as salmon, mackerel, and herring a day had a 15 percent improvement in symptoms in just six weeks.

These and other cold-water fish contain a type of fat called omega-3 fatty acids, which appear to reduce the body's production of prostaglandins and leukotrienes, compounds that can cause skin inflammation. While eating fish certainly won't cure psoriasis, it may provide added relief when you're already receiving other psoriasis treatments. Salmon is a particularly good choice because it's high in omega-3's.

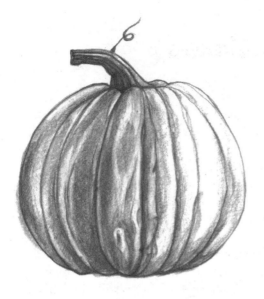

PUMPKIN
THE BETA-CAROTENE KING

HEALING POWER

CAN HELP:
Prevent macular degeneration

Boost immune system

Prevent heart disease and cancer

We have pumpkin at morning and pumpkin at noon.
If it were not for pumpkin, we should be undoon.

This is a poem that the early American colonists chanted whenever they were overcome with appreciation for this oversize orange squash. Pumpkin was a popular food back then, and the early settlers ate a peck of it in pumpkin soup, pumpkin pie, and even pumpkin beer.

It's a different story now. We usually buy pumpkin as a Halloween decoration and then throw away the meat. If we actually eat pumpkin at all, it's mainly in Thanksgiving and Christmas pies.

That's a darn shame, since pumpkin is more than just a giant winter squash and a whittler's delight. It's also filled with powerful carotenoids like beta-carotene, which can help stop cellular damage before it leads to disease.

GOOD FOR THE EYES—AND MORE

It's not just due to its size that pumpkin is called the king of squash. A half-cup of canned pumpkin has more than 16 milligrams of beta-carotene, 160 to 260 percent of the daily amount recommended by experts. Pumpkin is also a source of lesser-known carotenoids such as lutein and zeaxanthin.

Carotenoids, which create the orange color of pumpkin, help protect the body by neutralizing harmful oxygen molecules known as free radicals. "Lutein and zeaxanthin are very potent free radical scavengers," says Paul Lachance, Ph.D., professor of nutrition and chairman of the department of food science at Rutgers University in New Brunswick, New Jersey. A diet high in antioxidants can help prevent many of the diseases associated with aging, including heart disease and cancer.

Lutein and zeaxanthin aren't found only in pumpkin; they are also found in the lenses of the eyes. Studies suggest that eating foods high in these compounds may help block the formation of cataracts.

In one study, scientists at the Massachusetts Eye and Ear Infirmary in Boston compared the diets of elderly people who had advanced macular degeneration, a condition that leads to blurred vision, to the diets of those without the disease. The researchers found that those who ate the most carotenoid-rich foods had a 43 percent lower risk of getting this condition than folks who ate the least. Among people who already had macular degeneration, those who got the most carotenoids in their diets were less likely to develop a more serious form of the disease.

The beta-carotene in pumpkin helps protect the plant itself from diseases, from getting too much sunlight, and from other naturally occurring stresses. There's strong evidence that beta-carotene can help protect people from a variety of conditions as well. Research has shown, for example,

IN THE KITCHEN

Because of their size and perfect carvability, pumpkins have been destined to spend their lives on front porches rather than on dinner plates.

But pumpkins, despite their ornamental nature, are still squash, which means that they can be eaten whole, mashed, or cut into chunks for a hearty stew.

- To bake pumpkin, cut it in half (or, if it's large, into quarters), scoop out the seeds, and place the pieces, cut side down, in a baking pan. Add a little water to prevent scorching and bake at 350°F for 45 to 60 minutes, or until easily pierced with a knife.
- To speed cooking time, pumpkin can be cut into smaller pieces and either baked in the oven, steamed, or microwaved.
- When using pumpkin for a pie, soup, or stew, you have to remove the skin. The easiest way to do this is to prepare the pumpkin for baking, then bake in a 350°F oven until the flesh is slightly soft. When the pumpkin is cool enough to handle, scoop or cut out the flesh. Discard the skin and proceed with the recipe.

that getting more beta-carotene in the diet can help protect against a variety of cancers, including cancers of the stomach, esophagus, lungs, and colon. This protective effect is enhanced by phenolic acids, which are chemicals in pumpkin that bind to potential carcinogens and help prevent them from being absorbed.

The beta-carotene in pumpkin may play a role in preventing heart disease as well. Some research suggests that people with diets high in fruits and vegetables that contain beta-carotene have a lower risk of heart disease than those whose diets supplied less.

THE WHOLE PICTURE

In addition to its rich stores of beta-carotene and other phytonutrients, pumpkin contains generous amounts of fiber. For example, while 1 cup of cornflakes contains 1 gram of fiber, a half-cup of canned pumpkin contains more than 3 grams, 6 percent of the Daily Value.

Iron is another pumpkin mainstay. A half-cup of pumpkin provides almost 2 milligrams of iron, about 20 percent of the Recommended Dietary Allowance (RDA) for men and 13 percent of the RDA for women. This is particularly important for women, who need to replenish their iron regularly due to menstruation.

Even richer in iron than the flesh are the pumpkin's seeds. One ounce—which consists of about 140 seeds, a huge handful—contains about 4 milligrams of iron, about 40 percent of the RDA for men and 27 percent of the RDA for women. What's more, that ounce of seeds has as much protein—9 grams—as an ounce of meat, says Susan Thom, R.D., a resource spokesperson for the American Dietetic Association and a nutrition consultant in Brecksville, Ohio.

Of course, you don't want to eat too many pumpkin seeds, since about 73 percent of the calories (there are 148 calories in an ounce of seeds) come from fat. But when you have a taste for a crunchy, highly nutritious snack, pumpkin seeds, in moderation, are a good choice.

Getting the Most

Consider it canned. There's something about preparing a huge pumpkin that daunts even dedicated cooks and prevents them from utilizing its healing powers. An easy, convenient alternative is to buy canned pumpkin. Nutritionally, "it's almost equal to fresh," says Pamela Savage-Marr, R.D., spokesperson for the American Dietetic Association and a health education specialist at Oakwood Healthcare System in Dearborn, Michigan.

Buy it tender. When you have a taste for fresh pumpkin, be sure to shop for milder varieties, like the mini-sized Jack Be Littles. While large pumpkins are great for carving, they also tend to be tough and stringy, and most people don't enjoy them as much.

Temper the taste. Pumpkin is among the stronger-flavored squashes, and even people who like the taste can be overwhelmed by its potent presence. To get the most pumpkin into your diet, you may want to mellow the taste. One way to do this is to add about a tablespoon of orange juice or any other citrus juice during cooking, suggests Anne Dubner, R.D., a spokeswoman for the American Dietetic Association and a nutrition consultant in Houston.

Love your leftovers. There's no reason to force yourself to eat an entire pumpkin at one sitting—as though you could! Properly frozen, pumpkin retains virtually all its goodness and nutrition.

PUMPKIN MAPLE PUDDING

1 **can (16 ounces) pumpkin**

1 **can (12 ounces) evaporated skim milk**

¾ **cup maple syrup**

1 **egg**

2 **egg whites**

1 **tablespoon unbleached all-purpose flour**

2 **teaspoons ground cinnamon**

1¼ **teaspoons ground ginger**

⅛ **teaspoon salt**

¼ **cup chopped pecans**

PER SERVING

calories **229**
total fat **4.4 g.**
saturated fat **0.6 g.**
cholesterol **38 mg.**
sodium **163 mg.**
dietary fiber **3.8 g.**

Preheat the oven to 325°F. Coat a 2½-quart baking dish or soufflé dish with no-stick spray.

In a large bowl, combine the pumpkin, milk, maple syrup, egg, egg whites, flour, cinnamon, ginger, and salt. Whisk until smooth.

Pour into the prepared dish. Bake for 1 hour, or until almost set. (The pudding should still jiggle slightly in the center.)

Sprinkle with the pecans. Bake for 5 to 10 minutes, or until a wooden pick inserted in the center comes out clean. Remove to a wire rack to cool. Cover and refrigerate for several hours to chill.

Makes 6 servings

Cook's Note: For best results, serve the pudding the same day you bake it. Serve with nonfat whipped topping if desired.

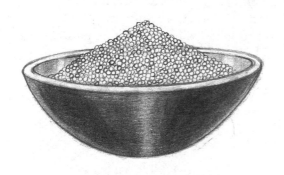

Quinoa
The Mother of All Grains

Healing Power
Can help:
Fight fatigue

Prevent anemia

Regulate blood pressure

High in the Peruvian mountains centuries ago, the Incas dined on a grain so important that they named it quinoa—literally, the "mother grain."

All grains are good for health, but quinoa stands head and shoulders above the rest. It contains more protein than any other grain, and it is such a rich and balanced source of essential nutrients that food experts have called it the supergrain for the future.

Packed with Protein

Quinoa is one of the best grain sources of protein. And unlike the protein found in most grains, quinoa's protein is complete, meaning that it contains all nine amino acids that the body must get from food, says Diane Grabowski-Nepa, R.D., a dietitian and nutritional counselor at the Pritikin Longevity Center in Santa Monica, California. This makes quinoa a choice grain for people who are limiting meat in their diets and may have trouble getting enough protein.

A half-cup of cooked quinoa delivers 5 grams of protein, 10 percent of the Daily Value (DV). "It's particularly high in the amino acid lysine," adds Grabowski-Nepa. Lysine is important for helping tissues grow and repair themselves.

In the Kitchen

While wheat, rice, and other grains are all prepared in similar ways, quinoa is smaller and more delicate and must be treated a little bit differently. Here's what chefs advise.

Wash it well. As quinoa grows it develops a natural, protective coating called saponin, which sometimes has a bitter taste. To wash away the residue, rinse quinoa before you start cooking.

Watch the time. Quinoa cooks more quickly than other grains, and because of its delicate texture, it can get twice as mushy when you overcook it. To get the proper consistency, bring 2 cups of water to a boil, add 1 cup of quinoa, reduce the heat to low and cook, covered, for 10 to 15 minutes, until the grains are tender and all the liquid has been absorbed.

Use a little, get a lot. Some folks balk at the price of quinoa, which is quite a bit more expensive than other grains. But because it plumps up a lot during cooking—up to four times its original volume—a little goes a long way.

A High-Energy Grain

For your blood to carry oxygen, it must have iron. When you don't get enough iron in your diet, red blood cells actually shrink, reducing the amount of oxygen they can carry. To make up the difference, the heart and lungs have to work harder. Over time, this extra exertion causes fatigue.

Quinoa can wake you up again. "Most grains have a little iron, but quinoa is a very good source," says Grabowski-Nepa. For example, a half-cup of cooked quinoa contains 4 milligrams of iron, 40 percent of the Recommended Dietary Allowance (RDA) for men and 27 percent of the RDA for women. Compare that to a similar amount of brown rice, which has only 1 milligram of iron.

Help for Circulation

Besides providing a mineful of iron, quinoa supplies two additional nutrients, magnesium and riboflavin, that help blood work more efficiently.

People who don't get enough magnesium in their diets have a higher risk of developing high blood pressure. In fact, doctors have found that when people low in magnesium start getting enough, their blood pressure improves, the blood is less likely to clot, and the heart beats more regularly.

Quinoa can help restore your magnesium to heart-healthy standards. A half-cup of cooked quinoa contains 90 milligrams of magnesium, 22 percent of the DV.

Getting the Most

Explore the possibilities. People often use grains only for side dishes because they're not sure what else to do with them. But quinoa is soft and somewhat bland, meaning that you can include it in almost any food. Adding quinoa to soups, pasta dishes, or stuffings makes it easy to get more of its nutritional power in your diet every day, says Grabowski-Nepa.

Keep it cold. While most grains are good keepers, quinoa spoils quickly. To preserve the nutrients and the good taste, it's best to buy quinoa only in small amounts and to store it in an airtight container in the refrigerator or another cool, dark place.

SOUTHWESTERN QUINOA AND CHICKPEA SALAD

1	**cup quinoa**
1¾	**cups water**
4	**teaspoons olive oil**
1	**cup rinsed and drained canned chickpeas**
1	**medium tomato, seeded and chopped**
3	**tablespoons fresh lime juice**
2	**tablespoons minced fresh cilantro**
½	**teaspoon ground cumin**
1	**clove garlic, minced**
⅛	**teaspoon salt**

PER SERVING

calories	**271**
total fat	**8.4 g.**
saturated fat	**0.9 g.**
cholesterol	**0 mg.**
sodium	**219 mg.**
dietary fiber	**6.4 g.**

Place the quinoa in a fine sieve and rinse well with cold water. Drain and transfer to a medium saucepan.

Add the water and bring to a boil over medium heat. Cover, reduce the heat to low, and simmer for 15 minutes, or until the quinoa is tender but still slightly crunchy. If all the water has not been absorbed, drain it through a fine sieve.

Place the quinoa in a medium bowl. Drizzle with the oil and toss to mix. Add the chickpeas, tomatoes, lime juice, cilantro, cumin, garlic, and salt. Toss thoroughly to mix.

Makes 4 servings

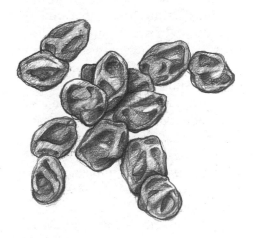

Raisins
Turn Down High Blood Pressure

Healing Power
Can help:
Improve digestion

Lower blood pressure

Keep blood healthy

Raisins may not be much to look at, but they do have an illustrious history. Prehistoric cave dwellers attributed religious powers to raisins. They made raisin necklaces and decorations and drew pictures of raisins on cave walls. As early as 1000 B.C., the Israelites used them to pay taxes to King David. Just try that with the IRS!

Raisins occupy a much humbler place in society today. But they're just as useful as ever. Backpackers and hikers appreciate raisins for being a high-energy, low-fat, very convenient snack. Raisins fit easily in a lunch box, and they don't get as mushy as bananas if you accidentally leave them in your desk drawer. And they almost never go bad, even when they're in the pantry for months at a time.

Raisins offer more than just convenience. Studies suggest that they can help lower blood pressure and cholesterol and even play a role in keeping digestion and blood healthy.

Lowering the Pressure

If you have high blood pressure—or even if you don't, but you want to make sure your pressure stays in a healthy range—raisins are one of the best snacks you can buy. They're a good source of potassium, a mineral that has been shown to lower high blood pressure.

In the Kitchen

There's very little nutritional difference between black and golden raisins. (The black variety has more thiamin, while the golden seedless type has a bit more vitamin B$_6$.) The main difference between them is the way they are dried.

- **Black, or sun-dried, raisins** are actually dried in the sun. This is what gives them their dark, shriveled look. They're used for both baking and snacking.
- **Golden seedless raisins** are dried by exposing them to the fumes of burning sulfur in a closed chamber, which gives them their golden hue. They're usually used for baking—in fruit cakes, for example—because of their attractive appearance.

Both types of raisins are extremely durable. As long as they are kept tightly wrapped, they will keep in the pantry for several months and for a year or more when stored in the refrigerator or freezer. You'll know they've gone bad if you spot white sugar crystals collecting on the surface.

It's common for raisins to dry out a bit during storage. Don't throw them out. Steaming them for about 5 minutes will restore much of the missing moisture and make them plumper. Or if you're going to use them for baking, let them sit in hot water or fruit juice for about 5 minutes, then add them to the recipe.

In one study, researchers at Johns Hopkins Medical Institutions in Baltimore gave 87 African-American men either potassium supplements or blank pills. Those who were given the potassium saw their systolic pressure (the higher number) drop almost 7 points, while their diastolic pressure went down almost 3 points. While the amount of potassium given in the study was quite high—you would have to eat about 3 cups of raisins to get the same amount—smaller amounts are also beneficial. Just ¼ cup of raisins contains 272 milligrams of potassium, almost 8 percent of the Daily Value (DV).

"All Americans, but particularly those who are over the age of 40, ought to be consuming a fair number of foods such as raisins that contain high levels of potassium," recommends Donald V. Schlimme, Ph.D., professor of nutrition and food science at the University of Maryland in College Park.

Iron and More

When we think of iron-rich foods, things such as red meat and liver usually come to mind. But raisins may be a better source of iron, particularly for people who eat little or no meat. "If someone were to ask me what food other than red meat I would recommend for high iron, I would say raisins," says Dr. Schlimme.

Iron is essential for the creation of hemoglobin in red blood cells, which the body uses to transport oxygen. Although iron is readily available in food, women who are menstruating or pregnant often need extra amounts of the mineral.

A quarter-cup of raisins has 0.8 milligram of iron, which is more than 8 percent of the Recommended Dietary Allowance (RDA) for men and 5 percent of the RDA for women.

Like other dried fruits, raisins are also a good source of dietary fiber, with nearly 2 grams of fiber in ¼ cup, about 8 percent of the Daily Value. Not only does fiber play a role in helping to prevent everyday problems such as constipation and hemorrhoids but it also lowers cholesterol and the risk of heart disease.

In one study, researchers at the Health Research and Studies Center in Los Altos, California,

asked people with high cholesterol levels to eat 3 ounces of raisins (a little more than a half-cup) a day as part of a high-fiber, low-fat diet. After a month, the participants' total cholesterol dropped an average of more than 8 percent, while their harmful low-density lipoprotein cholesterol levels dropped 15 percent.

Getting the Most

Have a raisin combo. Raisins contain a type of iron called nonheme iron, which is harder for the body to absorb than the heme iron found in meats. Eating raisins along with foods high in vitamin C, however, helps improve the absorption of nonheme iron.

Shop for convenience. To get the most raisins in your diet, nutritionists often recommend buying the snack-size packs. Due to their small size and the fact that raisins almost never go bad, they're perfect for tossing in your purse, glove compartment, or desk drawer and eating whenever you are in the mood for a quick snack.

RAISIN COFFEECAKE RING

Coffeecake

- **1** **pound frozen whole-wheat or white bread dough, thawed**
- **1½** **cups raisins**
- **½** **cup fresh orange juice**
- **2** **teaspoons vanilla**
- **¼** **teaspoon ground cinnamon**
- **2** **teaspoons unsalted butter**

Glaze

- **2** **tablespoons fresh orange juice**
- **3** **tablespoons confectioners' sugar**
- **1** **teaspoon unsalted butter**

PER SLICE

calories	**172**
total fat	**2.6 g.**
saturated fat	**0.6 g.**
cholesterol	**3 mg.**
sodium	**168 mg.**
dietary fiber	**3 g.**

To make the coffeecake: In a medium saucepan, combine the raisins, orange juice, vanilla, and cinnamon. Cook over medium heat, stirring frequently, for 5 to 7 minutes, or until the raisins have absorbed all the liquid. Remove from the heat. Stir in the butter. Cover and set aside.

Coat a baking sheet with no-stick spray. On a work surface, pat and stretch the dough into a 12″ × 6″ rectangle.

Spread evenly with the raisin mixture, leaving about ½″ uncovered along 1 long side. Starting with the other long side, roll the dough tightly. Pinch the edges together to seal them.

Transfer to the baking sheet, forming the dough into a ring. Pinch the ends together. Use a sharp knife to cut through the ring at intervals about 1½″ apart. (Cut almost all the way through the dough, leaving the center attached.) Spread the cuts out slightly so the filling is visible.

Cover loosely with plastic wrap. Set aside in a warm spot for 2 to 4 hours, or until doubled in bulk. Preheat the oven to 350°F. Remove the plastic wrap and bake for 20 to 25 minutes, or until golden. Remove and place on a wire rack.

To make the glaze: In a small microwaveable bowl, combine the orange juice, confectioners' sugar, and butter. Microwave on high for about 30 seconds, or until the butter melts. Whisk until smooth. Brush over the warm coffeecake. Remove the coffeecake carefully to a rack to cool.

Makes 12 slices

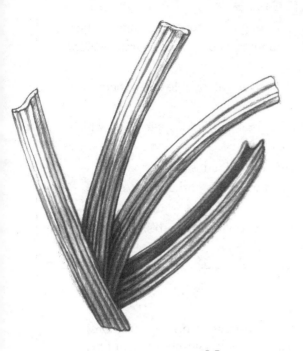

RHUBARB
RELIEF FROM CONSTIPATION

HEALING POWER

CAN HELP:
Lower cholesterol

Prevent cancer

Boost immunity

Ease digestive problems

Now *let us all praise the Rhubarb...*
Its roseate stalks are a treat
Especially when stewed or otherwise brewed
In concoctions delectably sweet.
"In Praise of Rhubarb"—Cynthia Francisco

Granted, not many of us get sufficiently excited enough about this tart, acidic plant to praise all of its virtues in verse. If you're suffering from constipation, however, rhubarb just might be able to give you something to sing about after all.

And you might not be the only one singing. Research shows that people with high cholesterol and low immunity may want to join the rhubarb chorus. Also, although more research needs to be done, evidence suggests that rhubarb may help fight certain cancers.

Before going any further, though, take heed of this critical caution. You should eat only the rhubarb stalks. Rhubarb leaves contain extraordinarily high levels of oxalates, which are mineral salts that the body cannot metabolize; for people who are sensitive to them, they can be toxic. When used properly, however, rhubarb is a wonderfully healthy food that you'll certainly want to try.

GARDEN-VARIETY LAXATIVE

It's folklore, but most experts agree: Eating rhubarb works against constipation because this member of the buckwheat family is a good source of fiber.

"People have historically used rhubarb for constipation by eating it stewed or in pies, but they didn't know why it worked," says Tapan K. Basu, Ph.D., professor of nutrition at the University of Alberta in Edmonton, Canada. "Today we know it's a good source of fiber."

The fibrous rhubarb stalks contain large amounts of dietary fiber—more than 2 grams in a half-cup serving—that add the bulk necessary to keep your bowels moving on a regular basis.

Ronald L. Hoffman, M.D., director of the Hoffman Center for Holistic Medicine in New York City and author of *Seven Weeks to a Settled Stomach*, offers this rhubarb recipe for when you're waiting for nature's call.

Chop three stalks of fresh raw rhubarb (removing and discarding the toxic leaves) and mix with 1 cup of apple juice, ¼ of a peeled lemon, and 1 teaspoon of honey. Put all the ingredients in a blender and puree until smooth. (Because raw rhubarb is very tart, you may want to add other juices to the recipe to soften the flavor.) Drink as necessary.

FLUSHING OUT CHOLESTEROL

Rhubarb, along with other fiber-rich foods such as oat bran and beans, can sop up cholesterol and flush it from your body before it gets a chance to stick to your arteries, clogging them up and contributing to heart disease.

In one study, researchers at the University of Alberta found that rhubarb fiber significantly reduces cholesterol, especially the harmful low-density lipoprotein (LDL) cholesterol, and also lowers triglycerides, which are potentially dangerous fats in the bloodstream. People who participated in the study consumed 27 grams of fiber-dense powdered rhubarb stalks a day for 30 days.

"How much rhubarb you need to eat to get the same effect, we don't know yet," says Dr. Basu, the study's lead researcher. "But we can say that rhubarb contains an effective kind of fiber, so eating it certainly can't hurt."

TUMOR-SQUELCHING POTENTIAL

Although the evidence is still preliminary, research indicates that rhubarb may contain compounds that can help prevent cancer.

In the only published study on rhubarb's effectiveness against cancer, researchers at the University of Mainz in Germany tested raw rhubarb juice, along with the juices of various other vegetables and fruits, against cancer-causing agents. They found that rhubarb ranked close to the top in preventing cell mutations that commonly lead to cancer.

Although this early research is promising, researchers still aren't sure if drinking rhubarb juice—or eating the whole stalk—will produce the same beneficial effects as those seen in test tubes.

A TART BURST OF PROTECTION

Rhubarb contains vitamin C, an antioxidant vitamin that attacks and immobilizes free radicals, oxygen molecules that are the damaging force behind heart disease, some cancers, and certain "symptoms" of aging, like wrinkles or eye damage.

In addition, vitamin C has been shown to help keep the bad LDL cholesterol in your body from oxidizing—the process that allows it to stick to artery walls. It also plays an important role in the formation of collagen, a protein that makes up skin and connective tissue and helps keep skin smooth. Plus, vitamin

C is a known immunity-booster, helping your body stave off colds and infections.

A half-cup of cooked rhubarb delivers almost 4 milligrams of vitamin C, nearly 7 percent of the Daily Value.

Getting the Most

Bet on red. Because of its tartness, most people would have a tough time downing more than a few bites of rhubarb. Here's a shopping tip that may help. Generally, the redder the stalk, the sweeter the taste, and the more you can eat with the least "pucker effect."

RHUBARB-ORANGE SAUCE

12　ounces rhubarb, trimmed and diced

¾　cup minced onions

¼　cup fresh orange juice

3　tablespoons honey

2　tablespoons golden raisins

2　teaspoons grated fresh ginger

PER ½ CUP

calories	**100**
total fat	**0.3 g.**
saturated fat	**0.1 g.**
cholesterol	**0 mg.**
sodium	**6 mg.**
dietary fiber	**2.4 g.**

In a large saucepan, combine the rhubarb, onions, orange juice, honey, raisins, and ginger. Bring to a boil over medium heat, stirring frequently. Reduce the heat to low and cook, stirring once or twice, for 5 minutes, or until the rhubarb is tender. Set aside to cool.

Makes 2 cups

Cook's Note: Serve the sauce over grilled chicken breast, roast turkey breast, or roast pork tenderloin.

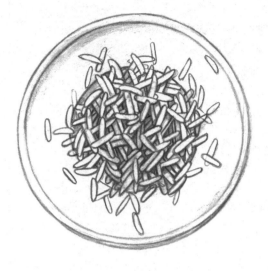

RICE
A GOOD GRAIN
FOR YOUR HEART

HEALING POWER

CAN HELP:
Reduce cholesterol

Lower the risk
of colon cancer

Keep digestion regular

If there were just one food in every cook's pantry, it would probably be rice. Rice is the main ingredient in cuisines around the globe, with an estimated 40,000 varieties available worldwide. In the United States you can buy basmati rice from India and Pakistan, arborio rice from Italy, Valencia rice from Spain, and "sticky" rice from Japan. (Wild rice, incidentally, is really a grass, not a rice at all.)

The most nutritious kind of rice is brown rice, which contains abundant amounts of fiber, complex carbohydrates, and essential B vitamins, says Maren Hegsted, Ph.D., professor of human nutrition and food at Louisiana State University in Baton Rouge. Plus, it contains a powerful compound that helps reduce the amount of cholesterol produced by the body. Since high cholesterol is one of the biggest risk factors for heart disease, brown rice can play a key role in any heart-protection plan.

STRIKE AT THE SOURCE

We often forget that the body actually needs small amounts of cholesterol for functions such as making cell walls, for example, and for manufacturing essential hormones. To supply the necessary amounts, the liver produces cholesterol every day. But when we eat a high-fat diet, the body churns out

IN THE KITCHEN

Manufacturers often promise that their rice will cook up perfect every time, which suggests that some rice, at least, is coming to the table sticky and wet, or, worse, dry and hard. Here's a strategy for making perfect rice every time, no matter what kind you buy.

Leave it alone. It's almost impossible for cooks not to stir or investigate a pot of rice while it cooks. The problem is, stirring rice frequently before it's done damages the grains and can make the finished product soft and gummy. (Arborio rice, however, is meant to be stirred during cooking.)

Choose your liquid. While rice is customarily cooked in plain water, many chefs prefer to use flavored liquids, which add depth and complexity to the finished dish. Chicken and beef broths are ideal cooking liquids. Or you can simply add a squeeze of lemon, a splash of flavored vinegar, or a sprinkling of herbs to the water.

Watch for separation. To prevent rice from overcooking, it's a good idea to check it just before you think it's done. If the rice still looks a little wet, it needs an extra minute or two (or more) to absorb excess water.

When it's done, the grains of long-grain varieties will separate easily, without being either dry or wet and sticky. Short- and medium-grain rice, however, will naturally clump together. Letting the rice stand for 15 to 20 minutes after cooking will help reducing the clumping.

---

more cholesterol than it can use. And that is when the risk of heart disease goes up.

Getting more brown rice, Dr. Hegsted says, can help keep this from happening. The outer layer of brown rice, called the bran, contains a compound called oryzanol that has been shown to reduce the body's production of cholesterol. In fact, this compound is chemically similar to cholesterol-lowering medications.

In a study at Louisiana State University, people ate 100 grams (about 3½ ounces) of rice bran a day for three weeks. At the end of the study, researchers found that their cholesterol levels had dropped an average of 7 percent. Better yet, levels of harmful low-density lipoprotein cholesterol went down 10 percent, while levels of beneficial high-density lipoprotein cholesterol stayed relatively high.

A 10 percent drop in cholesterol may not sound like much, but doctors estimate that for every 1 percent you lower your cholesterol, your risk of heart disease drops 2 percent. This means that the rice-eaters lowered their risk of heart disease by 20 percent in only three weeks.

"In combination with a low-fat diet, brown rice is one of the best foods you can eat for lowering cholesterol," says Dr. Hegsted.

A Digestive Sponge

Brown rice is darker and more chewy than its light-colored cousin because it's wrapped in a nutritious outer skin—the part of the grain that's highest in fiber, says Christine Negm, R.D., nutritionist and director of technical services for Lundberg Family Farms, which produces rice in Richvale, California. A half-cup of brown rice contains about 2 grams of fiber, she says.

The fiber in brown rice is the insoluble kind that acts like a sponge in the intestine, soaking up large amounts of water, says Dr. Hegsted. This causes stools to get larger and wetter, so they pass more easily. In addition, larger stools move more quickly through the colon. This means that any harmful substances that they contain have less time to damage cells in the colon wall, which can reduce the risk of cancer. Some researchers estimate that if people would increase the amount of fiber in their diets to 39 grams a day, the risk for colon cancer could drop 31 percent.

What's good for the colon is also good for the breasts. Since the fiber in brown rice binds with estrogen in the digestive tract, there's less of the hormone circulating in the bloodstream. This is important because high levels of estrogen have been shown to trigger changes in cells that can lead to breast cancer. A study by Australian and Canadian researchers found that women who ate 28 grams of fiber a day had a 38 percent lower risk of developing breast cancer than those getting half that amount.

Giving Nature a Hand

The problem with white rice is that the nutritious outer layers are stripped away during processing, leaving behind a tender but less healthful grain. To bring it up to speed, manufacturers do a nutritional sleight of hand. They replace some of the nutrients, like niacin and thiamin, that the processing took out. As a result, white rice may contain more of these nutrients than nature put in.

A half-cup of white rice has 0.2 milligram of thiamin, a B vitamin that's essential for converting food into energy, and 2 milligrams of niacin, which aids in metabolism. Brown rice, by contrast, has only 0.1 milligram of thiamin and 1 milligram of niacin. "White rice is fortified to the max," Negm says.

What white rice is lacking, however, is the fiber. A half-cup serving contains a scanty 0.2 gram of fiber, 10 times less than an equal amount of brown rice. So when you're trying to get the most nutritional bang for your buck, brown rice is usually a better choice.

Getting the Most

Keep it cool. Since brown rice is filled with oils, it quickly turns rancid when stored at normal room temperature, Dr. Hegsted says. To preserve the healing compounds, be sure to store brown rice in an airtight container in the refrigerator, where it will stay fresh for up to a year.

Save the water. Many of the important nutrients in brown and white rice leach into the water during cooking. To get these nutrients on your plate instead of pouring them down the drain, let rice cook until all the water is absorbed.

Use it "dry." Since the niacin and thiamin in fortified white rice are found on the outer layer of the grain, rinsing rice before cooking will wash these nutrients away. It's best to go straight from the bag into the cooking water, Negm says. The exception is when you're using imported rice, which may contain more impurities than the domestic kinds.

Fried Rice with Pork and Spinach

2⅓   cups water

1¼   cups long-grain brown rice

2   teaspoons canola oil

1   tablespoon grated fresh ginger

2   teaspoons minced garlic

6   cups loosely packed torn spinach leaves

1   cup finely diced cooked pork tenderloin

1   can (8 ounces) water chestnuts, drained and chopped

1   teaspoon dark sesame oil

¼   teaspoon salt

Per serving

calories	**341**
total fat	**7.3 g.**
saturated fat	**1.2 g.**
cholesterol	**27 mg.**
sodium	**203 mg.**
dietary fiber	**7.5 g.**

In a large saucepan over high heat, bring the water to a boil. Stir in the rice. Reduce the heat to low, cover, and cook for 40 to 50 minutes, or until the rice is tender and all the water is absorbed. Remove from the heat.

Uncover and let stand for 5 minutes, then fluff with a fork. Let stand to cool, fluffing occasionally with a fork, for 15 to 20 minutes. Place in a covered container and refrigerate for up to 2 days. The rice should be cold when you fry it.

In a large no-stick skillet over medium-high heat, warm the canola oil. Add the ginger and garlic. Cook for 30 seconds, or until fragrant. Add the rice, spinach, pork, water chestnuts, sesame oil, and salt. Cook, stirring and tossing, until the rice and pork are hot and the spinach is wilted.

Makes 4 servings

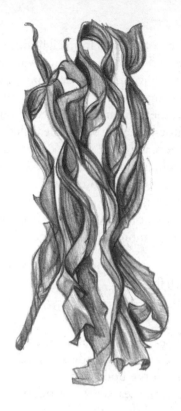

Sea Vegetables
Protection from the Deep

Healing Power
Can help:
Inhibit tumor growth

Boost immunity

Prevent macular
degeneration

When the Beatles were crooning "Octopus's Garden" back in 1969, they almost certainly weren't extolling the virtues of seaweed, or sea vegetables, as they're called by those who harvest and consume them today. But given what we've learned about these valuable plants, they probably should have been.

Eaten regularly, sea vegetables can be a valuable source of essential vitamins and minerals. In addition, they contain a variety of protective compounds that may help ward off some serious health threats, such as cancer.

A Traditional Cancer-Fighter

For hundreds, maybe thousands of years, sea vegetables have been used in Asian cultures to prevent and treat cancer. As is often the case, research now indicates that there is more than a little scientific evidence supporting these ancient healing methods. "We need more clinical studies, but so far there have been some interesting population and animal studies showing that sea vegetables can prevent tumors," says Alfred A. Bushway, Ph.D., professor of food science at the University of Maine in Orono, who believes that sea vegetables may be partially responsible for the lower cancer rates in countries like Japan, where the sea vegetable is as ubiquitous as our potato.

Japanese researchers studied the effects of extracts from eight different kinds of sea vegetables on cells that had been treated with potent cancer-causing agents. The results showed that sea vegetables may have tumor-squelching power.

Though scientists are unsure which compounds in sea vegetables are responsible, they suspect it may be beta-carotene, the same antioxidant compound found in such things as carrots and sweet potatoes. The sea vegetable called nori (also known as laver), which comes in dried sheets, is a good source of beta-carotene.

Researchers suspect that sea vegetables may have cancer-fighting compounds that simply aren't found in their land-loving counterparts. For example, a compound called sodium alginate, which is found in high concentrations in sea vegetables, could have cancer-fighting abilities, says Dr. Bushway. "But, again, this is a research area that needs to be more fully explored," he says.

KELP FOR YOUR HEART AND BLOOD

If you want your blood to have the strength of the sea itself, a dose of vegetables from its waters can help.

One ounce of kelp, a thin, tender sea vegetable often used in soups and stir-fries, provides 51 micrograms, 13 percent of the Daily Value (DV) of folate, a nutrient that helps break down protein in the body and aids in the regeneration of red blood cells. An ounce of nori, the sea vegetable frequently used in sushi, provides 42 micrograms, 11 percent of the DV of this vital nutrient.

Kelp also contains magnesium, a mineral that has been found to keep high blood pressure in check, especially among people who are sensitive to sodium. One ounce of kelp has more than 34 milligrams, or almost 9 percent of the DV of this heart-healthy nutrient.

A SEA OF IMMUNITY

You don't see too many whales swimming around with the sniffles. Maybe that's because of all the sea vegetables they're skimming off the ocean's swells.

Certain varieties of sea vegetables are packed with important vitamins that boost immunity and help fend off a host of diseases.

Topping this list is the nutritious nori. One ounce of raw nori contains 11 milligrams of infection-fighting vitamin C, more than 18 percent of the DV. Vitamin C is an antioxidant nutrient known for its ability to sweep up harmful, tissue-damaging oxygen molecules called free radicals.

An ounce of nori also delivers nearly 1,500 international units of vitamin A, 30 percent of the DV. Studies show that vitamin A not only builds immunity but also can safeguard against night blindness and vision problems associated with aging, like macular degeneration. In addition, vitamin A can protect against several kinds of cancer.

Good News for Vegans

If you're among the strictest of vegetarians, meaning that you don't eat meat, meat products, milk, or eggs, you may want to add some sea vegetables to your palette of land vegetables. It's a helpful way to ensure that you're getting adequate amounts of vitamin B_{12}, a nutrient most commonly found in meat.

Although there is some controversy about how much vitamin B_{12} sea vegetables provide, experts agree that those who regularly dine on these vegetables have higher levels of vitamin B_{12} in their blood than those who do not.

In one study of 21 strict vegetarians, researchers found that those who ate sea vegetables regularly had blood levels of vitamin B_{12} twice as high as those who didn't eat the vegetables.

Without adequate amounts of vitamin B_{12}, you can experience fatigue, memory loss, and nerve damage resulting in tingling in the feet and hands. Although few people are at risk for vitamin B_{12} deficiency, it can be a concern for strict vegetarians and for some elderly people who have trouble absorbing this vital nutrient.

Getting the Most

Rinse lightly. Since many of the valuable trace minerals in dried sea vegetables are on the surface, experts recommend using a light touch when rinsing them prior to

In the Kitchen

The first time you pull a flat, green sheet of dried nori from its wrapper, your reaction almost certainly will be, "How the heck am I supposed to eat this?"

Although seaweed, which is sold in health food stores and Asian markets, does look strange, it's surprisingly easy to work with. It's important, however, to know which kind you're getting, since each is handled somewhat differently.

Alaria. Also known as wakame, this is the seaweed traditionally used in miso soup. When using it for salads or pasta dishes, simply soften it in water for 2 to 3 minutes and cut it into slivers. Alaria can be quite chewy, but cutting away the stiff midrib will help make it tender.

Dulse. Dried dulse has deep red, wrinkled leaves, which can be eaten straight from the package. (It can be quite salty, however, so you may want to rinse it first.) Like nori, dulse is typically snipped and added to soups, stews, and pasta dishes. It is also available in ready-to-use flakes.

Hijiki. One of the stronger tasting seaweeds, hijiki (also spelled hiziki) resembles black angel hair pasta in its packaged form. To tame its wild briny flavor, soak it for 10 to 15 minutes, then drain; it will quadruple in size when hydrated. Chefs recommend simmering hijiki for about 30 minutes or until tender, then adding it to salads, vegetables, or bean dishes. It can also be drizzled with sesame oil and eaten as a side dish.

Kelp. Sold in wide, dried, dark green strips, kelp (similar to the Japanese kombu) is often added to soups and stews as a replacement for salt. To add seasoning to bean and grain dishes, chefs will sometimes add strips of kelp. Also, roasted kelp chips make a great garnish.

Nori. Also known as laver, nori is sold in paper-thin, green dried sheets. It has a mildly briny flavor and is generally used to wrap around sushi, float in soups, or accentuate salads and pasta. When adding nori to a dish, use scissors to cut it into strips. Or tear it with your hands and sprinkle it into the food, stirring to keep it from clumping.

cooking. "Some people soak and rinse the life out of their sea vegetables," says Dr. Bushway. "We just recommend light rinsing. Otherwise you'll lose a lot of the surface minerals, like potassium."

Invest in stock. The best way to retain the maximum amount of nutrients is to make soup out of your sea vegetables, says Dr. Bushway. "When sea vegetables are used in soups, some of the minerals are released in the broth," he says. "The remainder provide valuable fiber and unique phytochemicals, such as the alginate found in kelp."

Eat for variety. It doesn't take a lot of sea vegetables to get the benefits. "Nutritional studies indicate that as little as ¼ ounce of dried sea vegetables can make a significant nutritional contribution to your diet," says Dr. Bushway.

The best way to include more sea vegetables in your diet is to experiment. "Add small, bite-size pieces to salads, soups, stews, grain dishes, stir-fries, and sandwiches," says Carl Karush of Maine Coast Sea Vegetables in Franklin.

KELP AND POTATO CHOWDER

1   **tablespoon canola oil**

1   **large onion, diced**

7   **cups water**

4   **medium boiling potatoes, peeled and finely diced**

1   **cup finely crumbled dried kelp (about ¾ ounce)**

⅛   **teaspoon salt**

    Ground black pepper

PER SERVING

calories	**116**
total fat	**2.5 g.**
saturated fat	**0.2 g.**
cholesterol	**0 mg.**
sodium	**208 mg.**
dietary fiber	**2.7 g.**

In a Dutch oven over medium-high heat, warm the oil. Add the onions and cook, stirring frequently, for 8 to 10 minutes, or until the onions are golden.

Add the water, potatoes, kelp, and salt. Bring to a boil. Partially cover, reduce the heat to low, and cook for 30 to 35 minutes, or until the potatoes are tender. Season to taste with pepper.

Makes 6 servings

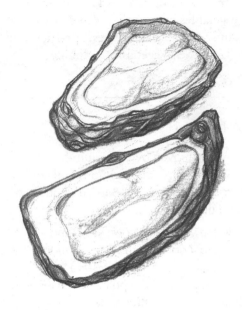

Shellfish
Health on the Half Shell

Healing Power
Can help:
Prevent anemia

Boost immunity

Prevent heart disease

For most folks, shellfish like lobster, shrimp, scallops, and oysters are luxuries—foods to be reserved for special occasions. For one thing, shellfish are expensive, often costing twice as much (or more) as other fish. Shellfish also have a reputation for containing boatloads of cholesterol and a sea of sodium, both of which health-conscious diners usually try to avoid.

While it's true that shellfish are high in cholesterol and sodium, these aren't the health threats that scientists once thought they were, says Robert M. Grodner, Ph.D., professor emeritus in the department of food science at Louisiana State University in Baton Rouge. In addition, shellfish contain generous amounts of vitamins, minerals, and other healthful compounds that more than offset their slight nutritional downside.

Good for the Heart

Ironically, the very thing that makes shellfish so healthful is the same stuff most of us are trying to avoid: the fat. Yet the kind of fat found in shellfish, known as omega-3 fatty acids, is very good for the heart. Researchers at the University of Washington in Seattle found that people who ate enough seafood to get almost 6 grams of omega-3's a month had half the risk of cardiac arrest, an

482

In the Kitchen

Shellfish are extremely perishable. Even when properly stored, they stay fresh for only a day or two. In addition, they cook very quickly. The difference between "just right" and "yuck" is often measured in minutes—or less. Here are a few tips for having the freshest catch every time.

Buy them live. Since shellfish go bad so quickly, it's best to buy them live and cook them the same day. To keep them fresh after bringing them home from the store, be sure to store them in the refrigerator until you're ready to start cooking.

Check for doneness. Few foods are less appetizing than undercooked shellfish. Lobsters and crabs turn bright red when they're done, usually in about 15 to 20 minutes. Clams, mussels, and oysters are nearly done when the shells open. Letting them cook for another 5 minutes will finish the job.

---

often fatal irregularity in heart rhythm, of those who ate none.

In fact, people who eat a lot of seafood fare even better than vegetarians when it comes to heart health. In one study, seafood-eaters with high concentrations of omega-3's in their blood had significantly lower blood pressure and lower levels of cholesterol and triglycerides—blood fats that in large amounts can increase the risk of heart disease—than vegetarians who didn't eat shellfish. Although many of the studies on omega-3's have focused on fish like salmon and mackerel, all fish, including shellfish, contain some omega-3's, says Dan Sharp, M.D., Ph.D., director of the Honolulu Heart Program.

The omega-3's in shellfish have a number of benefits. They strengthen the heart muscle, enabling it to beat steadily and soundly. They help lower blood pressure, keep cholesterol in check, and also reduce the tendency of platelets—tiny discs in the blood—from sticking together and causing clots.

Atlantic and Pacific oysters are particularly rich sources of omega-3's. Eating six medium oysters five to seven times a month will provide all the omega-3's your heart needs.

Multivitamins in a Shell

Aside from their role in protecting the heart, shellfish are incredibly rich sources of a variety of essential (and hard-to-find) vitamins and minerals. Shellfish contain large amounts of vitamin B_{12}, for example, which the body uses to keep nerves healthy and make red blood cells. When levels of vitamin B_{12} slip, the body (and mind) can literally short-circuit, causing memory loss, confusion, slow reflexes, and fatigue. In fact, what's sometimes thought to be senility in older people is sometimes nothing more than a lack of vitamin B_{12}.

Food Alert
Hazards on the Half-Shell

Shellfish are nutritious and delicious. But unless they're prepared with care, they can also be dangerous.

In order to eat and breathe, shellfish such as clams and oysters filter 15 to 20 gallons of water a day through their shells. When the water contains bacteria, like the potentially harmful *Vibrio vulnificus*, the shellfish become contaminated and have the potential to make you sick.

This doesn't mean that you can't eat shellfish safely. Since the bacteria are readily killed by heat, cooking your catch will prevent potential problems. While this is bad news for lovers of oysters-on-the-half-shell, there may be an alternative, at least in the future. Laboratory studies suggest that dousing raw oysters with hot sauce will kill the bacteria. Until further research is done, however, it's best to be safe and eat your shellfish cooked.

Three ounces of crab contains 10 micrograms of vitamin B_{12}, 167 percent of the Daily Value (DV). Clams are even better, with 3 ounces—about nine small steamed clams—providing 1,400 percent of the DV.

With the exception of shrimp, shellfish also contain a lot of zinc, which is essential for keeping the immune system strong. Oysters are the best source, with six oysters containing about 27 milligrams, almost 181 percent of the DV.

It's sometimes hard to get enough iron from foods, which is why about 20 percent of Americans are low in this important mineral. But if you can muster up enough muscle to lift a mussel to your mouth, you'll get much of the iron you need to help prevent iron-deficiency anemia. Three ounces of mussels provides about 6 milligrams of iron, 60 percent of the Recommended Dietary Allowance (RDA) for men and 40 percent of the RDA for women.

Finally, many shellfish are good sources of magnesium, potassium, and vitamin C. The vitamin C is a great bonus because it helps the body absorb more of the iron found in these foods.

A New Reputation

Although people are often nervous about eating shellfish because these foods contain large amounts of sodium and cholesterol, neither of these items is likely to cause problems for most folks.

"Unlike other cholesterol sources, such as red meat, shellfish contain almost no saturated fat," explains Dr. Grodner. Eating a diet high in saturated fat is much more likely to send your cholesterol soaring than eating the cholesterol itself, he says.

Then there's the sodium. As you would expect of creatures from the sea, shellfish contain quite a bit—about 150 to 900 milligrams in a 3-ounce serving, depending on the type. But unless your doctor has suggested that you reduce the amount of salt in your diet, shellfish shouldn't be a problem. One serving of shellfish is well within the DV of 2,400 milligrams of sodium.

Getting the Most

Eat them with vitamin C. Since your body is better able to absorb the iron in foods when you eat them with vitamin C, it's a good idea to include vitamin C–rich foods such as broccoli or peppers on the shellfish menu.

Mix and match. Because shellfish are usually considered a luxury item, most people eat only a handful or two at a time. An easy way to include more of them in your diet is to toss them together in one big, briny stew, says Dr. Grodner. "It can be a mighty healthful meal," he says.

OYSTERS WITH SWEET ONIONS AND WATERCRESS

1   **pint shucked oysters, rinsed and drained**
1   **bunch watercress**
⅓   **cup chopped Vidalia or other sweet onions**
    Ground black pepper
2   **tablespoons plain dry bread crumbs**
2   **teaspoons unsalted butter**
    Juice of 1 medium lemon
    Hot-pepper sauce

PER SERVING

calories	**135**
total fat	**4.6 g.**
saturated fat	**1.8 g.**
cholesterol	**59 mg.**
sodium	**152 mg.**
dietary fiber	**0.6 g.**

Preheat the broiler.

Coat a 12″ × 8″ baking dish with no-stick spray. Arrange the oysters in a single layer in the dish.

Trim and discard the thick stems from the watercress. Coarsely chop the leaves and sprinkle them over the oysters. Sprinkle with the onions, pepper, and bread crumbs. Dot with the butter.

Broil 6″ from the heat for 6 minutes, or until the oysters are cooked through and their edges curl slightly. Check by inserting the tip of a sharp knife into an oyster.

Sprinkle with the lemon juice. Serve with the hot-pepper sauce.

Makes 4 appetizer servings

SEAFOOD STEW

2 tablespoons olive oil

1½ cups chopped onions

1 tablespoon minced garlic

1 can (28 ounces) plum tomatoes with basil (with juice)

2½ cups water

1 cup reduced-sodium vegetable juice

¼ cup no-salt-added tomato paste

1 teaspoon dried oregano

8 ounces cooked Dungeness or blue crabmeat

9 ounces medium raw shrimp, peeled and deveined

8 ounces chopped clams (with juice)

1 tablespoon chopped fresh parsley

PER SERVING

calories	227
total fat	6.6 g.
saturated fat	0.9 g.
cholesterol	108 mg.
sodium	481 mg.
dietary fiber	2.7 g.

In a Dutch oven over medium heat, warm the oil. Add the onions and garlic. Cook, stirring frequently, for 5 minutes, or until the onions soften. Add the tomatoes (with juice). Break up the tomatoes with the back of a spoon.

Add the water, vegetable juice, tomato paste, and oregano. Stir to mix. Bring to a boil, then reduce the heat to low. Cover and cook for 30 minutes.

Meanwhile, pick over the crabmeat and discard any bits of shell. Place the crabmeat in a fine sieve. Rinse with cold water and drain.

Add the crabmeat, shrimp, and clams to the pot. Increase the heat to medium-high. As soon as the stew returns to a boil, remove it from the heat. Set aside for 5 minutes, or until the shrimp are opaque in the center. Test by cutting a shrimp in half.

Serve sprinkled with the parsley.

Makes 6 servings

Cook's Note: Serve the stew with plenty of whole-grain bread for dipping in the sauce.

SMOKING
OUTSMARTING THE EVIL WEED

Apparently there aren't a lot of smokers thumping melons or scrutinizing tomatoes at the local supermarket. Experts aren't sure why, but smokers don't eat as many fruits and vegetables as nonsmokers do. But the more fruits and vegetables you eat, studies show, the better your odds of escaping the ravages of the smoker's "big three"—heart disease, stroke, and cancer.

You don't have to eat boatloads of bananas or bushels of brussels sprouts to get the benefits. Eating just one fruit or a serving of vegetables a day may slightly cut your risk of lung cancer, and having nine or more servings a day can have a significant impact.

There are two reasons that fruits and vegetables should get top billing on a smoker's plate. First, they're packed with antioxidants, powerful nutrients that protect against smoking-related diseases like heart disease and cancer. Plus, produce is loaded with phytonutrients, compounds found in plants that show promise for preventing or even treating these diseases.

Of course, loading up on fruits and vegetables won't make up for a pack-a-day habit. The only way to truly cut the risk of smoking-related diseases is to stop smoking. But whether you've recently quit or plan on doing so, loading your plate with produce will offer substantial protection.

UNDERSTANDING THE DANGER

Bananas turn brown. Cooking oils turn rancid. Our bodies eventually decay. Yecch—it's not a pretty image. In all these cases, the damage is caused by the same thing: highly reactive, dangerous molecules called free radicals.

Although free radicals occur naturally, their numbers are greatly increased by such things as pollution and cigarette smoke. In large numbers, they may lead to age-related maladies like heart disease and cancer.

THE MAIN PLAYERS

Despite the potential ravages that can be caused by free radicals, nature provided a powerful defense: antioxidants. While some antioxidants, in the form of enzymes and other compounds, are found naturally in our bodies, others come from foods, particularly fresh fruits and vegetables.

The Best Protection

The U.S. Department of Agriculture recommends that we eat at least five servings of fruits and vegetables a day. But because tobacco smoke depletes valuable nutrients from the body, smokers "ought to eat at least twice that amount," says James Scala, Ph.D., a nutritionist and author of *If You Can't/Won't Stop Smoking*.

While it's always best to eat a wide variety of fruits and vegetables, some foods have been found to be especially protective.

Citrus fruit. Smoking one cigarette destroys between 25 and 100 milligrams of vitamin C, says pharmacist Earl Mindell, R.Ph., Ph.D., professor of nutrition at Pacific Western University in Los Angeles and author of *Earl Mindell's Food as Medicine*. "It would be a good idea to eat a fruit or vegetable that's rich in vitamin C for every cigarette you smoke," he says.

Cruciferous vegetables. Broccoli, cauliflower, and other members of this vegetable family contain compounds called indoles and isothiocyanates, which in laboratory studies have been shown to slow the growth of cancers.

Soy foods. Tofu, tempeh, and other soy foods contain a number of cancer-fighting substances, including genistein and protease inhibitors. In Japan (where people eat large amounts of soy), more than 60 percent of men over age 20 smoke, yet the incidence of lung cancer is much lower than it is here, says Dr. Mindell.

Strawberries, grapes, and cherries. These fruits are rich in ellagic acid, a phytochemical that has been shown to destroy hydrocarbons, potentially cancer-causing chemicals in cigarette smoke.

Tomatoes. Inside tomatoes is a substance called lycopene, which has powerful antioxidant abilities. In fact, tomatoes appear to provide more cancer protection than other fruits or green vegetables.

Antioxidants are of particular importance to smokers. The body pulls antioxidants out of the blood and into the lungs in a valiant attempt to neutralize free radical damage, says Gary E. Hatch, Ph.D., research toxicologist in the pulmonary toxicology branch of the Environmental Protection Agency. "The cells in the lungs of a smoker are loaded with a lot more antioxidants than those of a nonsmoker," he explains. "The antioxidants are trying to protect the airways from the onslaught of these noxious chemicals."

Antioxidants that have been linked with lower cancer rates include beta-carotene, vitamins C and E, and the mineral selenium.

Beta-carotene. Abundant in orange and yellow fruits and vegetables such as apricots, cantaloupes, carrots, pumpkins, and squash, beta-carotene seems to protect against "smokers' cancers"—those of the colon, kidneys, skin, and lungs, says James Scala, Ph.D., a nutritionist and author of *If You Can't/Won't Stop Smoking*. Study after study shows that low levels of beta-carotene are associated with a greater cancer risk, including the risk of lung cancer.

Vitamin C. Found in strawberries, papaya, citrus fruits, and many other foods, vitamin C has been found to protect against a variety of cancers as well as heart disease and stroke, says pharmacist Earl Mindell, R.Ph., Ph.D., professor of nutrition at Pacific Western University in Los Angeles and author of *Earl Mindell's Food as Medicine*.

Vitamin E. Concentrated in wheat germ and wheat-germ oil, vitamin E helps keep cell walls intact so it's harder for marauding free radicals to push their way in. More important, it also neutralizes free radicals, says Dr. Scala.

Selenium. Found in most fruits and vegetables, especially garlic, onions, and other bulb vegetables, selenium works with vitamin E to neutralize free radicals.

The Case for Produce

The evidence is strong (and getting stronger) that people who eat lots of fresh fruits and vegetables have a lower risk of developing lung and other cancers than people who eat less produce.

In a Japanese study, for example, researchers found that men who ate raw vegetables every day slashed their lung cancer risks by about 36 percent. Those who ate fruit every day reduced their risks of lung cancer by 55 percent.

Even the men who were smokers benefited. Smokers who ate fruit, raw vegetables, and green vegetables every day reduced their lung cancer risks by 59 percent, 44 percent, and 52 percent, respectively.

The benefits of produce aren't only in relation to lung cancer either. A high intake of fruits and vegetables has been linked to lower risks of just about every type of cancer.

Secondhand Protection

It's not only smokers who need extra dietary protection. Research has shown that secondhand smoke can be dangerous for those who live or work with those who light up. According to a study led by Susan Taylor Mayne, Ph.D., associate director of cancer prevention and control research at the Yale Cancer Center, eating 1½ additional servings of raw fresh fruits or vegetables a day may slash the risk of lung cancer from secondhand smoke by as much as 60 percent.

"Eating fruits and vegetables is associated with a decrease in risk, regardless of the amount of passive smoke that nonsmokers are exposed to," says Dr. Mayne. Particularly good choices are cantaloupes, carrots, and broccoli, which are loaded with beta-carotene.

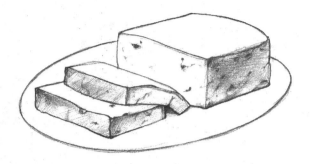

Soy Foods
Help for Your Hormones

Healing Power

Can help:
Prevent heart disease

Relieve menopause symptoms

Reduce the risk of breast and
prostate cancer

In a perfect world, milkshakes would lower cholesterol, burgers would help prevent cancer, and cheesecake would ease hot flashes, mood swings, and other uncomfortable conditions associated with menopause.

Sound far-fetched? Maybe not—if they were made with soy. According to researchers, all of these health benefits and more have been linked to this small bean that many Americans have never seen, let alone eaten—the common soybean.

Studies show that several compounds found in soybeans and in related foods like tofu, tempeh, and soy milk may help lower cholesterol, reduce the risk of heart disease and cancer, and ease some of the discomfort of menopause. Indeed, if early research proves fruitful, women in the future may use soy foods as a replacement for, or at least as a supplement to, estrogen replacement therapy.

Researchers speculate that the key to soy's healing power is a class of compounds called phytoestrogens. Phytoestrogens such as genistein and daidzein are weaker versions of the estrogen women produce naturally. They appear to help in a number of different ways, from blocking the negative effects of natural estrogens to supplementing them when they're running low.

Evidence of soy's health benefits is still preliminary, experts warn. Nonetheless, the possibilities are intriguing. "The data emerging on soy are really ex-

In the Kitchen

You've seen tofu in the produce section of your supermarket. But how do you eat this pale, spongy stuff?

Almost any way you want. The advantage of tofu is that while it has little taste of its own, it takes on the flavor of whatever it's cooked with. You can use it with meats, soups, vegetable dishes, and even desserts.

There are two main types of tofu, firm and soft. Which one you buy depends on how you're going to use it.

- **Firm tofu** has had much of the water removed, giving it a solid consistency. It's usually used when you want the tofu to keep its shape, as in recipes for stir-fries, casseroles, or mock meatballs.
- **Soft (also called silken) tofu** contains more water than the firm variety, giving it a soft, creamy texture. It's usually used for making dips, salad dressings, and desserts.

Both types of tofu should be rinsed with cold water before using. If you're not planning to use tofu immediately after opening the container, or if you buy it fresh from an open container at an Asian market, rinse it daily and keep it submerged in fresh water. You can also keep it frozen until you're ready to use it.

After rinsing, press out excess water with your hands or by placing the tofu between several layers of paper towels and pressing with your palm. Removing the excess water will help the tofu maintain its shape during preparation.

---

citing," says James W. Anderson, M.D., professor of medicine and clinical nutrition at the Veterans Administration Medical Center at the University of Kentucky College of Medicine in Lexington.

Good for Your Heart

High cholesterol is a major risk factor for heart disease. Putting more soy foods in your diet may play a role in sending cholesterol levels south.

As proof of the benefits of soy, researchers point to Asian countries, where people eat tofu, tempeh, or other soy foods virtually every day. Consider the Japanese: They live longer than people anywhere else in the world. Japanese men have the world's lowest rate of death from heart disease, with Japanese women coming in a close second. A possible reason is that the Japanese eat about 24 pounds of soy foods per person per year, which averages about 1 ounce a day. Americans, by contrast, eat an average of 4 pounds per person per year.

Researchers speculate that soy foods increase the activity of low-density

THE JOY OF SOY

Don't know tofu from tempeh? Here are some of the most common soy foods, along with a few suggestions for using them.

Meat substitutes. If you want to cut back on meat while getting more soy, look for "mock" meats, like cold cuts, bacon, sausage, franks, and burgers. These are mainly made from soy, and in some cases they are virtually indistinguishable from the real thing.

Soy flour. Made from roasted, ground soybeans, soy flour can be used to replace some of the wheat flour used for baking. Nutritionists advise buying defatted soy flour, which contains less fat and more protein than the full-fat variety.

Soy milk. A creamy, milklike drink made from ground, soaked soybeans and water, it's sold plain and in a variety of flavors. Some people prefer "lite" soy milk. It's lower in fat than the regular kind, but it may contain fewer of the protective phytoestrogens.

Tempeh. These chunky, tender cakes are made from fermented soybeans that have been laced with mold, giving them their distinctively smoky, nutty flavor. You can grill tempeh or add it to spaghetti sauce, chili, or casseroles.

Texturized soy protein. Made from soy flour, this meat substitute can replace part or all of the meat in meat loaf, burgers, and chili.

Tofu. A creamy white, soft, cheeselike food made from curdled soy milk. Tofu comes in firm and soft varieties and can be used in virtually anything from soups to desserts.

You will find soft and firm varieties of tofu at most supermarkets in the produce section. Other soy foods are available at specialty and health food stores.

---

lipoprotein (LDL) cholesterol receptors, "traps" on the surfaces of cells that seize harmful LDL molecules from the bloodstream and ship them to the liver, from which they're eventually excreted. Reducing the amount of LDL in the blood may help keep it from oxidizing and clogging the arteries leading from the heart.

In one large study, Dr. Anderson and his colleagues analyzed the results of 38 separate studies examining the relationship between soy and cholesterol levels. Their conclusion: Consuming 1 to 1½ ounces of soy protein (rather than animal protein) a day lowered total cholesterol by 9 percent and harmful LDL cholesterol by 13 percent.

TURNING DOWN THE HEAT

More than half of American women in menopause complain of hot flashes and night sweats. In Japan, there isn't even a phrase for "hot flash." Might Japanese women have fewer menopausal problems because they eat more soy?

"There are some preliminary data that suggest that soy reduces menopause symptoms such as hot flashes," says Mark Messina, Ph.D., former head of the National Cancer Institute's Designer Foods Program.

In one study, researchers at the Brighton Medical Clinic in Victoria, Australia, gave 58 postmenopausal women about 1½ ounces of soy flour or wheat flour every day. After three months, the women eating soy flour saw their hot flashes plummet by 40 percent. Women given wheat flour, by contrast, had only a 25 percent reduction.

"If these data are confirmed, then within a couple years we may be at a point where doctors are saying, 'Take 2 cups of soy milk per day' instead of recommending hormone-replacement therapy to relieve menopause symptoms," says Dr. Messina.

POWERFUL BREAST PROTECTION

Researchers believe that the phytoestrogens in soy, which mimic a woman's natural estrogen, may help reduce the effects of the hormone in the body. Since estrogen is thought to fuel the growth of breast tumors, lower activity in the body could mean a lower risk of developing breast cancer.

The estrogens in soy can help protect women in several ways, depending on the stage of life. In premenopausal women, for example, a diet high in soy foods may lengthen the menstrual cycle. This is important, since every woman experiences a surge in estrogen at the beginning of her cycle. Multiplied over a lifetime, these surges expose the body to large amounts of estrogen, which eventually could cause cellular changes that lead to cancer. Lengthening the menstrual cycle, experts say, reduces the frequency of these surges, and with it a woman's lifetime exposure to the hormone.

In one study, researchers at the National University of Singapore found that premenopausal women who consumed high amounts of soy foods, along with generous amounts of beta-carotene and polyunsaturated fats, had half the risk of developing breast cancer as women who consumed a lot of animal protein.

Curiously, in women who are postmenopausal, soy foods appear to provide an estrogen "lift" that helps make up for the body's low levels of the hormone. This lift appears to provide the protective benefits of estrogen (such as helping to prevent osteoporosis) without raising the cancer risk.

PROTECTION FOR MEN

While most research exploring the protective effects of soy foods has looked at women, experts agree that men can benefit as well.

It appears that a soy-rich diet may help reduce the harmful effects of the male hormone testosterone, which is thought to fuel the growth of cancerous cells in the prostate gland.

A study of 8,000 Japanese men living in Hawaii found that those who ate the most tofu had the lowest rates of prostate cancer. Even though Japanese men develop prostate cancer just as often as Western men do, they nonetheless have the lowest death rates from prostate cancer in the world. Experts suspect that soy foods, by inhibiting the effects of testosterone, help shut off the "fuel" that causes cancers to grow.

For both men and women, "what these studies suggest is that just one serving is enough to reduce cancer risk," says Dr. Messina. "If that's for real, then soy could have a tremendous public health impact."

Nutritional Extras

There's more to tofu, tempeh, and other soy foods than phytoestrogens. Soy foods are just plain good for you. "There are lots of reasons to add soy to your diet just from a basic nutritional perspective," says Dr. Messina.

For example, a half-cup of tofu provides about 20 grams of protein, 40 percent of the Daily Value (DV). The same half-cup supplies about 258 milligrams of calcium, more than 25 percent of the DV, and 13 milligrams of iron, 87 percent of the Recommended Dietary Allowance (RDA) for women and 130 percent of the RDA for men.

While soy foods are moderately high in fat, most of the fat is polyunsaturated. Soy foods contain little of the artery-clogging saturated fat found in meat and many dairy foods, says Dr. Messina.

Getting the Most

Add it last. When cooking with tofu or other soy products, always add them late in the cooking process. Researchers speculate that cooking at high heats for extended periods of time may reduce or eliminate many of the nutritional benefits.

Shop for power. While it's best to eat soy foods in their unadulterated form, there are times that you may have a taste for a ready-made vegetable burger or breakfast sausage. When buying processed soy foods, make sure that they contain "soy protein," "hydrolyzed vegetable protein," or "textured vegetable protein," which are all acceptable sources of phytoestrogens. By contrast, don't expect too much from products containing soy protein concentrates, says Dr. Anderson. "Unfortunately, most of the beneficial substances are extracted from these products," he says.

Look for full-fat. While it's usually a good idea to reduce the amount of fat in your diet, full-fat soy milk contains 50 percent more phytoestrogens than the low-fat kind, says Dr. Anderson. "Getting those extra phytoestrogens is a good trade-off for the extra fat," he says.

Soy-Fruit Smoothie

2 cups vanilla-flavored soy beverage, well-chilled

1 cup frozen sliced peaches

1 medium banana, cut into chunks

8 medium strawberries

¼ teaspoon ground cinnamon

In a blender, combine the soy beverage, peaches, bananas, strawberries, and cinnamon. Blend until smooth and creamy.

Makes 2 servings

Per serving

calories	**248**
total fat	**3.3 g.**
saturated fat	**0.6 g.**
cholesterol	**0 mg.**
sodium	**122 mg.**
dietary fiber	**4.8 g.**

Mocha Tofu Pudding

2 packages (10½ ounces each) silken tofu

⅔ cup packed light brown sugar

5 tablespoons cocoa powder

1¼ teaspoons vanilla

⅛ teaspoon ground cinnamon

2 teaspoons instant coffee powder

2 teaspoons boiling water

Drain the tofu and pat dry with paper towels. Place it in a food processor. Add the sugar, cocoa, vanilla, and cinnamon. In a cup, mix the coffee and water, stirring to dissolve the coffee. Add to the food processor.

Process until smooth, stopping occasionally to scrape down the sides of the container.

Spoon into small dessert dishes. Cover and refrigerate for at least 30 minutes, or until the pudding firms up.

Makes 6 servings

Per serving

calories	**133**
total fat	**3.6 g.**
saturated fat	**0.4 g.**
cholesterol	**0 mg.**
sodium	**43 mg.**
dietary fiber	**1.6 g.**

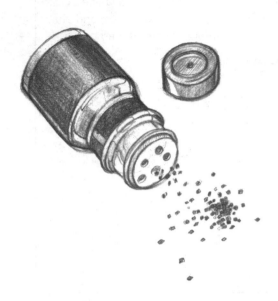

Spices
Protective Flavorings

Healing Power
Can help:

Protect against cataracts

Prevent cancer

Lower cholesterol
and triglycerides

Prevent excessive blood
clotting

In biblical times, mustard seeds were thought to cure everything from toothaches to epilepsy. (Some people even sniffed ground mustard seeds because sneezing was thought to purge the brain.) Saffron, black pepper, fenugreek, and many other spices were also prized for their healing powers.

As it turns out, the ancients had an uncanny sense of which spices were most likely to be effective. "Researchers have identified many substances in spices that offer health benefits," says Melanie Polk, R.D., director of nutrition education at the American Institute for Cancer Research.

The National Institute of Nutrition in India, for example, has found that turmeric contains compounds that may help prevent cancer. The research is so promising, in fact, that India's National Cancer Institute has proposed a public education campaign to promote greater use of this aromatic spice.

Unlike herbs, which come from the leaves of plants, spices are made from the buds, bark, fruits, roots, or seeds. The drying process doesn't appear to diminish their healing powers. When properly stored, spices can retain their active ingredients for months or even years.

Research into the world of spices is very new, Polk says, so scientists are only beginning to understand their healing potential. But what has been discovered so far is impressive.

Defense against Cancer

Spices contain an abundance of compounds called phytochemicals or phytonutrients, many of which may help prevent normal, healthy cells from turning into cancer. And the ways in which these compounds work are as varied as the spices themselves.

Many spices, for example, contain antioxidants, substances that block the effects of free radicals in the body. Free radicals are harmful oxygen molecules that punch holes in healthy cells, sometimes causing genetic damage that can lead to cancer.

Turmeric, for example, is a very rich source of antioxidants, including a compound called curcumin. In animal studies, curcumin has been shown to reduce the risk of colon cancer by 58 percent. Other research suggests that it may work against skin cancer as well.

What's more, some spices have the ability to help neutralize harmful substances in the body, taking away their cancer-causing potential. Nutmeg, ginger, cumin, black pepper, and coriander, for example, have been shown to help block the effects of aflatoxin, a mold that can cause liver cancer.

Finally, some spices appear to be capable of killing cancer cells outright. In laboratory studies, for example, compounds from saffron were placed on human cancer cells, including cells that cause leukemia. Not only did the dangerous cells stop growing, but the compounds appeared to have no effect on normal, healthy cells.

Since the research is still very new, researchers can't predict which spices or how much of different spices you might need to reduce your risk of getting cancer. "The best advice for now," Polk says, "is to use a variety of spices, especially for replacing salt and fat in your food."

Keeping Arteries Clear

The biggest health threat Americans face is heart disease. Much of the blame for heart disease can be placed squarely on cholesterol, the fatty stuff in the bloodstream that, in large amounts, can begin sticking to artery walls, slowing or even stopping the flow of blood to the heart.

There is good evidence that getting more spices in your diet can help keep the arteries clear. The reason, once again, is antioxidants. Some of the same compounds in spices that prevent free radicals from damaging healthy cells also prevent them from damaging cholesterol. This is important, because when cholesterol is damaged, it's much more likely to stick to artery walls.

Cloves, for example, contain a compound called eugenol, which is a powerful antioxidant. The curcumin in turmeric can also protect the arteries. Turmeric, incidentally, may provide double protection because it not only blocks

IN THE KITCHEN

Despite their robust appearance, spices don't last forever. And even when they're fresh, they're often reluctant to give up their full range of flavors. Here are a few ways to get the best tastes every time.

Stock up often. If you haven't bought spices since the last time you moved, it's probably time to throw out the old ones and start fresh. Ground spices lose their flavor quickly, usually in about six months. Whole spices, however, will keep their flavors for a year or two.

Store them carefully. Exposure to light, moisture, and air will quickly rob spices of their delicious flavors. To keep them fresh, store them in airtight containers in a cool, dry place, preferably away from direct light.

Cook them long. Unlike herbs, which flavor a dish almost instantly, spices are slow to reveal themselves. They are best used in long-simmering soups or stews, where they'll have ample time to release their flavors.

Boost the flavor. To make a spice's natural flavors stand out even more, toast it briefly in a dry skillet until it's slightly brown and aromatic.

free radicals but it has also been shown to lower levels of triglycerides—dangerous blood fats that, in large amounts, appear to raise the risk of heart disease.

Yet another way in which spices keep cholesterol levels down is by trapping cholesterol-containing substances in the intestine. Fenugreek, for example, contains compounds called saponins, which bind to cholesterol and cause it to be excreted from the body. In one study, for example, scientists found that animals given fenugreek had drops in cholesterol of at least 18 percent.

It's not only high cholesterol that can raise the risk for heart disease. Another potential problem is platelets—small, cell-like components in blood that aid in clotting. While platelets are essential for stopping bleeding, sometimes they get too active and begin forming excessive clots in the bloodstream. If a clot gets large enough to block an artery, the result can be a heart attack or even a stroke.

At least five spices—turmeric, fenugreek, cloves, red chili peppers, and ginger—have been shown to help prevent platelets from clumping. In fact, a compound in ginger called gingerol has a chemical structure somewhat similar to aspirin's, which is a proven clot-busting drug.

A PROMISING FUTURE

Since spices contain a large number of compounds, researchers have just begun mapping their healing powers. But research from around the globe indicates that the list of benefits will only keep growing.

Researchers at the National Cancer Institute, for example, have found that the curcumin in turmeric can help prevent HIV, the virus that causes AIDS, from multiplying. Research has shown, in fact, that when people with AIDS were given curcumin, the illness progressed at a slower rate.

Curcumin has also been shown to protect the eyes from free radicals, which are one of the leading causes of cataracts. In fact, a laboratory study found that curcumin was able to reduce free radical damage to the eyes by 52 percent.

Finally, researchers at the University of Wales College of Medicine discovered that a strain of black pepper called West African black pepper appears to produce changes in the brains of mice that can reduce the severity of seizures.

"We only have information on a few spices so far," Polk says. "But no doubt we'll be uncovering similarly exciting information about many others in the future."

INDIAN-STYLE SPICE MIX

8   teaspoons dry mustard
4   teaspoons ground fenugreek
4   teaspoons ground cumin
2   teaspoons ground turmeric
2   teaspoons ground ginger
2   teaspoons ground coriander
2   teaspoons ground cloves
½ teaspoon ground cinnamon

In a small bowl, combine the mustard, fenugreek, cumin, turmeric, ginger, coriander, cloves, and cinnamon. Mix well to blend. Store in a small, airtight jar in a cool, dark cupboard or the refrigerator.

Makes ½ cup

Cook's Notes: Ground fenugreek is available in Indian groceries, some specialty food shops, and health food stores.

Although you could easily cut the recipe in half, this spice mixture is delicious enough—and versatile enough—to keep on hand in the kitchen. It's excellent as a rub for broiled or pan-fried meats, fish, and poultry (rub the mixture over the food generously before cooking). Or use it as a flavoring for cooked cauliflower, carrots, onions, and other vegetables. To bring out the flavor, cook it for a few seconds in a dry skillet just before using.

SPICED POTATO CAKES

3 large baking potatoes
2 teaspoons canola oil
1 cup chopped onions
4 teaspoons Indian-Style Spice Mix (page 499)
¾ cup nonfat plain yogurt
¼ cup fat-free egg substitute
2 teaspoons unsalted butter
¼ teaspoon salt

PER SERVING
calories **243**
total fat **4.9 g.**
saturated fat **1.4 g.**
cholesterol **5 mg.**
sodium **171 mg.**
dietary fiber **3.9 g.**

Scrub the potatoes and pat dry with paper towels. With a fork, pierce each in 3 or 4 places. Arrange the potatoes, spoke fashion, in the microwave on top of a paper towel. Microwave on high power for 10 minutes. Turn the potatoes and rotate from the front to the back of the microwave. Microwave for 8 to 10 minutes, or until the potatoes are tender. Test for doneness by inserting the tip of a small, sharp knife in a potato. Let the potatoes stand for 5 minutes.

Halve the potatoes lengthwise. Use a large spoon to scrape all the flesh into a medium bowl; discard the skins. Mash with a fork and set aside.

In a large no-stick skillet over medium-high heat, warm the oil. Add the onions and cook, stirring frequently, for 5 minutes, or until they start to turn golden. Add the spice mix and cook for 30 seconds, or until fragrant.

Remove from the heat and transfer to a large bowl. Add the yogurt, egg substitute, butter, and salt. Stir to combine. Add the potatoes. Mix well.

Wipe the skillet with a paper towel and coat with no-stick spray. Warm over medium-high heat. Drop the potato mixture into the skillet in 4 mounds, patting the mixture with a spatula to make thick cakes. Cook for 5 minutes, or until golden on the bottom. Turn and cook for 3 minutes, or until golden.

Makes 4 servings

Cook's Note: You can serve these cakes topped with a dollop of nonfat plain yogurt and chutney.

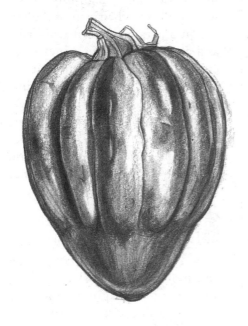

SQUASH
PACKED WITH BETA-CAROTENE— AND MORE

HEALING POWER
CAN HELP:
Prevent lung problems

Reduce the risk
of endometrial cancer

Judging from ancient remains found in Mexican caves, folks have been eating squash for at least 7,000 years. Squash was one of the nourishing "three sisters" in early Native American diets. (The other two were corn and beans.) And they were considered so important that they were often buried with the dead in order to provide them with nourishment on their final journey.

It has taken science a few thousand years to prove what early Americans knew from experience: Squash is almost overloaded with nourishing compound. In fact, squash contains such a rich array of vitamins, minerals, and other compounds that scientists have just begun to map its healing potential. "I don't think anybody really knows all the good substances there are in squash," says Dexter L. Morris, M.D., Ph.D., vice chairman and associate professor in the department of emergency medicine at the University of North Carolina School of Medicine at Chapel Hill.

When researchers talk about the healing powers of squash, what they're usually referring to is winter squash such as hubbard, acorn, and butternut, which are distinguished by their deep yellow and orange flesh colors. Pale summer squash, by contrast, while low in calories and a decent source of fiber, is generally regarded as a nutritional lightweight, at least unless future research proves otherwise.

In the Kitchen

Winter squash may be full of beta-carotene, vitamin C, and other healing compounds, but it doesn't readily give them up. The squash is encased in a tough, leathery skin, which requires a sharp knife and a strong hand to cut all the way through. And if your hand should slip—look out!

Here's how to make cutting it a little easier: Rather than trying to cut the raw, tough skin, partly bake the squash first. When the skin softens—usually after about 20 minutes at 375°F—cut the squash open and clean it out. Then put it back in the oven until it's tender.

"Not long ago I was saying that apples and onions didn't have much in them," admits Mark Kestin, Ph.D., chairman of the nutrition program at Bastyr University and affiliate associate professor of epidemiology at the University of Washington School of Medicine, both in Seattle. Then researchers discovered a variety of heart-saving flavonoids, and the produce suddenly looked rich. "Summer squash may have some incredible substance we haven't discovered yet," he says.

Color Them Healthy

The winter squash come in an enormous variety of shapes, sizes, and textures, ranging from baby acorn squash the size of walnuts to impossibly big hubbards the size of bowling pins. Yet there's one thing that they all have in common: strong, intense colors that indicate the presence of healing compounds within.

Two of the most popular winter squashes, the bumpy-skinned hubbard squash and the deeply tanned butternut squash, are both rich in vitamin C and beta-carotene, two antioxidant vitamins that have been shown in studies to help prevent cancer, heart disease, and certain age-related conditions such as problems with the eyes. Eating a half-cup of baked butternut squash will provide more than a quarter of the Daily Value (DV) for vitamin C. The same amount of squash delivers 40 to 66 percent of the amount of beta-carotene recommended by experts.

For people with asthma, squash and other foods rich in vitamin C can be powerful breath savers. It's easy to understand why. Modern life is filled with car exhaust, cigarette smoke, and other pollutants—scientists call them oxidants—that can damage tissues in the lungs, making it hard for them to work as efficiently as they should. Foods like squash, however, are rich in antioxidants, like vitamin C. Studies have shown that the more vitamin C you get, the lower your risk of getting asthma or other respiratory diseases.

"People who have more C in their diets over time have fewer lung ailments. The vitamin gets transported to the lining of the lung and serves as an antioxidant there," explains Gary E. Hatch, Ph.D., research toxicologist in the pulmonary toxicology branch of the Environmental Protection Agency.

Dr. Hatch recommends that everyone get at least 200 milligrams daily of dietary vitamin C, which is about the amount in 6½ cups of baked butternut squash.

On the beta-carotene front, "there are tons of studies showing that eating vegetables rich in beta-carotene" is good for you, says Dr. Morris. More is involved than just basic good nutrition. Doctors in Italy and Switzerland studied the diets of more than 1,000 of their country-women. Preliminary research suggests that women who got the most beta-carotene—5.5 milligrams a day, which is about the amount in 1 cup of baked winter squash—had half the risk of endometrial cancer of those who ate the least.

Beta-carotene is not the only carotene found in squash. A related compound, called alpha-carotene, is also present, though in smaller amounts. "It's very similar chemi-cally to beta-carotene, but there has not been a lot of work done on it yet," says Dr. Kestin.

Getting the Most

Shop for color. There's a huge variability in the amount of beta-carotene found in squash. It can range anywhere from about 0.5 milligram to about 5 milligrams, even in the same kind of squash.

As a rule, experts say, the darker the squash, the more beta-carotene it contains. The shell of an acorn

DELICIOUS CHOICES

When shopping for squash, most of us think of the old standbys, like acorn or spaghetti squash. But supermarkets these days often have many varieties to choose from. Here are some squashes you may want to try.

- **Buttercup squash** look like little drums wearing pale beanies, which match the stripes running down their green skin. About 3 pounds on the average, buttercup squash is mild and sweet, but sometimes dry.
- The giant **calabaza squash** from the West Indies wind up in markets cut into huge hunks that show off their neon-orange flesh. This is a sweet squash that is best pureed or cooked with other foods.
- **Delicata**'s skin is the color of heavy cream, but it's daubed and striped with green and sometimes orange, and the flesh is yellow and sweet.
- **Golden nugget** looks like Cinderella's carriage at midnight—a big pumpkin turned small. It's mildly sweet and only has enough flesh for one serving.
- Barely bigger than a good-size apple, **sweet dumplings** are cream-colored and scalloped with mottled green. They're often baked and served whole.

squash, for example, should be an intensely deep, dark green. Butternut squash should be a butterscotch tan, and hubbards should be almost glow-in-the-dark orange.

"The richer the color, the richer the nutrient content," says Susan Thom, R.D., a resource spokesperson for the American Dietetic Association and a nutrition consultant in Brecksville, Ohio.

Buy it ahead of time. The hard skin that makes winter squash such a challenge to cut also helps protect the flesh inside. This means that you can store it for a month or more in a cool, well-ventilated place before the nutrients start to diminish. In fact, storing squash actually causes the amount of beta-carotene to increase, according to Densie Webb, R.D., Ph.D., co-author of *Foods for Better Health*.

Try the summer kind. While zucchini and other kinds of summer squash don't have the rich nutrient stores of winter squash, they do contain a lot of fiber, but only if you eat the peel, says Pamela Savage-Marr, R.D., a spokesperson for the American Dietetic Association and a health education specialist at Oakwood Health Care System in Dearborn, Michigan. A half-cup of unpeeled, uncooked summer squash contains more than 1 gram of fiber.

ZUCCHINI WITH GARLIC AND OREGANO

$1^1/_2$ **pounds zucchini**

$1^1/_2$ **teaspoons olive oil**

4 **cloves garlic, minced**

1 **large tomato, seeded and diced**

$^3/_4$ **teaspoon dried oregano**

$^1/_4$ **teaspoon salt**

Pinch of ground black pepper

PER SERVING

calories	**48**
total fat	**1.9 g.**
saturated fat	**0.3 g.**
cholesterol	**0 mg.**
sodium	**141 mg.**
dietary fiber	**2.2 g.**

Trim the zucchini and cut into $^1/_4$" slices.

In a large skillet over medium heat, warm the oil. Add the garlic and cook for 30 seconds, or just until fragrant. Add the zucchini; toss to mix. Add the tomatoes and oregano. Toss well to mix. Reduce the heat to medium-low. Cover and cook for 5 minutes, or until the zucchini softens.

Add the salt and pepper and stir gently to mix.

Makes 4 servings

Cook's Note: If desired, sprinkle the zucchini with grated Parmesan cheese before serving.

ACORN SQUASH WITH BREAD STUFFING

2   **large acorn squash (about 1½ pounds each)**

4   **teaspoons olive oil**

1   **cup minced onions**

5   **slices stale bread, cut into ½" cubes**

¾   **teaspoon ground savory**

¼   **teaspoon ground black pepper**

¾–1   **cup water**

PER SERVING

calories	**256**
total fat	**6.2 g.**
saturated fat	**1 g.**
cholesterol	**0 mg.**
sodium	**182 mg.**
dietary fiber	**11.6 g.**

Preheat the oven to 375°F.

Cut each squash in half lengthwise. Scoop out and discard the seeds. Place the squash halves, cut side down, in a large baking dish. Add ½" of water. Bake for 25 to 30 minutes, or until the squash can be pierced with the tip of a sharp knife but is still fairly firm.

Meanwhile, in a large no-stick skillet over medium heat, warm the oil. Add the onions and cook for 5 minutes, or until softened. Add the bread, savory, and pepper. Stir to mix. Cook until the bread starts to brown slightly. Stir in ¾ cup of the water. Add up to ¼ cup of the remaining water to make the bread moist but not wet.

Remove the squash from the oven. Turn the halves over and spoon the bread mixture into the cavities. Pour enough hot tap water into the pan to return the level to about ½".

Bake for 20 to 30 minutes, or until the squash is tender and the filling is golden. Test for doneness by inserting the tip of a sharp knife into the squash.

Makes 4 servings

Cook's Note: Use stale wheatberry or multigrain bread for a really flavorful, nutritious stuffing.

Stomach Upset
Calming the Queasies

One of life's ironies is that many of the foods we like best, like creamy chocolate eclairs or a feast of roast turkey, stuffing, and gravy, are the same ones that our stomachs like least, at least when we overindulge. And overindulge we do—with family, friends, and co-workers—more than a few times a year. This is why our festive feasts sometimes end not with a glass of wine but with a spoonful of Pepto-Bismol.

Getting too much food in your system at one time is a common cause of stomach upset because your body has trouble handling the sudden increase in volume, says William Ruderman, M.D., a gastroenterologist in private practice in Orlando, Florida. Eating too much fat can also be a problem because it may trip the nausea sensor in the brain, which sends those miserable, queasy sensations down to the stomach.

High-fat foods are bad in yet another way. They temporarily weaken a small muscle at the base of the esophagus, the tube leading from the mouth to the stomach. This allows digestive juices, which normally stay in the stomach, to surge upstream, causing heartburn or nausea, says Marie Borum, M.D., assistant professor of medicine at George Washington University Medical Center in Washington, D.C. The combination of heartburn and that too-full feeling can take the cheerful bloom off any social evening.

Two of the best ways to keep your stomach calm is to eat a little bit less at meals and to cut back on fatty foods, especially fried meats, says Dr. Borum. But if your stomach's already upset, what you really need is something that will take the queasiness away fast. As it turns out, foods, especially bland foods, can do that, too.

"I recommend starting with water, then moving on to toast, broth, bland soup, or soft-boiled eggs," says Dr. Borum. "Naturally, you also want to avoid the hard-to-digest foods like ice cream or fried chicken."

When even bland foods are hard to get down, don't even try to eat, Dr. Borum adds. There's nothing wrong with going without food for 4 to 6 hours. Many people are reluctant to skip meals, but a temporary fast can actually be very soothing. In fact, that may be just the right thing to help your stomach recover.

One of the most popular remedies for an upset stomach is also one of the oldest. Studies show that ginger can sometimes work better than over-the-counter drugs to settle a somersaulting stomach. "Ginger is the one herbal treatment that's pretty widely accepted as effective," says Marvin Schuster, M.D., director of the Marvin M. Schuster Digestive and Motility Disorders Center at Johns Hopkins Bayview Medical Center in Baltimore.

While fresh ginger is effective, it's really too spicy to use to get the amounts that are necessary for healing. An easier strategy, says Dr. Schuster, is to brew a cup of ginger tea. Grate 2 teaspoons of fresh ginger and let it steep in hot water for 10 minutes. Strain the tea, then drink it until you feel better. For many people, just one cup is enough to do the trick.

Another beverage that may help settle your stomach is Coca-Cola. The ingredients in Coke are top secret, so no one really knows why so many people reach for the "real thing" when their stomachs are flip-flopping. Still, drinking Coke does seem to be helpful, says Dr. Borum. "Coke is also high in sugar, which is important if you've already been sick and need hydration," she adds.

One problem with having an upset stomach is that it's often difficult even to drink water without feeling sicker. To keep yourself from getting dehydrated, try keeping a small piece of ice in your mouth, Dr. Borum suggests. This will allow some water to enter your system, but not so much that it will upset your stomach even more.

MERRY, MERRY, QUITE CONTRARY

Good food, good drink, and good company—who doesn't like a good party? But making too many trips to the punch bowl can leave your stomach wishing you'd spent the night playing solitaire.

While there's no real cure for "morning-after stomach," there are a few foods that will help ease the discomfort of a hangover. Here are some examples that you can try.

Keep it plain. Having a slice of plain bread—without butter, peanut butter, or cream cheese—will help buffer acids in the stomach that can lead to nausea, according to Marie Borum, M.D., assistant professor of medicine at George Washington University Medical Center in Washington, D.C. In addition, bland foods like bread and pasta are very easy to digest, which can help keep an upset stomach calm.

Drink like a fish. Getting more water into your system can help relieve nausea and dehydration that may be caused by excessive drinking. If you've been drinking alcohol, in fact, it's a good idea to have plenty of water before going to bed at night because it can help prevent some of the discomfort you might experience the next morning.

STRESS
GETTING EASE WITH Bs

Late for work—grab a doughnut. The report's due—pour another cup of coffee. The children are yelling—take an ice cream break.

Stress is all around us, and food often provides a welcome, if momentary, break. Unfortunately, the foods we often turn to in times of stress, like coffee and sweets, have a way of making us feel even more frazzled later on.

It doesn't have to be this way. Research has shown that eating more of some foods and less of others can cause stress hormones in the body to decline. Making slight changes in your diet will produce physical changes in the brain that can make the world's problems just a little bit easier to handle.

CALMING CARBOHYDRATES

Mashed potatoes. Fresh-baked bread. A steaming plate of pasta. These are just a few of the "comfort foods" that many of us instinctively turn to in times of stress. As it turns out, our instincts are dead-on. Researchers have found that foods high in carbohydrates produce changes in the brain that can take the edge off stress.

During emotionally trying times, the brain quickly uses up its supply of serotonin, a chemical that imparts feelings of well-being. When serotonin levels fall, negative feelings tend to rise, says Joe Tecce, Ph.D., a neuropsychologist and professor of psychology at Boston College in Chestnut Hill, Massachusetts.

Eating foods that are high in carbohydrates, like pasta, bagels, or baked potatoes, can quickly raise low serotonin levels, making you feel less stressed and more relaxed, says Dr. Tecce. And here's a little carbohydrate bonus: As serotonin levels rise, appetite usually decreases, which means you're less likely to eat your way through hard times.

A ZOO STORY

Next time you visit the monkey house, take a moment to admire our swinging cousins. They turn somersaults, hang from trees, and generally appear to be having a great time. They don't have to deal with carpools or bills, which could explain their lack of stress. Then again, maybe it's all the bananas they've been eating.

Research suggests that foods high in vitamin B_6, such as bananas, potatoes,

508

and prunes, can relieve irritability and stress, making people (and maybe monkeys) feel just a little bit better. In one study Dr. Tecce and his colleagues at the Jean Mayer USDA Human Nutrition Research Center on Aging at Tufts University in Boston lowered vitamin B_6 levels in a group of volunteers. The people became increasingly irritable and tense.

The research is still preliminary, but it may be that vitamin B_6 improves mood by raising levels of dopamine, a chemical in the brain that is related to feeling good. When you don't get enough vitamin B_6 in your diet, dopamine levels fall, and you can experience negative feelings. In addition, people who don't get enough vitamin B_6 may produce too little serotonin, which will make them feel even worse.

It's not yet clear how much vitamin B_6 you might need to help keep stress levels down, says Dr. Tecce. It seems likely, however, that the Daily Value (DV) of 2 milligrams is probably enough. It's very easy to get this much vitamin B_6 in your diet. One banana, for example, has 0.7 milligram, 35 percent of the DV; a half-cup of chickpeas has 0.6 milligram, 30 percent of the DV; and a baked potato has 0.4 milligram, 20 percent of the DV.

THE CAFFEINE CRASH

Just about anywhere there are people hard at work, there will also be a coffeepot. And the more stress these people feel, the more likely they are to hit the joe. In a study of almost 300 people, for example, researchers at the University of Minnesota in Morris found that half of them drank more coffee or caffeine-containing soft drinks during high-pressure times.

Caffeine produces a quick zing that can momentarily make you feel more relaxed and confident. Fairly quickly, however, it stimulates the production of cortisol, a stress hormone that raises blood pressure and heart rate. This can make you feel more stressed than you did before, says William Lovallo, Ph.D., professor of psychiatry and behavioral sciences at the University of Oklahoma Health Sciences Center in Oklahoma City.

It doesn't take potfuls of coffee to rev up your stress levels, Dr. Lovallo adds. In a study of 48 men, Dr. Lovallo and his colleagues found that those drinking just 2 to 3 cups had a significant increase in blood pressure.

This doesn't mean that you have to give up your favorite drinks, Dr. Lovallo adds. But when the pressure's on, switching to drinks without caffeine will help keep you calmer and more in control.

And while you're filling your cup, put the lid back on the sugar. Within minutes after eating sweets, blood sugar levels start to fall. "When your blood sugar is going up and down, you are more susceptible to moodiness and irritability," says Peter Miller, Ph.D., executive director of the Hilton Head Health Institute in Hilton Head Island, South Carolina.

STROKE

A HEALTHY-BRAIN DIET

The most frightening thing about stroke is how suddenly it can strike. People who have had strokes say there's no warning, no sign—just a split-second sense that something has suddenly gone wrong.

But even though the stroke itself comes on suddenly, the problems that cause it can be years in the making. Stroke occurs when blood, and the oxygen and nutrients it contains, stop reaching parts of the brain. Anything that can interfere with blood flow, such as having high cholesterol or high blood pressure, makes strokes much more likely to occur.

Yet the factors that can cause a stroke are ones you can prevent by choosing the right foods. "Your diet plays a critical role in preventing stroke," says Thomas A. Pearson, M.D., Ph.D., professor and chairman of the department of community and preventive medicine at the University of Rochester in New York and a spokesman for the American Heart Association.

In a study of more than 87,000 nurses, for example, researchers at the Harvard School of Public Health found that women who ate the most fruits and vegetables were 40 percent less likely to have a stroke than those who ate the least. In another study, this one conducted at the University of California, San Diego, researchers discovered that people who ate a single serving of potassium-rich fruits or vegetables a day were also able to cut their risk of stroke by 40 percent.

What you don't eat can be just as important as what you do, adds Dr. Pearson. Research has shown, for example, that people getting the most fat in their diets—especially the saturated fat in meats and other animal foods—are much more likely to have a stroke than those eating more healthful foods. This is because a diet that's high in saturated fat raises cholesterol levels. Cholesterol, which is notorious for clogging arteries in the heart, can also block blood vessels in the brain.

"Reducing saturated fat intake is the most powerful dietary maneuver you can make to lower cholesterol levels," says John R. Crouse, M.D., professor of medicine and public health sciences at Bowman Gray School of Medicine of Wake Forest University in Winston-Salem, North Carolina.

For most people, limiting meat servings to 3 or 4 ounces a day, using less (or no) butter, switching to low-fat dairy foods, and avoiding high-fat snacks is all it takes to keep cholesterol at healthy levels.

Another way to control cholesterol is to eat more soy foods. Tofu, tempeh, and other soy foods contain two compounds, daidzein and genistein, that appear to lower cholesterol and help prevent it from sticking to artery walls. Studies suggest that eating about 47 grams of soy protein (about the amount in 10½ ounces of firm tofu) a day may lower total cholesterol by 9 percent and reduce dangerous low-density lipoprotein (LDL) cholesterol by almost 13 percent.

When you're at the supermarket, it's also important to shop in the produce section. When researchers from the well-known Framingham Heart Study group scrutinized the diets of more than 830 men, they found that for every three servings of fruits and vegetables people ate every day, their risk of stroke declined 22 percent.

There are several reasons that fruits and vegetables are so beneficial for preventing stroke. For one thing, they're high in fiber, which has been shown to lower cholesterol. And according to Michael Hertog, Ph.D., of the National Institute of Public Health and Environmental Protection in the Netherlands, these foods also contain powerful antioxidants, which help prevent the harmful LDL cholesterol from sticking to artery walls and blocking blood flow to the brain. Foods especially high in antioxidants include onions, kale, green beans, carrots, broccoli, endive, celery, and cranberries.

It doesn't take a lot of antioxidant-rich foods to get the benefits. In the Nurses Health Study, for example, Harvard researchers found that women who got as little as 15 milligrams of beta-carotene daily, about the amount in one large carrot, reduced their risk of stroke.

Another reason that fruits and vegetables are so beneficial is that they're often high in potassium, a mineral that has been shown to lower high blood pressure, a leading cause of stroke. Plus, potassium appears to make blood less likely to clot, which can reduce the risk of stroke even more. Good potassium sources include baked potatoes, dried peaches, cantaloupe, and spinach.

Along with fruits and vegetables, tea (both the green and black varieties) is an excellent source of flavonoids. When Dr. Hertog studied more than 550 men ages 50 to 69, he found that those who got most of their flavonoids from tea were able to reduce their risk of stroke by 73 percent, compared to those who got the least of these healthful compounds.

It doesn't take a huge amount of tea to get the benefits. Dr. Hertog found that those who drink at least 5 cups of tea daily can reduce their stroke risk by more than two-thirds, compared to those who drink less than 3 cups a day.

Milk is another beverage that appears to play a role in reducing the risk of stroke. In one large study, researchers from the Honolulu Heart Program found that men who did not drink milk were twice as likely to have a stroke as those who drank at least 16 ounces daily.

When reaching for the carton, however, be sure that it contains low-fat or skim milk, since the saturated fat in whole milk may offset its protective benefits.

FISH: FRIENDS OR FOES?

Many fish contain healthful fats called omega-3 fatty acids, which have been shown to raise levels of beneficial high-density lipoprotein (HDL) cholesterol, the kind that helps keep arteries clean. You would think that eating fish would be a smart choice for those trying to lower not only cholesterol or blood pressure but the risk of stroke as well.

The evidence, however, isn't quite so clear. While some studies have found that people who get more fish oil in their diets are less likely to have a stroke, other studies have found no connection at all. More seriously, some research has shown that people who eat a lot of fish actually may have a higher risk for stroke.

"This confusion is at least partly due to the fact that some studies don't take into account how fish oil influences the two different types of strokes," says James Kenney, R.D., Ph.D., nutrition research specialist at the Pritikin Longevity Center in Santa Monica, California.

Here's the story. Fish fats help prevent components in blood, called platelets, from clumping together in the bloodstream. While this can help prevent strokes caused by blood clots, it may increase the risk of strokes caused by leaky blood vessels, Dr. Kenney explains.

The best advice for now? "Don't hesitate to add a couple of fish meals each week to your diet, but only take fish oil capsules with a doctor's advice," says Dr. Kenney.

Among the best foods for preventing stroke are those that contain B vitamins. Many studies have shown that folate and vitamins B_{12} and B_6 can help reduce levels of a naturally occurring amino acid called homocysteine. This is important because when homocysteine levels rise, so does the risk of stroke, says Killian Robinson, M.D., a cardiologist at the Cleveland Clinic Foundation in Ohio.

The different B vitamins are found in a variety of foods. For folate, dark green, leafy vegetables like spinach and romaine lettuce are a good choice. Meats, low-fat dairy foods, and eggs contain vitamin B_{12}. And you can get vitamin B_6 in bananas, chicken, and wheat bran.

Not only what you eat but how much you eat can play a role in controlling stroke. Being overweight is perhaps the leading cause of high blood pressure, which vastly increases stroke risk. In fact, people with high blood pressure are five times more likely to have a stroke than those whose blood pressures are normal. In addition, being overweight makes you more likely to develop diabetes, which also increases the risk of stroke. "This is another important reason to shed unwanted pounds," says Dr. Pearson. You don't have to be model-thin to stay healthy, he adds. Just losing 10 to 20 pounds is often enough to lower blood pressure and with it, the risk of having a stroke.

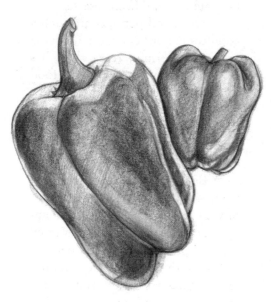

SWEET PEPPERS

PICK A PECK FOR HEALTH

HEALING POWER

CAN HELP:
Prevent cataracts

Reduce the risk
of heart disease

Due to the growing interest in ethnic cuisines, sweet peppers, which range in color from dark green to fire engine red, depending on how long they're left on the vine, aren't found only in salad bars anymore. They're also being used in soups, sauces, purees, and pasta dishes. Peppers do more than add a sweet high note to recipes. They're also filled with nutrients that have been shown to battle cataracts and heart disease. And unlike their fiery-tempered siblings, the chili peppers, sweet peppers are mild enough to eat in large amounts, so you can easily reap their health benefits.

STUFFED WITH ANTIOXIDANTS

Even though sweet peppers such as bell peppers, pimientos, and frying peppers don't get as much attention as broccoli, cauliflower, and other powerhouse foods, they're among the most nutrient-dense vegetables you can buy, especially when it comes to vitamin C and beta-carotene. (As a rule, the redder the pepper, the more beta-carotene it contains.)

Bite for bite, few vegetables contain as much beta-carotene (which is converted to vitamin A in the body) as the sweet red pepper. This is important because beta-carotene plays a key role in keeping the immune system healthy. It's also a potent antioxidant, meaning that it fights tissue-damaging oxygen molecules known

IN THE KITCHEN

Some like it hot—and some don't. If you prefer peppers that are sweet to those that make you sweat, here are a few varieties you may want to try.

- **Bell peppers**, which are available in almost every color of the rainbow, can be eaten raw, grilled, baked, or stir-fried.
- **Pimientos** are squat, heart-shaped peppers that aficionados claim are the best-tasting peppers you can buy. While they're often used commercially for stuffing olives, you can buy them fresh in some specialty produce markets from late summer to fall.
- **Frying peppers** have a mild, sweet taste, and their thin walls make them perfect for sautéing and using as a topping for toasted Italian bread.
- **Paprika peppers**, which are dried to make the spice, can also be fried, stuffed, or eaten raw.
- **Hungarian yellow wax (banana) peppers**, which resemble the fruit both in color and shape, have a mild, sweet taste and are often used in salads and sandwiches.

as free radicals, which scientists believe contribute to major health foes like cataracts and heart disease.

Sweet red peppers are such a good source of beta-carotene that a group of German researchers has classified them as a "must-eat" food for people trying to get more of this antioxidant. One pepper has 4 milligrams of beta-carotene, 40 to 66 percent of the recommended daily amount of 6 to 10 milligrams.

Both sweet red and green peppers also contain generous amounts of vitamin C, another powerful antioxidant. A half-cup of chopped green pepper (about half a pepper) contains 45 milligrams of vitamin C, 74 percent of the Daily Value (DV). Sweet red peppers are even better, with the same-size serving providing 142 milligrams of vitamin C, 236 percent of the DV. That's more than twice the amount that you'd get from a medium-size orange.

The combination of vitamin C and beta-carotene can provide potent protection against cataracts. In a study of more than 900 people, Italian researchers found that those who ate sweet peppers and other foods rich in beta-carotene regularly were significantly less likely to have cataracts than those who did not.

Getting the Most

Cook them lightly. Since vitamin C is fragile, it's readily destroyed during cooking. Eating peppers raw will provide the most of this nutrient. Beta-carotene, on the other hand, needs a little heat to release it from the pepper's fiber cells. To get the most of both nutrients, it's a good idea to steam, sauté, or microwave peppers until they're done but still have a little crunch.

Add some fat. In order for beta-carotene to be absorbed into the bloodstream, it needs to be accompanied by a little fat. Drizzling peppers with a touch of oil, before or after cooking, will help you get the most of this important compound. If you're eating raw peppers, dunking them in a bit of dip will also help the beta-carotene be absorbed.

Mix 'em up. Even though peppers are one of the healthiest vegetables going, few people eat enough of them to get the full benefit. The easiest way to get more peppers in your diet is to use them as an ingredient in other foods, says Dr. Bosland. You can use peppers to add a sweet punch to foods such as pasta, tuna salad, and green salad, for example.

Raise a glassful. Another way to get more peppers in your diet is to make them into juice. The juice from two green peppers contains 132 milligrams of vitamin C, three times the amount you'd get from the usual half-cup serving. Although pepper juice isn't very appetizing on its own, it adds a sweet zip to other juices, such as carrot juice. Try mixing four or five carrots with two green bell peppers in a juicer for a supercharged antioxidant cocktail.

SAUTÉED PEPPERS

1 **green pepper**
1 **sweet red pepper**
1 **sweet yellow pepper**
2 **teaspoons olive oil**
1 **tablespoon balsamic vinegar**
1/8 **teaspoon salt**
Ground black pepper

PER SERVING
calories **39**
total fat **2.4 g.**
saturated fat **0.3 g.**
cholesterol **0 mg.**
sodium **69 mg.**
dietary fiber **0.8 g.**

Cut the green, red, and yellow peppers in half lengthwise. Remove and discard the ribs and seeds. Cut the peppers lengthwise into 1/4"-wide strips.

In a large skillet over medium-high heat, warm the oil. Add the peppers and cook for 2 to 3 minutes, or until they just begin to soften. Remove from the heat and sprinkle with the vinegar and salt. Season to taste with the black pepper. Toss to combine. Serve warm.

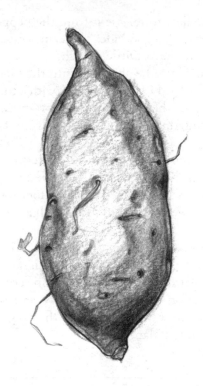

SWEET POTATOES
PACKED WITH ANTIOXIDANTS

HEALING POWER
CAN HELP:
Preserve memory

Control diabetes

Reduce the risk of heart disease and cancer

Have you ever wondered how Scarlett O'Hara maintained her 19-inch waist? One secret may have been sweet potatoes. Before Scarlett went to a barbecue, her nanny dished up sweet potatoes to keep her from filling up on fattening party fare. We can almost hear Scarlett's gentle protest—"Why, I can't eat a thing!"—as she pushed away temptation, filled up as she was by those sweetly nutritious, oddly shaped little roots.

Sweet potatoes are more than just a filling food, of course. A member of the morning glory family (except in name, they're not related to white potatoes), they contain a full trio of well-known antioxidants: beta-carotene and vitamins C and E. This means that they can play a role in preventing cancer and heart disease. And because sweet potatoes are rich in complex carbohydrates and low in calories—there are 117 calories in a 4-ounce serving—experts recommend them for controlling weight and weight-related conditions like diabetes.

A PACKAGE OF PROTECTION

Experts often recommend sweet potatoes for their high amounts of beta-carotene. A 4-ounce serving will provide more than 14 milligrams of beta-carotene. They are an easy way to get the heart-health and cancer-fighting benefits into your diet, says Pamela Savage-Marr, R.D., a spokesperson for the American Dietetic Association and a health education specialist at Oakwood Health Care System in Dearborn, Michigan.

As do vitamins C and E and other antioxidants, beta-carotene helps protect the body from harmful oxygen molecules known as free radicals, says Dexter L. Morris, M.D., Ph.D., vice chairman and associate professor in the department of emergency medicine at the University of North Carolina School of Medicine at Chapel Hill. Eating sweet potatoes and other foods rich in beta-carotene helps neutralize these molecules before they damage various parts of the body, such as the blood vessels or certain parts of the eye.

In a study of almost 1,900 men, Dr. Morris and his colleagues found that men who had the most carotenoids in their blood—not just beta-carotene but also such things as lutein and zeaxanthin—had 72 percent fewer heart attacks than those with the lowest levels. Even smokers, who need all the protection they can get, showed the benefits: Those who got the most of these protective compounds had 25 percent fewer heart attacks than those who got the least.

IN THE KITCHEN

Because they are cured (meaning that they are kept in high humidity and temperatures for about a week and a half) by growers before they are shipped to market, sweet potatoes are excellent keepers and will stay fresh for about a month after you bring them home from the store. It's important, however, to store them carefully to prevent them from going bad.

Keep them cool. Sweet potatoes should be stored in cellars, pantries, or basements, where temperatures stay around 45 to 55°F. (Don't put them in the refrigerator, since this shortens their shelf life.) When sweet potatoes are stored at room temperature, they'll keep for about a week.

Store them dry. Sweet potatoes will spoil once they get wet. That's why it's best to store them dry, then wash them only when you're ready to start cooking.

Treat them gently. Sweet potatoes spoil quickly when they get cut or bruised, so don't buy them if they look damaged. At home, treating them gently will help ensure their longevity.

Sweet potatoes are also a rich source of vitamin C, with a 4-ounce serving providing 28 milligrams, nearly half the Daily Value (DV). In addition, the same-size serving provides 6 international units of vitamin E, 20 percent of the DV. "That's a very difficult nutrient to get from natural sources," says Paul Lachance, Ph.D., professor of nutrition and chairman of the department of food science at Rutgers University in New Brunswick, New Jersey.

CONTROLLING BLOOD SUGAR

Since sweet potatoes are a good source of fiber, they're a very healthful food for people with diabetes. The fiber indirectly helps lower blood sugar levels by slowing the rate at which food is converted into glucose and absorbed into the bloodstream. And because sweet potatoes are high in complex carbohydrates, they can help people control their weight, which also helps keep diabetes under control.

The connection between weight and blood sugar levels is not a casual one. About 85 percent of people with Type II (non-insulin-dependent) diabetes are overweight, statistics show. Since sweet potatoes are so satisfying, you're less likely to reach for other, fattier foods.

The resulting weight loss can cause a dramatic improvement. In fact, even losing 5 or 10 pounds will help some people maintain normal blood sugar levels, says Stanley Mirsky, M.D., associate clinical professor of metabolic diseases at Mount Sinai School of Medicine in New York City and author of *Controlling Diabetes the Easy Way*.

GOOD FOR THE MIND

In addition to fiber and antioxidant vitamins, sweet potatoes also contain the B vitamins folate and B_6. These are the vitamins that may give the brain a boost in performing some of its functions, which can diminish as we age.

In a study at the Jean Mayer USDA Human Nutrition Research Center on Aging at Tufts University in Boston, researchers looked at the levels of folate and vitamins B_6 and B_{12} in the blood of 70 men ages 54 to 81. Men with low levels of folate and B_{12} had higher levels of an amino acid called homocysteine. High levels of homocysteine were linked to poorer performances on spatial tests such as copying a cube or a circle or identifying patterns.

Getting the Most

Shop for color. When buying sweet potatoes, always choose those with the most intense, lush orange color. The richer the color, the greater the jolt of beta-carotene, says Mark Kestin, Ph.D., chairman of the nutrition program at Bastyr University and affiliate assistant professor of epidemiology at the University of Washington School of Medicine, both in Seattle.

Have a little fat. While some vitamins dissolve in water, beta-carotene requires the presence of fat to get through the intestinal wall, says John Erdman, Ph.D., a beta-carotene expert and director of the division of nutritional sciences at the University of Illinois in Urbana. In most cases you'll get the necessary amount of fat, usually 5 to 7 grams, in other foods you'll be having with your meal, he explains.

Sweet Potatoes with Sesame

2 **pounds sweet potatoes**

2 **teaspoons sesame seeds**

1 **bunch scallions, chopped**

1 **tablespoon olive oil**

2 **cloves garlic, minced**

1 **tablespoon reduced-sodium soy sauce**

1 **tablespoon packed light brown sugar**

1 **teaspoon dark sesame oil**

Per serving

calories	**208**
total fat	**5.6 g.**
saturated fat	**0.8 g.**
cholesterol	**0 mg.**
sodium	**275 mg.**
dietary fiber	**4.7 g.**

Scrub the sweet potatoes and pat dry with paper towels. With a fork, pierce each in 3 or 4 places. Place the sweet potatoes, in spoke fashion and with the thinner ends pointing toward the center, on a paper towel. Microwave on high power for 5 minutes. Turn the sweet potatoes. Microwave for 5 to 8 minutes, or until the sweet potatoes can easily be pierced with the tip of a sharp knife but are still firm. Set aside until cool enough to handle. Peel, then cut into thick slices.

Place the sesame seeds in a large no-stick skillet. Stir over medium heat for 30 seconds, or until golden. Add the scallions, olive oil, and garlic. Stir to combine. Cook for 30 seconds, or until fragrant.

Add the soy sauce, sugar, and sesame oil. Cook for about 10 seconds, or until the sugar melts. Add the sweet potatoes and toss to coat. Cook for 1 minute, or until heated through.

Makes 6 servings

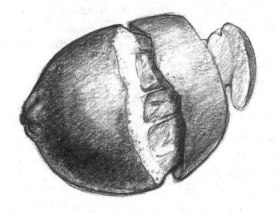

TANGERINES
PEEL A LITTLE PROTECTION

HEALING POWER
CAN HELP:
Prevent heart disease

Reduce the risk of cancer

At one time or another you've probably used canned mandarin oranges—tiny, doll-like sections of orange fruit that look precious and perfect. You can imagine them coming all the way from China, where most citrus fruits actually got their start.

Mandarin oranges are really small tangerines, or to be more precise, tangerines are really mandarin oranges, since tangerine isn't a formal botanical term. So mandarin oranges—we'll still call them tangerines—are actually no more exotic than a lunchbox fruit.

But their benefits are anything but commonplace. Tangerines contain an abundance of impressive healing compounds. Like oranges, they are rich in vitamin C. One tangerine has 26 milligrams, 43 percent of the Daily Value (DV). Tangerines also contain a compound called beta-cryptoxanthin, which turns into vitamin A in the body. Eight ounces of tangerine juice can provide up to 1,037 international units of vitamin A, more than 20 percent of the DV.

This combination is important, since both vitamins are antioxidants—that is, they can help stop harmful oxygen molecules called free radicals from causing cell damage in the body that can lead to everything from wrinkles and heart disease to cancer, says Bill Widmer, Ph.D., research scientist with the Florida Department of Citrus Research Center in Lake Alfred.

PROTECTION AGAINST CANCER

What makes tangerines really exciting to researchers are two compounds, tangeretin and nobiletin, which appear to be extremely potent against certain types of breast cancer. Researchers at the University of Western Ontario in London, Canada, found that each of these compounds was 250 times more potent against one type of human breast cancer cell than genistein, a powerful anti-cancer compound found in soy. When these compounds were combined, they were even more powerful, the researchers found.

In Japan, researchers at the Tokyo College of Pharmacy found that tangeretin could inhibit the growth of leukemia cells, essentially by causing them to program their own deaths. Better yet, the compound wasn't toxic to healthy cells, which is an important goal for any cancer treatment.

Getting the Most

Save the rind. While the flesh of tangerines contains a goodly share of healing compounds, most of the tangeretin and nobiletin are concentrated in the rind. To add more of these to your diet, use a zester to remove strips of the outer rind, then stir them into a glass of juice, mix them into rice and pasta dishes, or sprinkle them on salads. You'll get extra-zingy flavor along with the extra benefits.

Drink up. Although tangerines are in season only from October to May, you may want to enjoy tangerine juice during the off-season. When you go to the supermarket, look for ready-made juices or frozen concentrates that have had tangerine juice added to them.

IN THE KITCHEN

We often think of tangerines as being little more than small oranges, but they have a world of tastes and textures all their own. Here are some varieties you may want to try.

- **Fairchilds** are the first tangerines of the season, available mid-October through December, and they're wonderfully easy to peel.
- The **Dancy tangerine** has a sweet flavor, a loosely fitting peel, and a discomfiting number of seeds.
- **Satsumas** are also easy to peel. They're mild, sweet, juicy, and best of all, almost seedless.
- **Honey tangerines** are sweet enough to make you forget butterscotch. They're very juicy and can have an abundance of seeds.
- **Tangelos**, a cross between a tangerine and a grapefruit, often have a knob at one end like a little topknot. As you would expect, given their parentage, they're both tart and sweet, and very juicy.

Glazed Tangerines with Almonds

4 large tangerines
2 tablespoons chopped almonds
1 tablespoon packed light brown sugar
1 teaspoon grated fresh ginger

Per serving

calories	**70**
total fat	**2.3 g.**
saturated fat	**0.2 g.**
cholesterol	**0 mg.**
sodium	**2 mg.**
dietary fiber	**1.7 g.**

Preheat the broiler. Coat a broiler pan with no-stick spray.

Grate the rind from 2 of the tangerines and place it in a small bowl. Add the almonds, sugar, and ginger. Stir to mix.

Peel the tangerines and discard the peel. Separate the fruit into sections. Arrange close together on the broiler pan and sprinkle evenly with the almond mixture.

Broil 6" from the heat for 1 to 2 minutes, or until the topping bubbles and is lightly browned. Serve warm.

Makes 4 servings

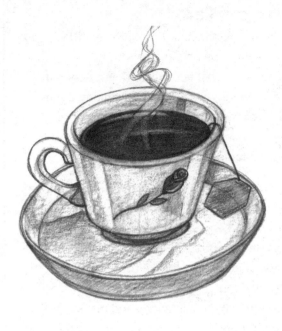

TEA
A CUP
OF GOOD HEALTH

HEALING POWER

CAN HELP:
Control cholesterol

Prevent stroke
and heart disease

Reduce tooth decay

Prevent intestinal cancer

What would you think if a man in a string tie and a long, black coat came up to you and said, "Psss-ss-st. Wanna buy a drink that stops cancer of the skin, lung, stomach, colon, liver, breast, esophagus, and pancreas? And cancer of the small intestine? And heart disease and strokes? And cavities—did I say cavities?"

"Snake oil salesman": That's what you'd think.

Well, Mister Snake Oil would be more right than wrong. Laboratory studies have shown that tea has indeed stopped tumors from forming. The risk of stroke and heart disease tumbles when you drink tea. And tea does have clout against cavities.

Tea contains hundreds of compounds called polyphenols. These compounds act like antioxidants—that is, they help neutralize harmful oxygen molecules in the body known as free radicals, which have been linked to cancer, heart disease, and a number of less serious problems, such as wrinkles.

"In general, polyphenols are very, very good antioxidants. But the best polyphenols are in tea, which has a lot of them," says Joe A. Vinson, Ph.D., professor of chemistry at the University of Scranton in Pennsylvania. "They make up nearly 30 percent of tea's dry weight."

This may help explain why tea is the most popular beverage in the world.

THE COLOR OF TEA

Green tea. Black tea. Vanilla maple tea. French vanilla tea. Raspberry tea. Black currant tea. Apricot tea. Which tea has the most healing polyphenols?

It doesn't matter. As long as it's real tea and not herbal tea, which doesn't contain leaves from *Camellia sinensis*, the tea plant, there's very little difference among them, says tea researcher Joe A. Vinson, Ph.D., professor of chemistry at the University of Scranton in Pennsylvania. After all, they all contain leaves from the same plant.

They're not identical, however. Here's a brief look at the various "real" teas.

- **Green tea** is the freshest and least processed. The taste is light and subtle, appreciated most deeply by tea drinkers in Asia and parts of North Africa.
- **Black tea**, with its strong and hearty taste, is green tea that has been fermented for 6 hours or so. Fermentation turns the green leaves black. It also transforms the polyphenols in green tea into other kinds of polyphenols, like theaflavine and thearubigen. "They're also very good antioxidants," says Dr. Vinson.
- **Semifermented oolong tea** is a compromise between green tea and black tea. Popular in Taiwan and parts of China, it's a bit more assertive than green tea, but still polite.

ARTERIAL PROTECTION

Blocked arteries, and the heart attacks, high blood pressure, and strokes they can lead to, don't happen all at once. They're typically preceded by years of steadily increasing damage, in which the body's dangerous low-density lipoprotein (LDL) cholesterol oxidizes and gradually clings to artery walls, making them stiff and narrow.

That's where tea can help. In studies Dr. Vinson found that the polyphenols found in tea were extremely effective in preventing cholesterol from oxidizing and fouling blood vessels. In fact, one of the polyphenols in tea, epigallocatechin gallate, was able to neutralize five times as much LDL cholesterol as vitamin C, the strongest of the antioxidant vitamins.

One reason that tea's polyphenols are so effective is that they can work in two places at once, blocking the harmful effects of oxidized LDL cholesterol both in the bloodstream and at the artery walls, "where LDL really produces atherosclerosis," says Dr. Vinson.

In a Dutch study of 800 men, researchers found that those who ate the most flavonoids, a large chemical family that includes tea's polyphenols, had a 58 percent lower risk of dying from heart disease than those who ate the least. When the results were further analyzed, it was revealed that the healthiest men were those getting more than half their flavonoids from black tea, with onions and apples contributing most of the rest.

You don't need to drink rivers of tea to get the benefits. In the Dutch study, the healthiest men drank about 4 cups of tea a day.

Just as tea helps protect arteries leading from the heart, it has a similar effect on those in or leading to the brain, says Dr. Vinson.

In another large study, Dutch researchers looked at the diets of 550 men ages 50 to 69. As in the heart study, the men who had the highest flavonoid levels—those who drank almost 5 cups of black tea a day or more—were 69 percent less likely to have a stroke than the men who drank less than 3 cups of black tea a day.

Help against Cancer

Every time you fry a hamburger, compounds called heterocyclic amines form on the surface of the food. In the body these chemicals turn into more dangerous forms, which can cause cancer, says John H. Weisburger, Ph.D., senior member of the American Health Foundation in Valhalla, New York.

Enter the tea polyphenols. Inside the body these compounds help prevent the formation of potential carcinogens, Dr. Weisburger says. In other words, they help stop cancer before it starts.

In experiments at Case Western University School of Medicine in Cleveland, Hasan Mukhtar, Ph.D., professor of dermatology and environmental health sciences, has seen tea stop cancer at each stage of its life cycle, arresting both its growth and spread. And where cancerous tumors have already formed, he has seen tea shrink them.

Studying the effects of green tea on sunburned skin in laboratory animals, Dr. Mukhtar found that the animals given tea developed one-tenth as many tumors as those given water. (Even when the tea-treated animals developed tumors, they were often benign, not cancerous.) What's more, tea was equally effective whether given as a drink or applied to the skin. Some cosmetics companies have started adding green tea to skin products for its potential protective benefits.

Good for the Teeth

Having a toothache generally isn't a big deal, unless it's your toothache. Tea can help prevent the pain, since it contains numerous compounds, polyphenols as well as tannin, that act as antibiotics. In other words, tea is great for mopping up bacteria that promote tooth decay.

Tea also contains fluoride, which provides further dental protection. When researchers at Forsyth Dental Center in Boston tested a variety of foods for their antibacterial qualities, they found that tea was far and away the most protective.

In the Kitchen

Perhaps the one thing the English love better than their gardens is a well-brewed cup of tea. Here's their strategy for having perfect tea every time.

1. Wash the teapot thoroughly with soapy water to remove bitter-tasting residues from the last batch.

2. Warm the pot by pouring in boiling water, swishing it around and then draining it out. This will help keep the tea from getting cold.

3. Put loose tea into the pot. Use 1 teaspoon of tea for every 6 ounces of boiling water.

4. Pour boiling water over the tea, cover the pot, and let steep for 3 to 5 minutes.

5. Unless you're going to drink the tea right away, remove the leaves from the pot using a slotted spoon or strainer. Otherwise, the tea will oversteep, giving the brew a bitter taste.

Japanese researchers at Kyushu University in Fukuoka, Japan, have identified four components in tea—tannin, catechin, caffeine, and tocopherol (a vitamin E–like substance)—that help increase the acid resistance of tooth enamel. This quartet of compounds was made even more effective with the addition of extra fluoride. The extra oomph made tooth enamel 98 percent impervious to the action of acids on the teeth.

Getting the Most

Steep three and see. When you brew tea, it takes 3 minutes for it to release the health-promoting compounds. That's also the amount of time researchers use in their studies on tea. Although longer steeping causes more compounds to be released, "those compounds are bitter. And a bigger dose doesn't necessarily put twice as much of them in the body," says Dr. Vinson.

Bag it. Tea aficionados always use loose tea. No easy tea bags for them. But the pulverized contents of tea bags actually release more polyphenols than the larger loose leaves. That's because the tiny particles in the bag yield more surface area for polyphenols to dissolve into hot water.

Pick your flavors. Although green tea has been more thoroughly researched than the black variety (mainly because the first studies were done in China and Japan, where green tea is the preferred brew), both kinds show equally salutary effects, says Dr. Vinson.

If you prefer decaffeinated tea, by all means drink up. The removal of caffeine has little effect on tea's polyphenol content, so little is lost in the translation, Dr. Vinson says.

The same goes for bottled teas, iced tea, and teas made from mixes, Dr. Vinson adds. In fact, some soft drink and juice companies have been so impressed with tea's benefits that they've begun fortifying their beverages with green tea. Check out your health food store for new products.

Hold the milk—at least for now. One preliminary study in Italy found that adding milk to tea, as the British do at tea time, blocked tea's antioxidant benefits. "There is some evidence that milk protein binds to some of the tea compounds and blocks their absorption. But those compounds could get unbound in the stomach. So we're not so sure milk is bad," says Dr. Vinson.

Keep it fresh. If you make your own iced tea, drink it within a few days, suggests Dr. Vinson. "And make sure you cover it to keep it fresh when you refrigerate it," he advises. "My experience tells me not to keep iced tea for more than a week because the concentration of compounds falls off. You get to the point where about 10 percent has been lost or changed."

Have tea with meat. Since tea's polyphenol compounds help block the formation of cancer-causing chemicals, it's a good idea to enjoy a tea party after eating fried or broiled meat.

TEA-POACHED FIGS

20	dried Calimyrna figs
3/4	cup water
1/2	cup apple cider
1	strip orange rind (1″ × 1/2″)
1	cinnamon stick (2″ long)
4	orange pekoe tea bags

PER SERVING

calories	**253**
total fat	**1.1 g.**
saturated fat	**0.2 g.**
cholesterol	**0 mg.**
sodium	**13 mg.**
dietary fiber	**8.7 g.**

Cut off and discard the stems of the figs. Pierce each fig in 1 or 2 places with the tip of a sharp knife.

In a medium saucepan, combine the water, cider, orange rind, and cinnamon. Bring to a boil over medium heat. Remove from the heat and add the tea bags. Let stand, stirring occasionally, for 5 minutes, or until the mixture looks like brewed tea. Press the tea bags with a spoon to extract the liquid. Discard the tea bags.

Add the figs. Cook over medium heat for 1 to 2 minutes, or until the liquid comes to a simmer. Reduce the heat to low and cook, stirring occasionally, for 5 minutes, or until the figs are plump and moist.

Transfer to a heatproof bowl. Discard the orange rind and cinnamon. Let cool. Serve the figs with the liquid.

Makes 4 servings

THYROID DISEASE
FOODS FOR HORMONAL HEALTH

Goiter. Bulging eyes. Overweight. Say "thyroid," and one of these words probably pops into your brain. Yet few of us know what this gland actually does until something goes wrong with it.

The thyroid is a butterfly-shaped gland that wraps around the windpipe and sits just below the Adam's apple. It produces hormones that help control the body's metabolism—how you burn calories and use energy. This means that the thyroid gland has a direct effect on your weight, energy levels, and your ability to absorb nutrients from food. When the thyroid produces the right amount of hormones, all is well. But when it produces either too much hormone or too little, it can interfere with all these bodily processes.

Thyroid disease is almost always treated with medications that regulate the amount of hormones the gland produces. But it can take several months for the medication to start working. During this time your body may not be able to adequately metabolize certain nutrients, such as iodine, calcium, fat, and protein. So your doctor may recommend adjusting your diet in the meantime.

"Once the medication has corrected the problem, you can follow a normal, healthy diet," says Robert Volpe, M.D., professor emeritus of endocrinology and metabolism in the department of medicine at the University of Toronto and director of the Endocrine Research Laboratory at Wellesley Hospital in Toronto.

A DELICATE BALANCE

As we've seen, the thyroid's main job is to regulate metabolism. When there's enough thyroid hormone in your blood, the thyroid "shuts off," just as an air conditioner turns off when a room reaches the right temperature. When your body needs more thyroid hormone, the gland kicks in again.

In people with thyroid disease, this internal switch doesn't work properly. If you have a condition called hypothyroidism, the gland doesn't produce enough thyroid hormone. The body stages a slowdown. You may feel cold or tired, your hair and skin may become dry, and you may gain weight. For reasons that aren't clear, women are 10 times more likely to develop this condition.

By contrast, people with a condition called *hyper*thyroidism produce too much thyroid hormone, causing the body to speed up. Common symptoms include weight loss, a pounding heart, and skin that's hot and sweaty. Again, women are far more likely than men to develop this condition.

Obviously, the different types of thyroid disease require different nutritional strategies while the medication is taking effect, says Dr. Volpe.

THE IODINE TIGHTROPE

The thyroid gland depends on iodine, which is found in food, to manufacture thyroid hormone. It doesn't take much. The iodine in your body makes up less than 0.00001 percent of your body weight. But your thyroid can't do its job without even this tiny amount of this trace mineral.

So hungry is the thyroid gland for iodine that when it doesn't get enough, it gradually grows larger as it tries to suck up as much iodine as it can. Eventually, it gets large enough to see from the outside. This swelling is called a goiter.

In developing countries, where iodine in the diet is in short supply, goiters are common. But in the United States, where there's plenty of iodine in food—not only in iodized salt but also in bread and milk—this type of goiter is rare.

But iodine still causes problems in this country. In fact, the average American consumes too much, says Dr. Volpe. This isn't a problem when the thyroid is working normally. But for those with thyroid disease, it can cause the gland to churn out too little (or not enough) of its essential hormones.

When you've recently started taking thyroid medication, your doctor may recommend that you avoid iodine-rich foods, like shellfish and spinach, says Dr. Volpe. Once the medication has fully taken effect, however, you can resume your normal diet, he adds.

Another food that you may want to avoid is kelp. While some alternative practitioners suggest eating kelp to treat thyroid problems, mainstream physicians generally advise against it. Kelp (a kind of seaweed) has large amounts of iodine, which could make things worse, says Dr. Volpe.

STAY REGULAR WITH FIBER

For people with an underactive thyroid, the entire body—including the digestion—slows down. This, in turn, can result in constipation, a common symptom in those with this condition.

To help keep digestion regular, it's wise to eat plenty of fiber-rich foods, advises Dr. Volpe. "The fiber in fruits, vegetables, and grains helps keep food moving through the system," he says.

Dr. Volpe recommends eating 20 to 35 grams of fiber a day. You don't have to make a science out of it. Eating 3 to 5 servings of vegetables (preferably raw), 2 to 4 servings of fresh fruits, and 6 to 11 servings of whole-grain bread, cereal, or grains every day should provide an adequate amount of fiber.

Bone Up with Calcium

We've been talking about people with underactive thyroids. Those with overactive glands have different concerns. One of the most significant is the risk of developing bone-thinning osteoporosis, says Deah Baird, a naturopathic doctor in private practice in Norwich, Vermont.

When the thyroid gland is overactive, calcium is removed from the blood and excreted in the urine, explains Dr. Baird. This is serious because the body compensates by removing calcium from the bones to make up the difference.

To prevent bone problems, it's important to eat a diet high in calcium, says Dr. Baird. Dairy foods, including milk, cheese, and yogurt, are all good sources, as are green leafy vegetables such as collard greens and spinach. Having 1 cup nonfat yogurt and 1 cup cooked greens, accompanied by a glass of skim milk, will provide you with the Daily Value of 1,000 milligrams of calcium. Since people with this condition frequently lose weight, it's important to eat a well-balanced diet with enough calories to maintain a healthy weight. For those who are allergic to dairy, it's a good idea to take a calcium supplement or add nondairy sources of calcium to the diet, she adds.

Feeding a Faulty Thyroid

If it weren't so dangerous, having an overactive thyroid gland might be considered the world's greatest weight-loss aid. "The severely hyperthyroid patient loses weight like a shot," says Dr. Volpe. "Since the metabolism speeds up, it can be hard to keep up with the amount of calories the body needs."

Most people with overactive thyroids need to eat 15 to 20 percent more calories than a person with a healthy gland, at least until the medication takes effect, says Dr. Volpe. Those with serious problems may need to eat twice as much—more than 3,000 calories a day—just to maintain the energy and weight they had before.

Dr. Volpe advises that his patients eat foods high in fat and protein to prevent their overactive metabolisms from burning away needed fat and muscle. Meat, fish, poultry, whole milk, cheese, butter, nuts, and seeds are good sources of both fat and protein.

Of course, this no-holds-barred eating strategy is only for the short term. Once the medication becomes fully active and the thyroid hormone levels are back to normal, "you'll need to eat fewer calories or you'll gain weight," says Dr. Volpe.

By contrast, people with an underactive gland may need only half the calories of other adults. They'll also want to limit their consumption of fatty foods. "People with underactive thyroids tend to have higher levels of cholesterol and triglycerides," says Dr. Volpe, which can increase their risk of cardiovascular disease. He recommends eating plenty of complex carbohydrates, such as whole-grain breads, cereals, fruits, and vegetables as well as skim milk and low-fat or nonfat cheese and yogurt.

Again, this special diet is only for the short term. "With the proper medication, thyroid levels will return to normal and you'll be able to eat as many calories as you did before you became hypothyroid," Dr. Volpe says.

The Benefits of Produce

We saw earlier how the fiber in fruits and vegetables can help relieve symptoms caused by an underactive thyroid gland. As it turns out, there are additional substances in vegetables, particularly cabbage, that may aid an overactive gland as well. Research suggests that these compounds may help the gland slow down naturally, says Dr. Baird.

Members of the brassica family of vegetables, including broccoli, cabbage, brussels sprouts, cauliflower, kale, mustard greens, and turnips as well as soybeans, peanuts, millet, and spinach, contain goitrogens—chemicals that block the thyroid's ability to use iodine. With less iodine, the gland naturally produces less thyroid hormone, Dr. Baird explains.

Since cooking may deactivate the goitrogens in vegetables, it's a good idea, when you're eating for thyroid disease, to have your vegetables raw. An alternative to eating raw vegetables is to drink them, since juices contain large amounts of the healing compounds. It's not clear how much you'd need to drink to have a positive effect on the thyroid. A good starting place would be to have an 8-ounce glass of juice every day.

Juices are very easy to make. Wash the vegetables well, cut them into pieces to fit the opening in the juicer, and drop them in. You can make a single-ingredient juice, or mix and match vegetables to create your own flavors. Many people include carrots and celery in their juices because these are considered "universal mixers."

Although it's usually a good idea to include a lot of vegetables in your diet, be careful eating too many brassica vegetables when you have an underactive thyroid—at least until your medication takes effect, says Dr. Volpe. "After that, they're fine," he says.

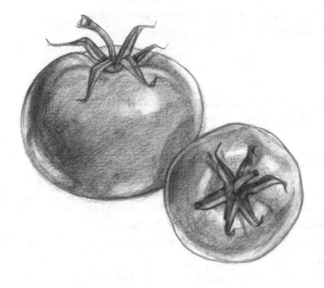

TOMATOES
PROTECTION FOR THE PROSTATE

HEALING POWER

CAN HELP:
Reduce the risk of cancer
and heart disease

Prevent cataracts

Keep older people active

If it weren't for Colonel Robert Gibbon Johnson, Americans might never have tasted tomatoes.

For centuries, tomatoes, which are members of the deadly nightshade family, were thought to be toxic, capable of causing appendicitis, cancer, and "brain fever." But Colonel Johnson, an admittedly eccentric gentleman, thought otherwise. After a trip overseas in the early 1800s, he returned to Salem, New Jersey, with tomatoes and a plan to liberate this lush, red fruit from its fearsome reputation.

Never one to miss a dramatic opportunity, Johnson announced to the townsfolk that on September 26, 1820, he would eat not just one but an entire basket of tomatoes. Public excitement was high, and some 2,000 spectators arrived to watch Johnson commit what they were certain would be suicide.

He lived, of course, and tomatoes went on to become our favorite fruit. Indeed, Americans eat more tomatoes, both fresh and processed, than nearly any other fruit or vegetable. It's really not surprising that tomatoes are among our favorite foods. They're incredible, versatile, and can be used for everything from sauces to main dishes. Better yet, tomatoes contain compounds that can help prevent a number of serious conditions, from heart disease and cancer to cataracts.

CELLULAR PROTECTION

Tomatoes contain a red pigment called lycopene. This compound appears to act as an antioxidant—that is, it helps neutralize cell-damaging oxygen molecules called free radicals before they cause damage. Until recently, lycopene's reputation for healing was overshadowed by its well-studied cousin, beta-carotene. But newer studies indicate that lycopene could have twice the cancer-fighting punch of beta-carotene.

In one large study of nearly 48,000 men, Harvard researchers found that men who ate at least 10 servings a week of tomatoes, whether raw, cooked, or in sauce, were able to cut their risk of developing prostate cancer by 45 percent. Ten servings sounds like a lot, but when they're spread out over an entire week, it's probably not much more than you're getting now. A single serving, after all, is only a half-cup of tomato sauce, which is about the amount of sauce on a slice of pizza.

"Lycopene is a very strong antioxidant," says Meir Stampfer, M.D., co-author of the study and professor of epidemiology and nutrition at the Harvard School of Public Health. "For some reason lycopene concentrates in the prostate. Men with high levels of lycopene in their blood are at lower risk for prostate cancer."

The benefits of tomatoes aren't limited to the prostate gland. In laboratory studies Israeli researchers found that lycopene is also a powerful inhibitor of breast, lung, and endometrial cancer cells.

Almost no one reaps more benefits from tomatoes than Italians, who eat them in one form or another virtually every day. Researchers in Italy found that people who ate seven or more servings of raw tomatoes a week had a 60 percent lower chance of developing stomach, colon, or rectal cancers than folks who ate two servings or less. Once again, lycopene is thought to account for at least some of the protective effects.

Research also suggests that getting more lycopene in the diet may help older people stay active longer. In a study of 88 nuns ages 77 to 98, researchers found that those who got the most lycopene were the ones least likely to need help with daily activities such as getting dressed and walking.

NEW DISCOVERIES

In the not-too-distant future, doctors may be recommending tomatoes as a way of preventing lung cancer. Tomatoes contain two powerful compounds, coumaric acid and chlorogenic acid, that may help block the effects of nitrosamines, which are cancer-causing compounds that form naturally in the body and "are the most potent carcinogen in tobacco smoke," says Joseph Hotchkiss, Ph.D., professor of food chemistry and toxicology at

Cornell University in Ithaca, New York.

Until recently, scientists believed that it was the vitamin C in fruits and vegetables that helped neutralize these dangerous compounds. But a study conducted by Dr. Hotchkiss and his colleagues revealed that tomatoes blocked the formation of nitrosamines even after the vitamin C was removed from the fruit.

The protective coumaric and chlorogenic acids found in tomatoes are also found in other fruits and vegetables, like carrots, green peppers, pineapples, and strawberries. Dr. Hotchkiss speculates that these compounds may be one of the reasons that people who eat more fruits and vegetables have a lower risk of developing cancer.

ADDITIONAL PROTECTION

Lemons and limes are not the only fruits that are high in vitamin C. Tomatoes also contain loads of this powerful vitamin, which has been shown to help relieve conditions ranging from cataracts and cancer to heart disease. One medium-size tomato provides almost 24 milligrams, or 40 percent of the Daily Value (DV) for vitamin C.

Tomatoes are also a good source of vitamin A, a vitamin that has been shown to boost immunity and help prevent cancer. One medium tomato provides 766 international units of vitamin A, 15 percent of the DV.

In addition, a tomato provides 273 milligrams of potassium, 8 percent of the DV. Each one also contains about 1 gram of iron, 7 percent of the Recommended Dietary Allowance (RDA) for women and 10 percent of the RDA for men. While the amount of iron is relatively small, your body is able to absorb it very efficiently when it's taken with vitamin C, which tomatoes have in abundance.

Getting the Most

Shop for color. When buying fresh tomatoes, look for a brilliant shade of red. Red, ripe tomatoes can have four times more beta-carotene than green, immature ones.

Shop for convenience. You don't have to buy fresh tomatoes—or those pale impostors that hit the supermarket come February—to get healing benefits. Lycopene can withstand the high heats used in processing, so canned tomatoes and tomato sauce both contain their full complement of this helpful compound.

Cook them a bit. The lycopene in tomatoes is located in the cell walls. Cooking tomatoes in a little bit of oil causes the cell walls to burst, releasing more of the healing lycopene.

Have a little fat. "If you eat a tomato with a little bit of fat, like olive oil, you'll absorb the lycopene better," says Dr. Stampfer.

CLASSIC TOMATO SAUCE

2 teaspoons olive oil

1 cup chopped onions

2 cloves garlic, minced

1 can (28 oz.) crushed tomatoes in puree

2 tablespoons no-salt-added tomato paste

1½ teaspoons dried basil

½ teaspoon dried thyme

PER CUP
calories	**111**
total fat	**2.4 g.**
saturated fat	**0.3 g.**
cholesterol	**0 mg.**
sodium	**495 mg.**
dietary fiber	**4.4 g.**

In a Dutch oven over medium-low heat, warm the oil. Add the onions and garlic. Cook, stirring occasionally, for 8 minutes, or until the onions soften. Add the tomatoes, tomato paste, basil, and thyme.

Partially cover and cook over medium heat for 30 minutes, or until the tomatoes are softened.

Makes about 4 cups

Cook's Note: This sauce is perfect served over pasta, couscous, rice, or baked potatoes.

GAZPACHO

8 medium tomatoes

¼ cup diced red onions

2 tablespoons chopped fresh cilantro

2 teaspoons extra-virgin olive oil

1 tablespoon red-wine vinegar

2 cloves garlic, minced

¼ teaspoon salt

1 small sweet yellow pepper, finely diced

PER SERVING
calories	**87**
total fat	**3.2 g.**
saturated fat	**0.4 g.**
cholesterol	**0 mg.**
sodium	**157 mg.**
dietary fiber	**3.5 g.**

Core the tomatoes and cut into chunks. Place in a blender or food processor. Add the onions, cilantro, oil, vinegar, garlic, and salt and process to make a chunky puree.

Transfer to a bowl. Stir in the pepper. Cover and refrigerate for at least 2 hours to allow the flavors to blend.

Makes 4 servings

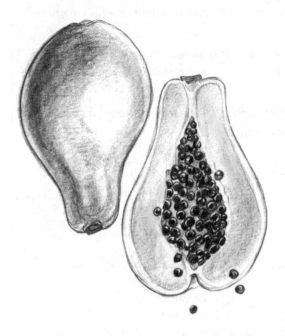

TROPICAL FRUITS
EXOTIC HEALING

HEALING POWER
CAN HELP:
Aid in digestion

Prevent heart disease
and cancer

The next time you're pushing your shopping cart past the pineapples, pause for a moment to check out their tropical neighbors. In June you'll find luscious mangoes. Guavas, masquerading as oversized lemons and limes, make their appearance in summer and again in winter. And all year long you'll find papayas, which look like pears on steroids.

Despite their unfamiliar appearance, tropical fruits offer many of the same benefits as their homegrown kin—and then some. Not only are they high in fiber, but they also contain an array of powerful compounds that can help fight heart disease and even cancer.

While dozens of tropical fruits are grown worldwide, the ones you're most likely to find in this country are mangoes, papayas, and guavas.

MANGO MAGIC

You don't really chew a mango—you slurp it up. But even though this exceedingly juicy fruit, which tastes like peach and pineapple mixed together, only sweeter, is messy to eat, it's well worth the effort.

Mangoes, like many fruits, contain large amounts of vitamin C. What makes them really special is that they also contain a lot of beta-carotene. Both vitamin C and beta-carotene are antioxidants—meaning they can block the effects of harmful oxygen molecules called free radicals. This is important because free radicals can damage healthy tissues throughout the body. What's more, they also damage the body's low-density lipoprotein (LDL) cholesterol, making it more likely to stick to artery walls and increase the risk of heart disease.

One mango contains almost 5 milligrams of beta-carotene, 50 to 83 percent of the recommended amount of 6 to 10 milligrams, and 57 milligrams of vitamin C, 95 percent of the Daily Value (DV). It's a very healthful mix. In an Australian study, people were given juice containing both beta-carotene and vitamin C every day for three weeks. Researchers found that the LDL cholesterol in the juice-drinkers suffered less damage than before they started drinking up.

It's not only antioxidants that make mangoes good for the heart. They're also high in fiber, with one mango supplying almost 6 grams of fiber—more than you'd get in 1 cup of cooked oat bran. What's more, nearly half of the fiber in mangoes is the soluble kind. Study after study has shown that getting more soluble fiber in the diet can help lower cholesterol and reduce the risk of heart disease, high blood pressure, and stroke. The insoluble fiber in mangoes is also important, because it causes stools—and any harmful substances they contain— to move through the body more quickly. This means that eating more mangoes can play a role in reducing the risk of colon cancer.

THE POWER OF PAPAYAS

On the outside they look like yellow or orange avocados. On the inside, you'll find beautiful yellow-orange flesh that hints at the healing power within.

Papayas are packed with carotenoids, natural plant pigments that give many fruits and vegetables their beautiful hues. But carotenoids do much more than pretty up a plate. They can, quite literally, save your life.

The carotenoids in papayas are extremely powerful antioxidants. Studies have shown that people who eat the most carotenoid-rich foods like papayas have a significantly lower risk of dying from heart disease and cancer.

Many fruits and vegetables contain carotenoids, but papayas are way ahead of the pack. In one study, German researchers rated 39 foods according to their carotenoid content. Papayas came out on top, with half a fruit providing almost 3.8 milligrams of carotenoids. By contrast, grapefruits (which came in second) have 3.6 milligrams, and apricots have 2.6 milligrams.

Papaya also contains a number of protease enzymes, such as papain, which are very similar to enzymes produced naturally in the stomach. Eating raw papaya during or after a meal makes it easier for the body to digest proteins, which can help ease an upset stomach, says Deborah Gowen, a certified nurse-midwife with the Harvard Community Health Plan in Wellesley, Massachusetts.

Papaya may play a role in preventing ulcers as well. In a laboratory study, animals given high doses of stomach-churning drugs were less likely to get ulcers when they were fed papaya for several days beforehand. While similar research hasn't been done in people, it seems likely that having a little papaya each day could help counteract the irritating effects of aspirin and other anti-inflammatory drugs.

GREAT GUAVAS

It's not always easy to find guavas in the supermarket, but these pink or yellow, lemon-size fruits, which are often available in gourmet, Hispanic, or Indian markets, are definitely worth the search.

What makes guavas so special is a carotenoid called lycopene. For a long time, lycopene took a backseat to a related compound called beta-carotene. But studies now suggest that lycopene may be even more powerful than its more-famous kin. In fact, lycopene is one of the strongest antioxidants, says Paul Lachance, Ph.D., professor of nutrition and chairman of the department of food science at Rutgers University in New Brunswick, New Jersey.

In laboratory studies, Israeli scientists found that lycopene was able to quickly block the growth of lung and breast cancer cells. And in a large study of almost 48,000 men, Harvard researchers found that men who got the most lycopene in their diets had a 45 percent lower risk of developing prostate cancer than those getting the least. While tomatoes have long been admired for their high lycopene content, guavas are a far better source, with at least 50 percent more lycopene in a single fruit.

Finally, when it comes to dietary fiber, guava is truly a superstar, containing about 9 grams per cup. That's more fiber than you'd get in an apple, apricot, banana, and nectarine combined. This has drawn the attention of heart researchers, since getting more fiber in the diet is one of the best ways to lower cholesterol, and with it the risk for heart disease.

In a study of 120 men, Indian researchers found that those who ate five to nine guavas a day for three months had a drop in total cholesterol of almost 10 percent. Better yet, their levels of healthful, high-density lipoprotein cholesterol actually rose 8 percent.

Getting the Most

Pass the cans. Even though frozen tropical fruits retain their nutrients, the canned kind doesn't fare so well. A study in Spain, for example, found that canned papaya lost many of its protective carotenoids during processing.

Add a little fat. The lycopene in guavas is absorbed more efficiently when it's eaten with a little fat. Spooning yogurt on sliced guava, for example, will help you get the most lycopene, while adding a hint of richness to this tangy fruit.

Keep the heat down. Tropical fruits are often used as ingredients in recipes such as sauces for meat dishes. Unfortunately, the heat used in cooking destroys some of the vitamin C, says Donald V. Schlimme, Ph.D., professor of nutrition and food science at the University of Maryland in College Park. To get the most vitamins, he recommends eating tropical fruits raw—the way nature intended.

Store them carefully. Tropical fruits that are exposed to air and sunlight will quickly give up their vitamin C. Keeping the fruits in a cool, dark place will help keep them fresh while preserving this vital nutrient.

MANGO-PAPAYA SALAD

2 ripe medium mangoes
1 ripe medium papaya
1 tablespoon fresh lemon juice
1 teaspoon vanilla
1/8 teaspoon ground allspice

PER SERVING

calories	**100**
total fat	**0.4 g.**
saturated fat	**0.1 g.**
cholesterol	**0 mg.**
sodium	**5 mg.**
dietary fiber	**4.3 g.**

Slice through the mangoes on all sides of the pit to remove the flesh. Cut the flesh into strips, then run a knife between the flesh and the peel to remove the peel. Discard the peel and cut the mango into 1/2" pieces. Place in a medium bowl.

Cut the papaya in half lengthwise. Scoop out and discard the seeds. Cut off the peel, then cut the papaya into 1/2" pieces. Add to the bowl. Add the lemon juice, vanilla, and allspice. Toss gently to mix. Cover and let stand for 30 minutes for the flavors to blend.

Makes 4 servings

GUAVAS WITH SWEET LIME DRESSING

10 **ripe guavas (about 1½ pounds)**
 1 **tablespoon fresh lime juice**
 1 **tablespoon granulated sugar**
 ¼ **cup confectioners' sugar**
 ⅛ **teaspoon vanilla**
    Pinch of ground cinnamon

PER SERVING
calories	**112**
total fat	**0.8 g.**
saturated fat	**0.2 g.**
cholesterol	**0 mg.**
sodium	**4 mg.**
dietary fiber	**7.4 g.**

Set a fine sieve over a large bowl.

Peel the guavas and cut in half lengthwise. With a sharp spoon, scoop out the seedy inner flesh and place it in the sieve.

Cut the resulting guava shells in half lengthwise. Place in a large bowl. Add the lime juice and granulated sugar. Toss to mix.

With the back of a large spoon, press the guava flesh through the sieve until only the small seeds remain. Discard the seeds. Add the confectioners' sugar, vanilla, and cinnamon. Stir to mix.

Divide the guava shells among dessert plates. Drizzle with the puree.

Makes 4 servings

Cook's Note: Serve the guavas for dessert or as a side dish at brunch.

ULCERS
EATING FOR RELIEF

Gone are the days when doctors treated ulcers by putting people on a bland diet consisting of milk, cream, and eggs. The idea was that this bland fare would somehow neutralize excess stomach acid, which was caused, it was thought, by stress or frequent meals of three-alarm chili, and allow the ulcers to heal.

As it turns out, most ulcers are caused by bacteria, which is why the bland diets didn't help. Still, if you have an ulcer, what you eat and drink does affect how you feel, says Isadore Rosenfeld, M.D., clinical professor of medicine at New York Hospital–Cornell Medical Center in New York City and author of *Doctor, What Should I Eat?* Some foods, like coffee (including decaf), stimulate the secretion of stomach acid, which can delay healing and make the pain of ulcers worse. On the other hand, a number of foods have a strengthening effect on the stomach's protective lining, making it less vulnerable to attack. Choosing the right foods, in fact, can help ulcers heal faster and make them less likely to return.

THE HEAD HEALER

Cabbage is one of the oldest folk remedies for ulcers, dating back to Roman times. In 1949, a group of researchers at Stanford University School of Medicine decided to put this virtuous vegetable to the test. In the study, 13 people with ulcers drank 1 liter (about a quart) of raw cabbage juice every day. They healed six times faster than people whose only treatment was the standard bland diet.

Cabbage contains glutamine, an amino acid that increases blood flow to the stomach and helps strengthen its protective lining.

It's an extremely effective ulcer treatment, says Michael T. Murray, a naturopathic doctor in Bellevue, Washington, and author of *Natural Alternatives to Over-the-Counter and Prescription Drugs.* The healing usually takes place in less than one week, he adds.

During an ulcer flare-up, Dr. Murray says, you should drink the juice from half a head (about 2 cups) of cabbage each day. If you prefer to chew your medicine, eating the same amount of cabbage is equally effective. Don't cook the cabbage, however, since heat destroys its anti-ulcer abilities.

A Sweet Solution

When ulcer pain hits, most people are more likely to reach for a bottle of antacid than a spoonful of honey. But a dose of honey goes down a lot easier than that chalky white stuff, and it may do more than a bit of good.

Honey has been used in folk medicine for all kinds of stomach troubles. Researchers at King Saudi University College of Medicine in Saudi Arabia found that raw, unprocessed honey strengthens the lining of the stomach. And a laboratory study at the University of Waikato in New Zealand found that a mild solution of honey made from the nectar of the manuka flower, native to New Zealand, was able to completely stop the growth of ulcer-causing bacteria. The reason is that honey contains substances that appear to build up the stomach's protective lining. They also appear to have potent antibacterial abilities, says Patrick Quillin, R.D., Ph.D., vice president of nutrition for the Cancer Treatment Centers of America.

Dr. Quillin recommends using only raw, unpasteurized honey for easing an ulcer, since heat-processed honey doesn't contain any of the beneficial substances. Try taking 1 tablespoon of raw, unprocessed honey at bedtime on an empty stomach. You can do this every day to help the ulcer heal. Continue this sweet treatment indefinitely to help prevent them from coming back, he adds.

Healing Cultures

Yogurt is one of the great healing foods. It has been used successfully for treating yeast infections, easing lactose intolerance, and boosting immunity. There's reason to believe that it may play a role in preventing ulcers as well.

Yogurt's healing ability stems from the living stowaways it contains—live, healthful bacteria in every creamy cupful. "These are friendly bacteria that will compete with the bacteria that cause ulcers," says Dr. Quillin. The helpful bacteria in yogurt, such as *Lactobacillus bulgaricus* and *L. acidophilus*, hustle for elbow room inside the stomach. Get enough of these beneficial bacteria in your system, and the ulcer-causing bacteria will find themselves outnumbered and unwelcome.

In addition, a natural sugar in yogurt called lactose breaks down into lactic acid during digestion. This helps restore a healthful acidic environment in the intestines, says Dr. Quillin.

When you have an ulcer, try eating 1 cup of yogurt three or four times a day for a couple of weeks, recommends Dr. Rosenfeld.

When you combine yogurt therapy with any medical treatment you may be using, you can expect to shorten the course of your ulcer by about a third, says Dr. Quillin.

Incidentally, when buying yogurt, look for brands labeled "live and active cultures," which contain the beneficial live bacteria.

A Whole-Diet Plan

Even though you can help heal an ulcer by eating specific, healing foods, there's really no substitute for an overall healthful diet. Regardless of whether you're taking medication, "good nutrition will put the wind at your back when it comes to treating an ulcer," says Dr. Quillin.

For starters, help yourself to a plantain. This cousin to the banana contains an enzyme that stimulates mucus production in the stomach lining, strengthening its natural defenses. When buying plantains, look for those that are green and slightly unripe, because these are thought to contain more of the healing enzymes.

It's also a good idea to take advantage of fiber. Getting lots of fruits, whole grains, legumes, and vegetables in your diet can help prevent or even heal ulcers. This is because these foods contain generous amounts of dietary fiber, which encourages the growth of the stomach's protective mucous layer. Dr. Rosenfeld recommends getting at least 35 grams of fiber every day.

Even though doctors once recommended milk as the cornerstone of anti-ulcer diets, it was bad advice. Milk not only increases stomach acid production, but some people are allergic to it, and food allergies may cause ulcers, according to Dr. Murray.

While you're making basic changes in your diet, don't forget to look at some of the obvious problem areas. Even though the caffeine in coffee doesn't cause ulcers, it can make you more susceptible to getting them. Along with cigarettes and alcohol, it can also make existing ulcers worse, says Dr. Rosenfeld.

Urinary Tract Infections
Flushing Out the Plumbing

For a long time, doctors dismissed food cures for urinary tract infections (UTIs) as being nothing but folklore. But there's increasing evidence that what you drink can play a role in preventing and even treating these painful conditions.

UTIs occur when bacteria take up residence in the bladder or urethra (the tube through which urine flows), causing painful or frequent urination. More common in women than men, UTIs are usually treated with antibiotics, which can clear up the problem in a few days.

Research suggests, however, that drinking cranberry juice will not only help prevent UTIs but also speed recovery if you're already sick. In one study, researchers in Boston gave 153 women either 10 ounces of cranberry juice or 10 ounces of a look-alike fluid every day for six months. They found that women drinking the cranberry juice were 58 percent less likely to develop UTIs than those drinking the phony fluid.

Researchers believe that women who are prone to UTIs may have "stickier" cells in the urethra, making it easier for bacteria to hold on. It appears that cranberries contain a substance, which hasn't yet been identified, that acts like a no-stick coating for these cells, making bacteria more likely to slip away.

Incidentally, it's not only cranberry juice that works against UTIs. Scientists believe that blueberry juice may have similar effects.

While you might get some benefit from eating whole berries, juices are a more convenient way to get more of the protective compounds. That's why doctors recommend that women who frequently get UTIs should drink 10 ounces of cranberry juice—or, if you can find it, blueberry juice—every day.

Wash Away Infection

Even if you don't have juice in the refrigerator, there's another liquid strategy for preventing UTIs. Drinking eight 8-ounce glasses of water a day will help your body wash away bacteria before they cause infection.

THE ACID TEST

When scientists first started investigating cranberry juice as a cure for urinary tract infections (UTIs), they suspected that its high acid content was probably responsible. Acidic urine, they reasoned, would provide a less hospitable environment for bacteria.

Soon people were trying to ease infections with other high-acid substances, such as vitamin C or large amounts of oranges and tomatoes.

As it turns out, acid may not be the answer. In fact, some doctors believe that creating a high-acid environment just irritates an already-inflamed bladder.

It still isn't certain whether women with UTIs should eat, avoid, or simply not worry about having acidic foods. But doctors do recommend listening to your body. If you have an infection and find that certain foods, like citrus fruits, tomatoes, aged cheese, spicy foods, and coffee, make it more painful to urinate, you're better off leaving them alone until the infection has gone away.

Drinking water is particularly important when it's time for your annual pelvic exam. Many women get UTIs after the exam, possibly because the instruments can irritate the vagina and push bacteria nearer to the urethral opening, where they're more likely to cause infection. Having two big glasses of water—one before the exam and one after—and then using the bathroom will help keep the urinary tract free of bacteria.

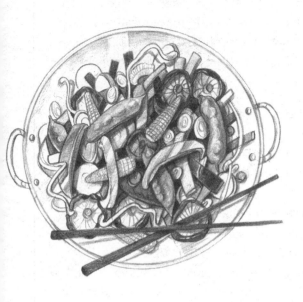

VEGETARIAN DIETS
EATING FOR A LONG LIFE

HEALING POWER

CAN HELP:
Lower cholesterol levels

Prevent vision loss

Reduce the risk of cancer
and heart disease

When people first started experimenting with meatless cooking in the 1960s, meals were often colorless, tasteless, or both. After all, there's only so much you can do with brown rice-and-lentil loaf or plain tofu on a bed of alfalfa sprouts.

But the "nuts-and-berries" approach of the early years has pretty much gone the way of the Volkswagen minibus. With over a quarter-century's experience to learn from, cooks today are combining fruits, vegetables, grains, and legumes in exciting new ways. The tastes are so good, in fact, that even large restaurant chains are now offering meatless meals.

Although vegetarian menus have changed, one thing has stayed the same. A plant-based diet—which is low in saturated fat and high in fiber, antioxidant vitamins, and a powerful array of protective chemicals—is the ultimate prescription for a longer, healthier life, says Virginia Messina, R.D., a dietitian in Port Townsend, Washington, and co-author of *The Vegetarian Way*.

Nearly 40 years ago, a large study of 27,530 Seventh-Day Adventists, whose religion advocates a meatless diet, provided the first scientific link between vegetarian diets and better health. Researchers were amazed to discover that among the vegetarian Adventists, death rates from cancer were 50 to 70 percent lower than among other Americans.

Since then, study after study has shown that people who eat little or no meat have much lower rates of heart disease, diabetes, and gallstones. Vegetarians are less likely to be overweight than meat-eaters. They're also less likely to suffer from high blood pressure or stroke.

In China, for example, where people eat little or no meat, diseases such as heart disease, breast cancer, and diabetes are far less common than in this country. "If we had diets similar to this in America, they could prevent 80 to 90 percent of the chronic, degenerative diseases that people get before age 65," says T. Colin Campbell, Ph.D., a nutritional biochemist at Cornell University in Ithaca, New York.

NATURALLY LEAN

One thing that makes vegetarian meals so healthful is what they *don't* have—all the saturated fat and cholesterol that come from meat. In fact, while most Americans get about 36 percent of their total calories from fat, vegetarians get less, usually between 30 and 34 percent. And most of the fat they do get is the healthier, polyunsaturated and monounsaturated kinds, and not the dangerous, saturated fat that comes from animal foods.

In one study, researchers put 500 people on a vegetarian diet. After 12 days, cholesterol levels had dropped an average of 11 percent, says John A. McDougall, M.D., medical director of the McDougall Program at St. Helena Hospital in Napa Valley, California, and author of *The McDougall Program for a Healthy Heart.*

It's not just the lack of saturated fat that makes vegetarian meals so healthful. It's also the "good" fats that are used to replace it. Studies have shown, for example, that both polyunsaturated and monounsaturated fats, which are found in olive oil, nuts, seeds, and many other plant foods, can lower levels of cholesterol when they're used to replace saturated fat in the diet.

THE POWERS OF PLANTS

For years doctors have been pleading with Americans to eat more fruits, vegetables, whole grains, and legumes, the same foods that vegetarian meals include in abundance. Most plant foods are loaded with antioxidants, such as beta-carotene and vitamins C and E, which are essential for protecting the body from disease. In addition, many plant foods contain an abundance of phytonutrients, natural plant compounds that appear to lower the risk for cataracts, heart disease, and many other serious problems.

In one study, for example, researchers found that people who got the most carotenoids, the plant pigments that are found in spinach, collards, and a variety of deep-orange fruits and vegetables, had half the risk of developing macular degeneration (the leading cause of irreversible vision loss in older adults) of people getting less.

But even if you took all the nutrients out of plant foods, the vegetarian diet would still have an edge because of all the dietary fiber it contains. The average American gets only about 12 grams of fiber a day, while vegetarians get as much as three times that amount, Messina says.

It's almost impossible to exaggerate the importance of getting enough dietary fiber. Because it isn't absorbed by the body, fiber passes through the digestive tract, adding bulk to stools and helping them move more swiftly. This does more than prevent constipation. The more quickly stools and any harmful substances they contain move through the colon, the less likely they are to do cellular damage that could lead to cancer.

In addition, one type of fiber, called soluble fiber, forms a gel in the intestine that helps prevent fat and cholesterol from passing through the intestinal wall and into the bloodstream. In a study of more than 43,000 men, for example, researchers found that those who added just 10 grams of fiber a day to their diets—about 25 percent of the amount vegetarians get each day—decreased their risk of heart disease by almost 30 percent.

STAYING IN BALANCE

A vegetarian diet can provide all the nutrients your body needs, including protein. This is even true for strict vegetarians, who may avoid eggs, milk, or other animal foods entirely. The proteins in meats are complete, meaning that they contain all the amino acids you need. The proteins in legumes and grains, however, may be low in one or more of the amino acids. But because legumes and grains contain some amino acids, eating these foods throughout the day will provide the proper balance.

Apart from protein, there is one nutrient that people following a strict vegetarian diet have to be aware of. Vitamin B_{12}, which the body uses to make red blood cells, is found only in animal foods. People who don't get enough vitamin B_{12} get tired and weak, a condition doctors call pernicious anemia.

But you can get plenty of vitamin B_{12} by eating foods fortified with this nutrient, such as fortified cereals, fortified soy milk, or B_{12}-enriched nutritional yeast.

BRAISED VEGETABLE MEDLEY

4 teaspoons olive oil

4 medium potatoes, cut into large chunks

6 ounces small button mushrooms

16 baby carrots

1 package (9 ounces) frozen artichoke hearts

4 cloves garlic, sliced

1½ cups vegetable broth or water

¼ teaspoon salt

1½ tablespoons minced fresh dill

Ground black pepper

In a Dutch oven over medium heat, warm the oil. Add the potatoes, mushrooms, and carrots. Cook for 5 minutes, or until the vegetables begin to lightly brown.

Add the artichokes, garlic, broth or water, and salt. Cover and reduce the heat to low. Cook for 30 to 35 minutes, or until the potatoes and carrots are very tender. Add up to ¼ cup more water if the vegetables begin to dry out.

Add the dill. Season to taste with pepper. Stir gently to mix.

Makes 4 main-dish servings

Cook's Note: For a heartier meal, serve the vegetables over cooked couscous.

PER SERVING

calories	**181**
total fat	**5.3 g.**
saturated fat	**0.8 g.**
cholesterol	**0 mg.**
sodium	**187 mg.**
dietary fiber	**7.1 g.**

Spiced Tofu with Spinach and Tomatoes

16   **ounces firm regular tofu**

2   **teaspoons canola oil**

1³/₄   **cups chopped onions**

1   **tablespoon minced garlic**

1¹/₂   **tablespoons grated fresh ginger**

1¹/₂   **teaspoons ground cumin**

2   **medium tomatoes, cut into 8 wedges each**

¹/₃   **cup water**

1   **bag (6 ounces) washed and trimmed spinach, torn into bite-size pieces**

¹/₄   **teaspoon salt**

Per serving

calories	**163**
total fat	**8.3 g.**
saturated fat	**1 g.**
cholesterol	**0 mg.**
sodium	**174 mg.**
dietary fiber	**4 g.**

Cut the tofu into 1″ cubes. Place on several layers of paper towels, then cover with several more paper towels. Press down lightly to remove some of the liquid. Set aside.

In a large no-stick skillet over medium heat, warm the oil. Add the onions. Cook, stirring frequently, for 6 to 8 minutes, or until golden.

Increase the heat to medium-high. Add the tofu, garlic, ginger, and cumin. Cook for 3 to 4 minutes, or until the tofu starts to brown. Add the tomatoes and stir to mix. Cook for 1 minute. Add the water.

Add the spinach, a handful at a time; add more spinach as the first batch starts to cook down. Cook just until the spinach is wilted. Sprinkle with the salt.

Makes 4 main-dish servings

Cook's Note: Serve with cooked rice or toasted pita bread.

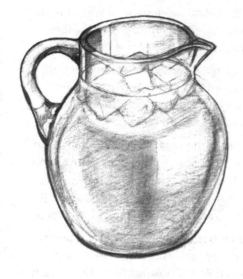

WATER
WASH AWAY
KIDNEY STONES

HEALING POWER
CAN HELP:
Reduce the risk
of kidney stones

Restore energy

Prevent constipation

Run your car without water in the radiator and it will come to a steaming halt. Yet people who wouldn't dream of letting their cars run dry often walk around without enough water in their own radiators. And because every cell in the body requires fluids to dissolve and transport vitamins, minerals, sugar, and other chemicals, not drinking enough water can leave you feeling like a run-down Ford.

The average person loses about 2 percent of her body weight (about 1½ quarts of water) in urine, perspiration, and other body fluids every day. To replace these fluids, doctors advise drinking at least eight glasses of water, milk, or juice a day—more if you're a large person, over age 55, sick with a cold, or simply active.

To make sure you drink enough, the brain has special sensors in a part of the brain called the thalamus, which monitor blood levels of sodium. When concentrations of sodium rise, it means that water levels are low. The brain then sends a signal, in the form of thirst, that says it's time to head to the water cooler.

This system usually works well. As we age, however, the thirst sensor gets less sensitive, so we don't always drink enough, says Lucia Kaiser, R.D., Ph.D., assistant professor of nutrition and cooperative extension specialist at the University of California, Davis. Plus, sometimes we get so busy we don't take time to drink. That can cause serious problems, ranging from kidney stones and constipation to fatigue. Let's take a look at a few of the ways in which water can keep you healthy.

Stopping Stones

Men say it's the worst pain they've ever known. Women say they'd rather have the pain of childbirth. Both men and women agree that once you've had a kidney stone, you never want to get another one.

Getting enough water, doctors say, will help ensure you never do. Normally, many of the wastes in the body are dissolved in fluids and carried out in the urine. But when you don't drink enough water, the wastes may become concentrated, forming crystals that can bond together and form kidney stones.

"I tell people to think of the insides of their bodies as they would their kitchens," says Bernell Baldwin, Ph.D., applied physiologist at Wildwood Lifestyle Center and Hospital in Georgia and science editor of *Journal of Health and Healing*. "You can't expect your body to be able to clean up its dishes without giving it enough water."

Here's an easy test to tell if you're getting enough water. Look at your urine. Except in the morning, when you haven't had fluids all night, it should be pale yellow or even clear. If it's dark, that means wastes are too concentrated and you should be drinking more water.

Fluid Movements

Another way in which water helps remove wastes from the body is by keeping the stools soft, which helps prevent constipation, says Dr. Baldwin. When you don't drink enough, stools become hard and dry, and it takes longer for them to move through your system.

Constipation isn't merely uncomfortable, Dr. Baldwin adds. Studies have shown that constipation may lead to other problems, such as hemorrhoids, diverticular disease, or even colon cancer.

"You should drink two glasses of water about a half-hour before eating breakfast," Dr. Baldwin advises. "This not only hydrates your body but also primes your system, flushing out wastes and getting it ready for food."

Wash Away Fatigue

We think of fatigue as being caused by not getting enough sleep or working too hard. But in many cases, the problem is even more basic: not getting enough water.

Here's what happens. When you don't drink enough, cells throughout your body start getting a little dry. To quench their thirst, they draw water from the most convenient place—the bloodstream. This leaves the blood thick, sludgy, and harder to pump. The extra work involved in pumping the blood can cause energy levels to decline, Dr. Baldwin says.

You don't have to run completely dry to feel the effects. In a small study of cyclists, researchers found that their performance levels dropped when they lost as little as 2 percent of their body weight in fluids—the equivalent of about six glasses of water.

WASH AWAY WEIGHT

One of the nicest benefits of drinking more water is that it can help you lose weight. For one thing, many of us think it's time to eat when, in fact, we're merely thirsty. Drinking water is a great way to quell hunger pangs. In addition, when you drink with meals, you're more likely to take in fewer calories, says Dr. Kaiser.

Water can help in yet another way. When you drink cold water (40°F or cooler) you actually burn calories, because the body has to raise the temperature of the water to 98.6°F. In the process, it burns slightly less than 1 calorie per ounce of water. So if you toss back eight glasses of cold water a day, you'll burn about 62 calories. That adds up to 430 calories a week, according to Ellington Darden, Ph.D., author of *A Flat Stomach ASAP*.

Getting the Most

Eat for drink. Drinking isn't the only way to get more water in your diet. Many foods are also very high in moisture. Having soups or stews, for example, can be a big help toward getting your daily water allowance, says Dr. Kaiser. "For even more fluid, add some crunchy vegetables like celery and peppers to these dishes," she says.

Pick some fruit. Juicy fruits like watermelons, cantaloupes, oranges, and grapefruits are mostly water, so they're an excellent (and convenient) way to get more water in your diet, Dr. Kaiser says.

Choose your drinks carefully. Though juices and decaffeinated tea count toward your daily water total, caffeine-containing drinks like coffee and cola do not. In fact, along with alcohol, caffeinated drinks are diuretics, meaning they pull more water out of your body than they put in. Drinking a glass of water for every caffeine- or alcohol-containing drink will help you break even.

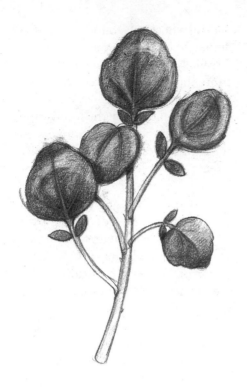

WATERCRESS
A BOUQUET OF PROTECTION

HEALING POWER
CAN HELP:
Reduce the risk
of lung cancer

Prevent heart disease

Decrease the risk
of cataracts

Prevent wrinkles

Looking for something special to make for Valentine's Day? Give your sweetie a special treat by saying "sayonara" to chocolates, "arrivederci" to lobster, and "hello" to a fresh bouquet of watercress.

This delicate green, with dime-size leaves and a pungent, peppery flavor, is more than just a celebration salad. First, it's a cruciferous vegetable (meaning that its flowers have four petals, resembling a cross). The crucifers, including broccoli and cauliflower, are well-known for their cancer-fighting potential. Watercress is also a dark green, leafy vegetable, meaning that it's packed with beta-carotene, a nutrient that helps ward off heart disease and diseases associated with aging, such as cataracts.

SNUFFING OUT CANCER

Population studies show that people who eat plenty of cruciferous vegetables, like watercress, have lower rates of cancer. Watercress researchers will tell you that this crucifer is particularly potent against lung cancer caused by smoking or breathing secondhand smoke. Scientists have found that when they included phenethyl isothiocyanate (PEITC), a natural compound found in watercress, in the daily diets of laboratory animals and exposed them to cancer-

In the Kitchen

With its tiny, delicate leaves and thick stems, watercress looks quite a bit different from other salad greens. But with a little care, you can use this lively member of the mustard family the same way you would any leafy green.

To keep watercress fresh, refrigerate it in a plastic bag. Or refrigerate it stems-down in a glass of water and cover it with a plastic bag. It will keep for up to five days.

When using watercress, unless you're adding it to soup stock, use only the leaves and the thinner stems. Otherwise, the pungent, peppery flavor may be overpowering.

Incidentally, this is one green you don't want to skimp on. Watercress shrinks substantially during cooking, and what may look like a big pile on the counter may almost disappear on the plate. Plan on cooking one bunch per person.

causing chemicals found in tobacco smoke, the animals were 50 percent less likely to develop lung cancer tumors than animals given their regular diet, sans PEITC.

Encouraged by the results, the scientists recruited 11 smokers to see if watercress would have similar effects in people as it did in the laboratory.

It did. "We got results with humans that were consistent with what we saw in laboratory animals," says Stephen Hecht, Ph.D., professor of cancer prevention at the University of Minnesota Cancer Center in Minneapolis.

The catch, of course, is that you have to eat a lot of watercress for it to be effective. And watercress won't necessarily protect you from other cancer-causing chemicals in tobacco smoke, adds Dr. Hecht.

"The volunteers in our study ate 2 ounces of watercress at each meal, three meals a day. That's a pretty hefty sandwich or a large salad—more than you would normally eat at one sitting. And you would have to do it several times a day," says Dr. Hecht.

Of course, no one is telling you that eating watercress is going to wash away smoke's toxic effects. No food on the planet can. But adding watercress to your daily diet may be a step in the right direction while you work on clearing the smoke from your life.

Other Benefits

Along with keeping cancer cells at bay, watercress also helps fight another major public health enemy—heart disease.

Like other dark green, leafy vegetables, watercress is packed with beta-carotene, an antioxidant nutrient that has been linked to lower rates of heart disease. As a bonus, a 1-cup serving of watercress also provides 24 percent of the Daily Value for vitamin C, another valuable disease-fighting antioxidant vitamin.

The antioxidants, which include beta-carotene and vitamins C and E, help sweep up cell-damaging oxygen molecules from your body. Keeping lots of beta-carotene in your bloodstream seems to be the ticket to lowering your risk of heart attack, certain cancers, and lots of ailments associated with aging, such as cataracts and wrinkles.

Getting the Most

Eat it raw. Watercress is best eaten in its natural state, fresh and crisp. When cooked, it loses its ability to release PEITC. "Fortunately, most people don't cook it," says Dr. Hecht. "Your dose of that active ingredient is less in a cooked vegetable than a raw one."

Use it often. Chances are that you'll never eat the 6 ounces of watercress a day that you need to extract the maximum healing benefit, says Dr. Hecht. But you can put a hefty amount in your diet simply by using it more often. For example, it makes a tasty replacement for lettuce in sandwiches and salads.

WATERCRESS SALAD

4 **bunches (about 1 pound) watercress**

2 **tablespoons brown mustard**

2 **tablespoons red- or white-wine vinegar**

2 **tablespoons nonfat plain yogurt**

1½ **tablespoons honey**

1 **tablespoon olive oil**

Ground black pepper

Rinse the watercress under cold water. Cut off and discard the thickest stems. Pat dry with paper towels. Place in a large bowl.

In a small bowl, combine the mustard, vinegar, yogurt, honey, and oil. Whisk until smooth. Season to taste with the pepper.

Pour over the watercress. Toss gently to coat.

Makes 4 servings

PER SERVING

calories	**76**
total fat	**3.8 g.**
saturated fat	**0.5 g.**
cholesterol	**0 mg.**
sodium	**139 mg.**
dietary fiber	**1.7 g.**

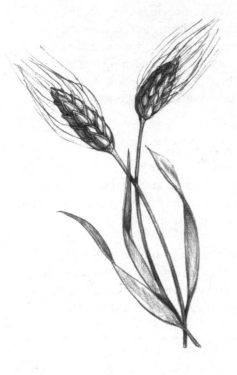

WHEAT
The E Grain

HEALING POWER
CAN HELP:
Improve digestion

Reduce the risk of heart
disease and cancer

Forget corn, oats, rice, or rye. For Americans wheat is by far the number one grain. The average American, in fact, eats 148 pounds of wheat, in the form of pasta, bread, bagels, and cereals, a year.

One reason that we eat so much wheat is that it's a remarkably versatile grain. Even if you don't care for bread, there are literally dozens, if not hundreds, of common recipes that call for wheat. It has a light flavor that works well in all kinds of foods, from the flakiest biscuits to the heartiest polentas.

It's our good fortune that wheat is nutritious as well as delicious. In fact, it's one of the most healthful foods you can buy. Like all grains, wheat is rich in vitamins, minerals, and complex carbohydrates.

But what makes wheat truly special is that it contains one thing that many foods do not: vitamin E. This is important because vitamin E is mainly found in cooking oils such as safflower and canola oils. As a result, getting the Daily Value (DV) of 30 international units of vitamin E can be tricky unless you choose your foods carefully, says Susan Finn, Ph.D., director of nutrition services at Ross Laboratories in Cleveland.

Eating more wheat makes it just a little bit easier. It's worth doing, Dr. Finn adds, because vitamin E may play a direct role both in lowering cholesterol and in preventing it from sticking to artery walls, which can help reduce the risk of heart disease.

A Vitamin for the Heart

Every day, the body produces an enormous number of free radicals, which are harmful oxygen molecules that have lost an electron. As a result, these molecules go zipping through the body, grabbing extra electrons wherever they can find them. In the process they damage cholesterol in the bloodstream, making it sticky and more likely to stick to artery walls—the first step in causing heart disease.

Research has shown that eating more wheat can help stop this process from getting started. In a study of 31,000 people, for example, researchers found that those who ate the most whole-wheat bread had a much lower risk of heart disease than those who ate white bread.

Doctors speculate that the vitamin E in wheat causes the liver to produce less cholesterol, says Michael H. Davidson, M.D., president of the Chicago Center for Clinical Research. In one study, for example, people with high cholesterol were given 20 grams (about a quarter-cup) of wheat germ a day for four weeks. (Most of the vitamin E in wheat is concentrated in the germ layer.) Then, for 14 weeks after that, they upped the amount to 30 grams. At the end of the study, researchers found that their cholesterol levels had dropped an average of 7 percent.

Wheat germ is a very concentrated source of vitamin E, with a little less than 2 tablespoons providing 5 international units, about 16 percent of the DV. Oat bran and whole-wheat breads and cereals also contain vitamin E, although in smaller amounts than the germ.

A Fiber Find

If you remember the oat bran frenzy of a few years ago, you already know that this grain is prized for its high fiber content. But Mr. Ed's favorite breakfast isn't the only way to get a lot of fiber in your diet. Wheat bran, in fact, contains more than 1½ times the fiber of oat bran, and that's good news for your health.

The type of fiber that is in wheat, called insoluble fiber, absorbs large amounts of water as it passes through the intestine, causing stools to get larger and heavier. The larger stools pass through the body more quickly—which means that any harmful substances they contain have less time to damage cells in the colon, says Beth Kunkel, R.D., Ph.D., professor of food and nutrition at Clemson University in South Carolina.

When researchers analyzed more than 13 international studies involving more than 15,000 people, they found that those who got the most fiber had a substantially lower risk of developing colon cancer. The researchers estimated that if people would increase the amount of fiber in their diets to 39 grams a day, their risk of colon cancer might drop as much as 31 percent.

One serving of All-Bran cereal, which is made from wheat, has close to 10 grams of fiber. That's almost 40 percent of the DV, all in one bowl. Wheat germ is also a good fiber source, with a little less than 2 tablespoons providing more than 1 gram. Bulgur, whole-wheat pasta, and cracked wheat (which is used to make taboulleh) are other good fiber finds, says Dr. Finn.

Getting the Most

Buy it whole. To get the most vitamin E and fiber from wheat, it's important to buy foods containing wheat germ or whole wheat, which contain the outer, more-nutritious parts of the grain. Once wheat has been processed—when making white bread or "light" cereals, for example—most of the protective ingredients are lost, says Dr. Finn.

Check the labels. Some foods that say "whole wheat" on the package contain only a smattering of whole wheat inside. To be sure you're getting the real thing, read the label, says Dr. Finn. When you see "whole wheat" or "whole-wheat flour" at the top of the ingredient list, you know you're making a good choice.

WHOLE-WHEAT PANCAKES

1¼ cups whole-wheat flour

¼ cup toasted wheat germ

1½ teaspoons baking powder

½ teaspoon ground cinnamon

⅛ teaspoon salt

1½ cups skim milk

¼ cup fat-free egg substitute

1 tablespoon unsalted butter, melted

PER 3 PANCAKES

calories	**221**
total fat	**4.5 g.**
saturated fat	**2.1 g.**
cholesterol	**10 mg.**
sodium	**325 mg.**
dietary fiber	**5.5 g.**

In a large bowl, combine the flour, wheat germ, baking powder, cinnamon, and salt. Stir to mix. Add the milk, egg substitute, and butter. Mix just until the ingredients are blended. Do not overbeat.

Coat a large no-stick skillet with no-stick spray. Warm over medium-high heat until a drop of water dropped into the skillet sizzles. Using a ¼-cup measuring cup as a ladle, scoop out slightly less than ¼ cup of batter for each pancake. Drop the batter into the pan, being careful not to crowd the pancakes.

Cook for 2 minutes, or until the edges begin to look dry. Flip and cook for 1 minute, or until browned on the bottom. Remove from the pan.

Take the skillet off the heat and coat it with more no-stick spray. Continue until all the batter is used.

Makes 12

Cook's Note: Place the pancakes on a baking sheet in a 175°F oven to keep them warm until all are cooked. Serve with maple syrup or honey.

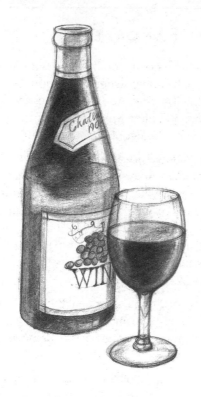

WINE
THE SECRET TO A HEALTHY HEART

HEALING POWER

CAN HELP:
Prevent heart disease
and stroke

Control intestinal bacteria

Ever since man discovered the fruits of fermentation, wine has been a welcome guest, not just at the dinner table but also at weddings, religious rituals, and even doctors' offices.

Only recently, however, have scientists begun to investigate the actual health benefits of sipping Chianti with your ziti. And the findings they've uncorked are enough to make any wine-lover raise his glass and say, "Salut!"

Used in moderation, wine, particularly the red varieties, can help lower cholesterol and fight hardening of the arteries and heart disease. In addition, studies suggest that it can kill bacteria that cause food poisoning and traveler's diarrhea. Obviously, experts don't recommend that people start guzzling wine rather than sipping it or that people who don't drink should suddenly start. Rather, what the evidence suggests is that moderate drinking can be a helpful addition to a healthy diet.

FRUIT OF THE VEIN

For years researchers looked with amazement across the Atlantic as their French allies indulged in cigarettes, buttery croissants, and fat-laden pâtés—and were still 2½ times less likely to develop heart disease than their supposedly healthier American counterparts.

Researchers are still investigating the so-called French Paradox, but it appears likely that the French have healthier hearts at least partly because of their penchant for red wines. These wines are rich in compounds that help lower cholesterol and prevent harmful low-density lipoprotein (LDL) cholesterol from sticking to artery walls—the process that leads to heart disease. Red wines also help keep blood platelets from sticking together and forming dangerous clots.

DUAL-ACTION HEART PROTECTION

The ways in which red wine keeps your pump primed are complex. There is more than one chemical compound at work, and some of these compounds have more than one benefit, say researchers.

For starters, the alcohol in red wine may be beneficial. For example, people who drink small amounts of alcohol seem to have increased protection from heart disease, studies show.

The reason, say researchers, is that ethanol, or alcohol, in spirited drinks raises levels of good, heart-protecting high-density lipoprotein (HDL) cholesterol.

But if raising HDL cholesterol were the only benefit, drinking red wine wouldn't be any more effective than, say, quaffing a shot of scotch or a mug of beer. And that's not the case.

The reason wine seems to offer superior protection is that it contains powerful flavonoids such as quercetin. Along with other potentially protective compounds like resveratrol, it apparently helps prevent the body's dangerous LDL cholesterol from oxidizing. This, in turn, makes LDL cholesterol less likely to stick to artery walls, causing them to become blocked and to harden.

"Flavonoids in red wine are more powerful than vitamin E, which everyone knows is an important antioxidant," says John D. Folts, Ph.D., professor of medicine and director of the coronary thrombosis laboratory at the University of Wisconsin Medical School in Madison.

Keeping LDL cholesterol in check is a good start against heart disease, but that's not all the quercetin in wine does, says Dr. Folts. It also helps prevent platelets in blood from sticking together. Indeed, a study led by Dr. Folts and his colleagues found that when red wine was given to laboratory animals, it eliminated potentially dangerous clots.

"Red wine performs double duty, giving you two major benefits in one place," says Dr. Folts.

COLOR COUNTS

When researchers talk about the healing benefits of wine, they're usually referring to red wine. When it comes to heart health, researchers say, light wines

THE BENEFiTS
WiTHOUT THE BOOZE

For every connoisseur of fine bouquets and vintages, there's someone who would just as soon skip the sherry and sip something sans alcohol.

If nonalcoholic wine is your toast of choice, you're in luck. Except for the alcohol, which is extracted during processing, these beverages contain the same active ingredients as "real" wines, including quercetin and resveratrol, two compounds that show healing potential.

When drinking for health, experts say, pick nonalcoholic wines the same way you do their spirited counterparts, by the darkness of their hue. Many of the protective compounds are also the ones that give the beverage its crimson color.

pale in comparison to their robust red brethren.

In a laboratory study at the University of California, Davis, for example, researchers found that red wines could prevent anywhere from 46 to 100 percent of LDL cholesterol from oxidizing, while white wines were not as protective. Similarly, laboratory studies suggest that white wine lacks the clot-blocking ability of red, says Dr. Folts.

Why is red wine so much superior to its paler counterpart? It's all in the making, say experts.

When vintners make wine, they throw everything in the vat—not just grapes but also the skins, seeds, and stems. They're all mashed up to create a chunky mixture called must, which is where the healthy flavonoids reside.

"The longer the must ferments in the alcohol, the more of these compounds release into the wine, says Dr. Folts. With white wine, the must is taken out early so that the wine never darkens. With red wine, the must is kept in a long time, and the wine picks up a lot of flavonoids."

WINE AGAINST INFECTION

When you were a kid, you probably ran into your share of bacteria that resulted in nasty bouts of the runs. At the same time, you probably spent a lot of time running away from your mother as she chased you with drippy pink spoonfuls of bismuth subsalicylate, better known as Pepto-Bismol.

Even today, experts advise taking a shot of the pink stuff while traveling to help prevent bacterial infections that can cause traveler's diarrhea. If only it didn't taste so bad! Wouldn't it be nice if you could exchange that chalky, neon liquid for something a bit more palatable—like a nice glass of chardonnay?

You might be able to, say scientists from Tripler Army Medical Center in Honolulu. Intrigued by the use of wine as a digestive aid throughout history, the researchers tested red wine, white wine, and bismuth subsalicylate against some of the meanest intestinal germs, including shigella, salmonella, and *Es-*

cherichia coli. They found that both red and white wine were more effective than the drug for wiping out harmful bacteria.

More research needs to be done, but it appears likely that sipping a little wine with your vacation meals could help bolster your intestinal health so that you aren't slowed down by a case of the runs.

Getting the Most

Know when to say when. The most important tip for getting the maximum health benefits from your wine cellar is knowing when to put your glass down, say the experts. The daily limit is one 5-ounce glass a day for women and two 5-ounce glasses a day for men.

Go for the gusto. When you're scanning the shelves for the wine with the highest levels of heart-healthy compounds, go for the full-bodied, robust varieties, advises Andrew L. Waterhouse, Ph.D., assistant professor in the department of vitriculture and enology at the University of California, Davis.

"There is a close relationship between the level of tannin, the substance that makes wine dry, and the level of healing compounds in red wines," says Dr. Waterhouse. Three of the most heart-healthy wines are cabernet sauvignon, petite sirah, and merlot.

FOOD ALERT
THE GRAPES OF WRATH

Everyone knows that having a glass too many of red wine can leave you wishing your head were attached to someone else's body.

But for some people with a tendency toward migraine headaches, even a little wine can cause a lot of headache. Red wine contains substances called amines, which cause blood vessels in the brain to constrict and then expand. In sensitive people, this can result in eye-popping headaches.

Although white wine contains fewer headache-producing amines than the red varieties, it doesn't contain as many healing compounds either. So if headaches are a problem for you, you may want to ask your doctor if a nonalcoholic wine will allow you to enjoy the great tastes without the pain.

WOUND HEALING
REPAIRING THE DAMAGE

No one makes it through the bumper-car ride of life without getting cuts and scrapes along the way. In fact, doctors estimate that Americans get more than 12 million cuts and other wounds every year.

If you happen to be among the walking wounded, you can count yourself fortunate that the skin is usually able to heal itself in deft displays of regeneration. But for healing to occur, you have to eat the right foods. Nutrients such as protein, vitamin C, and zinc are the building blocks for new skin. If you don't get enough of them in your diet, it takes longer for wounds to heal, says Judith Petry, M.D., medical director of the Vermont Healing Tools Project in Brattleboro.

A STRONG FOUNDATION

Protein is essential for healing cuts and wounds, but it isn't always available where you need it most. Only about 10 percent of the body's protein is found in the skin, while the rest is used elsewhere in the body.

"Protein gets used for energy before it goes to healing," says Michele Gottschlich, R.D., Ph.D., director of nutrition services for the Shriners Burns Institute in Cincinnati.

When your body goes into healing mode, the need for protein can double. Suppose, for example, that you normally get 50 grams of protein a day. After burning yourself, you may need to increase that amount to 100 grams in order to heal properly, Dr. Gottschlich says. This means increasing your daily intake of protein-rich foods to 8 to 10 servings instead of the usual 4 to 6 servings that nutritionists recommend for general well-being. The amount of protein your body needs for healing depends largely on the severity of the wound.

Meats are among the best sources of protein. A 3-ounce serving of flank steak, for example, has 23 grams of protein, about 46 percent of the Daily Value (DV). If you don't want to eat meat, you can also get protein from fish, beans, nuts, and grains.

"Tofu is also an impressive source of protein," adds Dr. Gottschlich. A 4-ounce serving has more than 9 grams, about the same amount you'd get from 1¼ ounces of ground beef.

Seize the Vitamin C

Orange juice is a favorite home remedy for colds because the vitamin C it contains helps strengthen immunity. What works for sniffles will work for wounds as well. If you aren't getting enough vitamin C in your diet, your susceptibility to infection quickly increases.

In addition, vitamin C is essential for strengthening collagen, the tissue that holds skin cells together. When you don't get enough vitamin C in your diet, collagen gets weaker and wounds heal more slowly. "Tissue integrity, the actual strength of the skin, relies on vitamin C," says Vincent Falanga, M.D., professor of medicine and dermatology at the University of Miami School of Medicine.

In a study at the Burn Center of Cook County Hospital in Chicago, researchers found that laboratory animals that got extra vitamin C in their diets had better blood circulation and less wound swelling than those getting less.

Whether you have a cut, a burn, or any other kind of wound, it's a good idea to get at least 500 milligrams of vitamin C a day, about eight times the DV of 60 milligrams, says Dr. Falanga. In fact, it doesn't hurt to get even more—up to 1,000 milligrams a day, he says. This is particularly true for older folks and those who smoke, since these people are often low in vitamin C.

It's easy to get a lot of vitamin C from foods. A half-cup serving of sweet red peppers, for example, has 95 milligrams of vitamin C, 158 percent of the DV, while an orange has nearly 70 milligrams, 116 percent of the DV. For a superb vitamin C kick, grab a guava. One guava contains 165 milligrams of vitamin C, 275 percent of the DV.

Think Zinc

Many Americans don't get enough zinc, a mineral that helps tissues grow and repair themselves. In fact, slow wound healing is often a telltale sign that you're not getting enough of this important mineral.

The DV for zinc is 15 milligrams. This doesn't sound like a lot, but getting enough zinc can be a bit tricky, since only about 20 percent of the zinc in foods is absorbed during digestion, says Ananda Prasad, M.D., Ph.D., professor of medicine at Wayne State University School of Medicine in Detroit. However, eating zinc-rich foods along with protein from animal foods will help the absorption of zinc, he says.

An excellent source of zinc is oysters, with ½ cup providing 8 milligrams, 54 percent of the DV. Wheat germ is also good, with 1⅔ tablespoons containing about 2 milligrams, 13 percent of the DV.

YEAST INFECTIONS
HEALING CULTURES

For a long time, women have been telling each other how effective yogurt is for clearing up yeast infections. Doctors have always been skeptical, but that's about to change.

In a small study at Long Island Jewish Medical Center in New York, women who got frequent yeast infections were given 1 cup of yogurt every day for six months. At the end of the study, researchers found that the rate of yeast infections had dropped by *75 percent.*

The yogurt used in the study contained live cultures of bacteria called *Lactobacillus acidophilus,* which are "friendly" bacteria that help control the growth of yeast in the intestines and vagina, explains Paul Reilly, a naturopathic doctor in Tacoma, Washington, and an adjunct instructor at Bastyr University in Seattle. Eating yogurt helps restore the vagina's natural environment, so yeast infections are much less likely to recur, he adds.

For most women, the amount of yogurt used in the study—1 cup a day—is plenty, Dr. Reilly adds. The one challenge may be finding yogurt that contains *L. acidophilus* bacteria, since most national yogurt brands contain other types of organisms. In fact, even when you do find a supermarket yogurt that contains *L. acidophilus,* the concentration may be too low for it to be effective. Your best bet, says Dr. Reilly, is to buy the yogurt at health food stores, which usually have a good selection to choose from.

NATURE'S PENICILLIN

Through the ages, garlic has been used for disinfecting wounds, stopping dysentery, and even treating tuberculosis. Here's another feather in its cap. Research suggests that garlic can help cure yeast infections as well as prevent them from coming back.

Garlic contains dozens of chemical compounds, among them ajoene, allicin-alliin, and diallyl sulphide, that have proven power against fungal infections. In a laboratory study at Loma Linda University in California, animals with yeast infections were given either a placebo (inactive) saline solution or a solution made with aged garlic extract. Two days later, animals in the saline group were still infected. Those in the garlic group, however, were completely free of the fungus.

Garlic has been shown to kill the yeast fungus on contact. In addition, garlic appears to stimulate the activity of neutrophils and macrophages, immune system cells that battle infection.

Even though the animals in the study were given aged garlic extract, fresh garlic is also effective, says Dr. Reilly. For treating and preventing yeast infections, he recommends eating anywhere from several cloves to a bulb of garlic a day. You don't have to eat it raw to get the benefits, he adds. Garlic retains some of its strength when it's baked, microwaved, or sautéed. To be most effective, however, the cloves should be crushed or chopped, since this releases more of the active compounds.

BOOSTING YOUR DEFENSES

The research is still preliminary, but evidence suggests that eating more foods containing beta-carotene and vitamins C and E can help prevent yeast infections.

Researchers at Albert Einstein College of Medicine in the Bronx found that women with yeast infections had significantly less beta-carotene in their vaginal cells than women without the infections. The researchers speculate that women with higher levels of beta-carotene may be more resistant to the fungus.

Foods that are high in vitamins C and E can also play a protective role, Dr. Reilly says. "These vitamins stimulate the immune system to activate specialized cells, which are a primary defense against things like yeast," he says.

You can get plenty of beta-carotene and vitamin C simply by eating a variety of fruits and vegetables. Vitamin E, however, is found mainly in vegetable oils. To get more vitamin E in your diet without all the fat, Dr. Reilly recommends having several servings a day of nuts and seeds, which are high in vitamin E. An even better source of vitamin E is wheat germ.

A SWEET PROBLEM

For women who frequently get yeast infections, sugary foods can be a real problem because yeast, it appears, likes sweets just as much as we do, Dr. Reilly says.

Research has shown that women who eat a lot of honey, sugar, or molasses get more yeast infections than women who eat less. It makes sense because eating sugar raises the amount of sugar in the bloodstream, which provides a perfect medium for yeast to thrive. For some women, even the natural sugars in fruit and milk can be a problem, says Carolyn DeMarco, M.D., a physician in Toronto and author of *Take Charge of Your Body: Woman's Health Advisor*.

"I tell women who are susceptible to yeast infections to think about cutting back on their intake of fruits and to avoid fruit juices completely," Dr. DeMarco says.

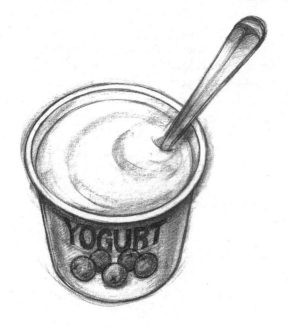

YOGURT
THE BENEFITS OF BACTERIA

HEALING POWER
CAN HELP:

Prevent yeast infections

Boost immunity

Heal and prevent ulcers

If someone suggested that you swallow a spoonful of live organisms, you wouldn't do it on a bet. But what if they told you that every spoonful would provide dramatic improvements in your health?

Millions of Americans willingly eat millions of live organisms every day when they open containers of yogurt. Yogurt is positively brimming with bacteria—the live and active cultures that you read about on the label. Research has shown that these "friendly" bacteria can strengthen the immune system and help ulcers heal more quickly. The bacteria also may help prevent recurrent yeast infections, says Eileen Hilton, M.D., an infectious disease specialist at Long Island Jewish Medical Center in New York. And even if you took the bacteria out of yogurt, it would still be a super source of calcium—better, in fact, than a serving of low-fat milk.

STOPPING THE YEAST BEAST

If you've ever had a yeast infection, you know that you never want to get another one. Eating more yogurt, Dr. Hilton says, may help prevent them from occurring.

Yeast infections occur when a fungus that normally lives in the vagina suddenly multiplies, causing itching, burning, and other uncomfortable symptoms. A study at Long Island Jewish Medical Center suggests that eating live-culture yogurt, especially yogurt containing bacteria called *Lactobacillus acidophilus*, may help keep the fungus under control.

In the study, women who frequently had yeast infections were asked to eat 8 ounces of yogurt a day for six months. At the end of the study, the rate of yeast infections had dropped significantly. The women were so satisfied, in fact, that when researchers asked them to stop eating yogurt, many of them refused to give it up.

The Long Island researchers speculate that eating yogurt helps keep the vagina's natural bacterial environment in balance, making it harder for the yeast fungus to thrive. Additional studies need to be done, Dr. Hilton adds, but in the meantime, women who are trying to prevent yeast infections may want to try eating 1 cup of yogurt a day—the same amount that was used in the study.

It's important, however, to eat yogurt that contains live cultures, Dr. Hilton adds. Yogurt that has been heat-treated doesn't contain bacteria and probably won't be effective. Read the label to find out if your brand has been heat-treated.

HELP FOR IMMUNITY

You probably remember the television commercials for yogurt that featured hearty, 100-year-old Russians hiking up rocky peaks with energy to spare. The ads were an exaggeration, of course, but yogurt's healthful reputation is not.

The same bacteria in yogurt that help prevent yeast infections can also strengthen the immune system. In one study, for example, researchers at the University of California, Davis, found that people who ate 2 of cups yogurt a day for four months had about four times more gamma interferon, a protein that helps the immune system's white blood cells fight disease, than people who did not eat yogurt. "Gamma interferon is the best mechanism the body has to defend itself against viruses," says Georges Halpern, M.D., Ph.D., professor emeritus in the department of internal medicine at the University of California, who was author of the study.

There's some evidence that yogurt may work against bacterial infections as well. In a laboratory study conducted by researchers at the Netherlands Institute for Dairy Research, animals given yogurt had much lower levels of salmonella bacteria, a common cause of food poisoning, than animals given milk. What's more, the bacteria that did survive had little impact on the animals given yogurt, while those given milk got much sicker.

It's not entirely clear why yogurt helped protect the animals from disease. Apart from its immunity-boosting effects, researchers speculate that yogurt's high calcium content may create an unfavorable environment in which the bacteria can't thrive.

ULCER RELIEF

Since most ulcers are caused by bacteria, the usual treatment is to give large doses of antibiotics. But there's good evidence that eating plenty of live-culture yogurt can keep ulcer-causing bacteria under control, says Patrick Quillin, R.D., Ph.D., vice president of nutrition for the Cancer Treatment Centers of America.

When you eat yogurt, the beneficial bacteria take up residence inside the digestive tract. Once in place, they begin competing with the harmful bacteria that cause ulcers, Dr. Quillin explains. This makes it more difficult for the ulcer-causing germs to thrive.

In addition, yogurt contains a natural sugar called lactose, which breaks down into lactic acid during digestion. The lactic acid helps restore a healthful environment in the intestine, says Dr. Quillin.

Even if you already have an ulcer and are taking medication, eating yogurt will make the treatment more effective, says Khem Shahani, Ph.D., professor of food science and technology at the University of Nebraska in Lincoln. "The organisms that are in many yogurts tend to act like antibiotics in the stomach," he explains.

If you have an ulcer, try eating between 1 and 4 cups of yogurt a day, recommends Isadore Rosenfeld, M.D., clinical professor of medicine at New York Hospital–Cornell Medical Center in New York City and author of *Doctor, What Should I Eat?* Just be sure to buy yogurt that says "live and active cultures" on the label.

CALCIUM WITHOUT PAIN

Even though the large amounts of calcium in low-fat milk make it one of the most healthful foods you can find, many people simply can't drink a lot of it. In fact, doctors estimate that more than 30 million Americans don't have enough of the enzyme (lactase) needed to digest the sugar (lactose) in milk.

Yogurt, however, is an easy-to-digest alternative. Even though yogurt does contain lactose, the live bacteria help the body break it down, so it's less likely to cause discomfort, says Barbara Dixon, R.D., a nutritionist in Baton Rouge, Louisiana, and author of *Good Health for African Americans*. And when it comes to calcium, yogurt is a super source, with 1 cup of plain low-fat yogurt providing 414 milligrams, more than 40 percent of the Daily Value. Compare that to low-fat milk, with just 300 milligrams per serving.

Getting the Most

Eat it cold. Since the bacteria in yogurt can't withstand high heat, it's best to eat your yogurt cold. When you do use yogurt for cooking—when making a sauce, for example—add it when the dish is finished cooking and has been removed from the heat.

Buy it fresh. Fresh yogurt contains about 100 million bacteria in a single gram. After a few weeks on the shelf, however, that number quickly dwindles. To get the most of these healing cultures, try to buy yogurt that's less than a week old. Your best bet is to get it from health food stores. Since these stores usually sell a lot of yogurt, you have a much better chance of getting it fresh off the truck.

HERBED YOGURT CHEESE DIP

2 **cups nonfat plain yogurt**

2 **ounces reduced-fat cream cheese**

1½ **tablespoons minced fresh chives**

1 **tablespoon minced fresh basil**

¼ **teaspoon coarsely ground black pepper**

PER 2 TABLESPOONS

calories	**42**
total fat	**1.6 g.**
saturated fat	**1 g.**
cholesterol	**6 mg.**
sodium	**54 mg.**
dietary fiber	**0 g.**

Line a sieve with 2 layers of cheesecloth and set over a large bowl. Spoon the yogurt into the sieve. Cover and refrigerate for at least 12 hours, or until the yogurt is the consistency of cream cheese. You should have about 1 cup of yogurt cheese and 1 cup of drained liquid. (Discard the liquid or use as directed in the note below.)

Place the yogurt cheese, cream cheese, chives, basil, and pepper in a food processor. Process until well-blended. Spoon into a small bowl. Cover and refrigerate for at least 1 hour to allow the flavors to blend.

Makes 1 cup

Cook's Notes: Use yogurt that does not contain gums as thickeners; they will prevent it from draining.

The liquid drained from the yogurt (called whey) can be used in place of milk in pancake, muffin, and quick-bread batters.

Serve the dip with raw vegetables or pretzels or use it as a spread on low-fat crackers.

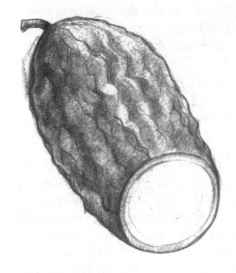

YUCCA
THE BLOOD-BUILDER

HEALING POWER

CAN HELP:

Prevent heart disease

Reduce the risk of cancer

Prevent cataracts

Keep skin smooth

Everyone knows about tapioca, but you may not have heard of manioc, cassava, or yucca. Don't let the strange names confuse you. They're all the same food, although the name is different in different parts of the world.

In the United States, what we call yucca is a long, brown, tropical vegetable (a tuber, actually) with rough skin. It's not much in the looks department, but inside is a mild, crisp, white flesh that resembles a potato's. The tapioca we make into pudding is made from dried, ground yucca. Yucca can also be boiled and mashed just like a potato.

Yucca is the world's number two vegetable crop, after potatoes. In the United States, it's still little-known outside ethnic supermarkets. But it's starting to attract a following. For one thing, this tuber is as tough as nails—it's uniquely full of iron, plus the vitamin C that helps your body absorb it. It's also a very good source of magnesium, which is needed to protect your bones, heart, arteries, and blood pressure.

HELP FOR IRON MAIDENS

Iron is an essential mineral that helps your cells get enough oxygen. Men rarely have a problem getting enough iron in their diets. But women of childbearing

IN THE KITCHEN

With its unfamiliar looks and foreign pedigree, yucca can be a daunting presence when you're cooking it for the first time. Don't be intimidated—it's no more complicated than cooking a potato.

- To peel yucca, first cut it into 2- or 3-inch sections. Using a paring knife, slit the skin (both the upper and lower layer), then work the blade underneath to loosen it. Grab the loose skin with your fingers and peel it off.
- Slice each piece in half lengthwise and remove the tough fiber that runs down the middle.
- Put the pieces in a deep pot and cover with cold water. Bring the water to a boil, then lower the heat to maintain a steady simmer.
- After 20 minutes, test for doneness using a thin, sharp knife. When it penetrates the flesh easily, the piece is done. (Not all pieces will cook at the same rate, so you may want to check them individually.)
- Drain and serve as you would potatoes: in pieces, mashed, or with your favorite toppings.

age lose a lot of iron due to menstruation. In fact, 30 percent of women in this country may have low iron stores, says Sally S. Harris, M.D., clinical faculty member at Stanford Medical School. Having low iron levels makes you feel tired and run-down. Over time it can lead to iron-deficiency anemia.

Although iron is easy to get from meat, most of us are trying to eat less meat these days. There's simply not a lot of iron in vegetables, and the type of iron they do contain (called nonheme iron) isn't readily absorbed by the body unless it's also accompanied by vitamin C.

Yucca, however, is a veritable iron mine. A half-cup of cooked yucca contains more than 2 milligrams of iron, 13 percent of the Recommended Dietary Allowance (RDA) for women and 20 percent of the RDA for men. And because it also contains large amounts of vitamin C—almost 21 milligrams, 35 percent of the Daily Value—the iron is much easier to absorb.

ADDITIONAL BENEFITS

The vitamin C in yucca does more than help contribute to your iron stores. It's also a powerhouse vitamin that has been shown to help prevent heart disease, cancer, and age-related conditions such as cataracts. Vitamin C plays a role in forming collagen, the stuff that keeps skin supple. It has also been shown to reduce the duration and severity of colds and other viral infections.

Yucca appears to have additional healing powers apart from its vitamin content. In parts of the Amazon, yucca is made into a poultice and used to relieve chills and fever. It has also been used in the Amazon to soothe sore muscles, and when mixed in a bath, to treat sterility in women.

GARLICKY YUCCA

1 **medium yucca (about 1¾ pounds)**

¼ **cup skim milk**

¼ **teaspoon salt**

2 **tablespoons extra-virgin olive oil**

4 **cloves garlic, minced**

Juice of ½ lime

Ground black pepper

Ground red pepper (optional)

PER SERVING

calories	**201**
total fat	**7.2 g.**
saturated fat	**1 g.**
cholesterol	**0 mg.**
sodium	**150 mg.**
dietary fiber	**1.9 g.**

With a large knife, cut the yucca into 2″ cross-sections. With a paring knife, slice the peel from each section, using the inner "ring" just under the peel as a guide. Cut the pieces lengthwise into quarters, then slice off the tough fiber that runs down the middle. Discard the peel and fiber.

Place the yucca in a large saucepan and add cold water to cover. Add the milk and salt. Stir to mix. Bring to a simmer over medium heat, then reduce the heat to low.

Simmer for 25 to 35 minutes, or until tender when pierced. Yucca does not cook evenly, so some pieces may be done before others. Start checking at 25 minutes by inserting the tip of a sharp knife. The yucca will look starchy and slightly translucent around the edges. Drain. Slice into smaller pieces, if desired.

In a large no-stick skillet over medium-high heat, warm 1 tablespoon of the oil. Add the garlic, then the yucca. Cook, tossing, for 5 minutes, or until the yucca starts to brown. Remove from the heat. Drizzle with the remaining 1 tablespoon oil. Sprinkle with the lime juice. Season to taste with the black pepper and red pepper (if using).

Makes 4 servings

Cook's Note: Served like potatoes, this makes a delicious accompaniment for black bean stew and other spicy legume dishes.

Index

Underscored page references indicate boxed text. **Boldface** references indicate tables. Prescription drug names are denoted with the symbol Rx.

B vitamins. *See also specific types*
    for Alzheimer's disease, 7–8
    deficiency of, in older adults, 5–6
    for insomnia, 303
    in meat, 330–31
    for memory problems, 347–48
    sources of, 303
        cereal, 135
        mushrooms, 367–68
        poultry, 443–44
        sweet potatoes, 518
    for stroke prevention, 512

C

Cabbage
    Bok Choy with Mushrooms, 105
    getting the most from, 104
    health benefits of, 102–4
    neutralizing odor of, 104
    Red Cabbage and Kohlrabi Slaw, 105
    for treating ulcers, 542
Caffeine
    calcium absorption blocked by, 399
    for constipation prevention, 160
    depression from, 180
    as diuretic, 554
    fatigue from, 196
    fibrocystic breasts from, 207
    for headache relief, 271
    infertility and, 299
    memory problems and, 349
    premenstrual symptoms and, 450
    stress and, 509
    ulcers and, 544
Cakes
    Chocolate Mint Pudding Cake, 324
    Raisin Coffeecake Ring, 468
Calcium
    absorption of, 398–99
    Daily Value for, 355
    in dairy vs. plant foods, 41, 263
    for dental health, 176
    interfering with iron absorption, 11
    kidney stones and, 311, 312, 313
    loss of
        boron for preventing, 414
        from eating meat, 42–43

        in menopause, 350
        soy foods for preventing, 42–43
    for lowering blood pressure, 84, 354
    in menopause, 350, 352
    for preventing
        headaches, 270
        muscle cramps, 364
        osteoporosis, 396–98
        premenstrual problems, 452–53
    sources of, 6, 270, 314, 352, 364
        broccoli, 87–88
        buttermilk, 354
        celery, 131
        cheese, 397–98
        greens, 263
        milk, 355, 396–97
        soy foods, 352
        tofu, 494
        yogurt, 572
    supplements, 398
    for thyroid disease, 530
Calcium-channel blockers, grapefruit
        interacting with, 254
Cancer. *See also specific types*
    from free radical damage, 233
    Laetrile for treating, 27
    preventing, with
        acerola, 2
        antioxidants, 107–8
        apples, 22
        asparagus, 46
        barley, 60
        basil, 62–63
        beans, 67–68
        beets, 71–72
        berries, 74–75
        beta-carotene, 307–8
        broccoli, 86–87
        brussels sprouts, 91
        buckwheat, 94–95
        bulgur, 98–99
        cabbage, 102–3
        cantaloupe, 111, 112
        carotenoids, 114–15, 425
        carrots, 119–20
        cauliflower, 125–26
        celery, 130–31
        cherries, 138

Garlic *(continued)*
  for preventing
    colds and flu, 157
    yeast infections, 297, 568–69
  roasting, 239
  Zucchini with Garlic and Oregano,
    504
Gas
  basil for relieving, 63
  causes of, 243–44
    fiber, 205
  with irritable bowel syndrome, 304,
    305
Gazpacho, 536
Ginger
  Double-Ginger Gingerbread, 249
  getting the most from, 247–48
  Ginger Chicken and Snow Peas,
    248
  Gingered Lentils, 70
  health benefits of, 245–47
  preparing, 247
  for relieving
    headaches, 271
    heartburn, 272
    motion sickness, 245–46, 361
    stomach upset, 246, 361, 507
Glucose tolerance, impaired, oats for
    controlling, 377
Gluten, hidden sources of, 133
Gluten-free flours, 132–33
Gluten sensitivity. *See* Celiac disease
Gout, 250–52
  from cauliflower, 126
  cherries for relieving, 140, 252
  in women, 251
Grains. *See also specific types*
  whole, fiber in, 20, 205
Grapefruit, 255
  drug interactions with, 254
  getting the most from, 256
  health benefits of, 253–55
  Honey-Marinated Grapefruit,
    256
Grape juice
  Grape Slush, 259
  health benefits of, 257–59
Grapes, for smokers, 488

Greens
  Beef and Spinach Stir-Fry, 333
  calcium in, 398
  Creamed Swiss Chard with Onions,
    265
  Fried Rice with Pork and Spinach,
    476
  health benefits of, 260–64
  kidney stones from, 264
  Mustard Greens with Smoked Turkey,
    265
  preparing, 261, 264
  Spiced Tofu with Spinach and
    Tomatoes, 551
  Spinach-Mushroom Salad, 266
Grilling meat, cancerous compounds
    and, 331
Guavas, 539–40
  Guavas with Sweet Lime Dressing,
    541
Gum
  irritable bowel syndrome and,
    304
  sugarless
    diarrhea from, 190
    gas from, 244

H

Halcion (Rx), grapefruit interacting
    with, 254
Hangover, relieving, 507
Hardening of the arteries. *See*
    Atherosclerosis
Hay fever, 267
HDL cholesterol. *See* High-density
    lipoprotein
Headaches, 268
  carbohydrates and, 269
  migraine *(see* Migraines)
  relieving, with
    caffeine, 271
    calcium, 270
    ginger, 271
    iron, 270–71
    magnesium, 270
  triggers for, 268–69
    wine, 565

iron, 270–71
magnesium, 270
vitamin B$_6$, 270
triggers for, 268–69
wine, _565_
Milk
buttermilk, _354_
calcium in, 396–97
Creamy Potato Soup, _357_
getting the most from, 356–57
health benefits of, 353–56
for herpes sores, 288
low-fat, _321_, 353
adjusting to, 356–57
soy, _492_, 494
for stroke prevention, 511
in tea, 527
ulcers and, 544
Millet
getting the most from, 360
health benefits of, 358–59
Millet-Cranberry Muffins, _360_
preparing, _359_
Millet flour, 360
Mineral deficiencies. _See_ Nutritional deficiencies
Mineral supplements, 11, 228–30, _398_
Mint
Chocolate Mint Pudding Cake, _324_
Minty Pears, _286_
Vegetable Pitas with Creamy Mint Sauce, _341_
Monosodium glutamate (MSG), migraines from, 269
Monoterpenes, health benefits of, **426–27**, 429
Mood swings
carbohydrates for, 180
premenstrual
foods aggravating, _450_
preventing, 180, 453
Motion sickness
preventing, 245–46, 361–62
unusual remedies for, _362_
MSG, migraines from, 269
Muffins
fat in, _320_
Millet-Cranberry Muffins, _360_

Muscle cramps, 363–64
Muscle soreness, vitamin E for, 18
Mushrooms
Barley-Mushroom Soup, _61_
Bok Choy with Mushrooms, _105_
Braised Vegetable Medley, _550_
getting the most from, 368
Glazed Shiitake Mushrooms, _368_
health benefits of, 365–68
raw, toxins in, _367_
shiitake, preparing, _366_
Spinach-Mushroom Salad, _266_
Mustard greens
Mustard Greens with Smoked Turkey, _265_
vitamin C in, 264

N

Nasal congestion. _See_ Congestion, nasal
Nausea, 506–7. _See also_ Motion sickness; Seasickness; Stomach upset
ginger for, 245–46
Nervous system, poultry for strengthening, 444
Neural tube defects, folate for preventing, 45, 79, 343
Niacin
deficiency of, pellagra from, 175
for insomnia, 303
memory problems and, 347, 348
for Parkinson's disease, 405
sources of, 175, 303, 348, 405
meat, 331
mushrooms, 367
poultry, 444
rice, 475
Night blindness, preventing, with carrots, 120
Nitrates, harmful effects of, 98–99
Nitrites
harmful effects of, 98–99, 100–101
garlic for counteracting, 240
migraines from, 269
Noodles
Asian Noodles with Vegetables, _44_
Spicy Chicken Noodle Soup, _144_

Wheat germ, <u>560</u>
Whole grains, fiber in, 20, 205
Whole wheat. *See also* Wheat
    Whole-Wheat Pancakes, <u>561</u>
Wine
    getting the most from, 565
    hay fever and, 267
    health benefits of, 562–65
    migraines from, <u>565</u>
    nonalcoholic, <u>564</u>
    for preventing
        diarrhea, <u>189</u>
        heart disease, 258, 339, 563–64
Wound healing, 566–67
    promoting, with
        acerola, 2
        honey, 289–90
        millet, 359

Y

Yeast infections, 297, 568–69, 570–71
Yogurt
    getting the most from, 572–73
    health benefits of, 570–72
    Herbed Yogurt Cheese Dip, <u>573</u>
    for lactose intolerance, 133, 189, 244,
        314, 572

for ulcers, 543
for yeast infections, 568, 570–71
Yucca
    Garlicky Yucca, <u>576</u>
    health benefits of, 574–76
    preparing, <u>575</u>

Z

Zest, citrus
    health benefits of, 316, 317
    removing, <u>316</u>
Zinc
    for calcium absorption, 399
    deficiency of, in older adults, 5
    for improving fertility, 300
    for infection prevention, 298
    sources of, 5, 300, 399, 567
        buckwheat, 96
        meat, 329–30
        poultry, 446–47
        shellfish, 484
    for wound healing, 567
Zostrix, for pain relief, <u>146</u>
Zucchini
    Poached Cod with Mixed Vegetables,
        <u>323</u>
    Zucchini with Garlic and Oregano, <u>504</u>